BIOCHEMISTRY RESEARCH TRENDS

MINERAL WATER

FROM BASIC RESEARCH TO CLINICAL APPLICATIONS

Biochemistry Research Trends

Additional books and e-books in this series can be found on Nova's website under the Series tab.

BIOCHEMISTRY RESEARCH TRENDS

MINERAL WATER

FROM BASIC RESEARCH TO CLINICAL APPLICATIONS

MARIA JOÃO MARTINS, PHD
EDITOR

nova science publishers
New York

DOI: https://doi.org/10.52305/IVAQ8581

Library of Congress Cataloging-in-Publication Data

ISBN: 978-1-68507-458-6

Published by Nova Science Publishers, Inc. † New York

To my parents.
To my family and friends, who helped me through the COVID-19 pandemic.

Contents

Foreword ix
Maria Augusta Vieira Coelho

Preface xi

Acknowledgments xiii

Chapter 1 **Natural Mineral Waters: Concept and Classifications** 1
Francisco Armijo and Francisco Maraver

Chapter 2 **Clinical and Immunological Effects of Inhaled Thermal Waters in Chronic Obstructive Pulmonary Disease** 29
Luís Taborda-Barata and Marco Contoli

Chapter 3 **Thermal Waters in Otorhinolaryngology** 73
João Filipe Simões, Helena Castro, Maria João Martins and António Miguéis

Chapter 4 **Spa Therapies and Rheumatic Diseases** 115
Bruno Miguel Fernandes and Miguel Bernardes

Chapter 5 **Mineral Water Consumption and Diet-Induced Acid Load: Putative Relevance for Bone Health** 133
Cidália D. Pereira, Cátia Pontes, Vânia Ribeiro and Maria João Martins

Chapter 6 **Mineral Waters in Dermatology** 165
Carmen Lisboa

Chapter 7 **Water - A New Non-Pharmacological Therapeutic Agent Against Metabolic Dysfunction Through Gut Microbiota Modulation?** 187
Christophe Espírito Santo, Maria João Martins and Inês Brandão

Chapter 8 **Influence of Mineral Waters Upon Membrane Transporters** 227
Fátima Martel

About the Editor 255

List of Contributors 257

Index 261

FOREWORD

Water resources are a wealth of essential value for the life of our planet. The recognition that climate changes are related to the negative impact of human activity, particularly on water resources, makes the study and knowledge of mineral waters an extremely relevant subject. In fact, as is clear from the goals of the World Health Organization 2030 agenda, water is at the heart of sustainable development and its three dimensions - environmental, economic and social. This edition is thus aligned with these objectives and also puts in focus the mineral water as a rehabilitation, therapeutic and preventive vehicle in medicine.

This book brings together basic concepts of Hydrology, such as the classification of natural mineral waters, to laboratorial and clinical evidence of the therapeutic effects of mineral waters in a wide spectrum of pathologies, namely respiratory, ear, rheumatological, bone, dermatological, metabolic, and intestinal diseases. The essential concepts and the most interesting results are presented and discussed objectively and faithfully to scientific methods.

The Faculty of Medicine from the University of Porto has been offering, for several decades, the Course in Climatology and Hydrology. In this context, I foresee a huge interest in this book for technicians, students, physicians and researchers in the field of thermal medicine.

Maria Augusta Vieira Coelho
Department of Biomedicine, Pharmacology and Therapeutics Unit,
Faculty of Medicine, University of Porto, Porto, Portugal

PREFACE

Mineral water: from basic research to clinical applications, written by a multi-disciplinary group of educators, researchers and medical doctors, gathers a timely review on the effects of mineral waters upon several aspects of human biology and pathophysiology, as it gives an overview of how mineral waters may provide a positive impact on different settings, namely health promotion and disease prevention as well as rehabilitation and therapy. A major advantage of this book is the gathering of up-to-date information on the benefits, and associated mechanisms, of mineral waters through different routes of internal and external exposure.

Concept and classifications of mineral waters are disclosed.

The relevance of Spa therapies in Chronic Obstructive Pulmonary Disease, Otorhinolaryngology, rheumatic diseases and Dermatology is addressed.

The mitigation of diet-induced acid load by mineral waters consumption and its putative relevance for bone health is discussed.

The importance of mineral waters consumption against metabolic dysfunction through gut microbiota modulation is argued.

Modulation of membrane transporters by mineral waters is reviewed.

Mineral water: from basic research to clinical applications aims to target health professionals (medical doctors, nurses, physiotherapists, nutritionists and dietitians), educators and students (in the aforementioned subject areas) as well as health science researchers (biochemists, biologists and pharmacists), beverage companies and policy-makers.

Maria João Martins
Department of Biomedicine, Biochemistry Unit,
Faculty of Medicine, University of Porto, Porto, Portugal
i3S-Instituto de Investigação e Inovação em Saúde, University of Porto, Porto, Portugal

Acknowledgments

Firstly, I would like to acknowledge Professor Pedro Cantista and Professor Rosário Monteiro for the help given in structuring the proposal that led to this book.

Then, I would like to acknowledge the effort done by all authors in writing their book chapters during a period of time with increased workload in their pedagogical, scientific and medical activities due to the COVID-19 pandemic.

At last, I would like to acknowledge the publisher, editors and support staff at Nova Science Publishers, they were very helpful in the various stages of development and production of this book.

In: Mineral Water
Editors: Maria João Martins
ISBN: 978-1-68507-458-6

Chapter 1

NATURAL MINERAL WATERS: CONCEPT AND CLASSIFICATIONS

Francisco Armijo, PhD
and Francisco Maraver*, MD, PhD
Professional School of Medical Hydrology,
Complutense University, Madrid, Spain

ABSTRACT

The water substance, due to its peculiar structure, can dissolve many products and give rise to different types of water. The waters have very diverse uses, among which their beneficial actions for health stand out. In this field those that have an underground origin, are microbiologically healthy and have a constant composition, that is to say, natural mineral waters, are used, either bottled or directly, in the Health Resort Medicine. Therefore, tap water is not included, nor are bottled spring waters or prepared drinking waters, which have their own legislation. The natural mineral waters are classified mainly based on their temperature, dry residue, and chemical composition. In this chapter the most important natural mineral water classifications are shown, from the point of

* Corresponding Author's E-mail: fmaraver@ucm.es.

Medical Hydrology, which can predict their possible beneficial effects for the organism.

Keywords: bottled water, classifications, concept, health resort medicine, medical hydrology, natural mineral water

Introduction

As the universal solvent, water –defined as a macroscopically connected, random network of hydrogen bonds, with frequent strained and broken bonds, that is continually undergoing topological reformation– is able to dissolve different substances depending on conditions of pressure and temperature [1].

While ionic solids and polar molecules readily dissolve in water, some non-polar molecules are also dissolved provided they are sufficiently small to fit in the cavities of its network, and even lipophilic substances dissolve when water reaches its supercritical state [2-6].

This means that in natural waters we may find many substances in smaller or higher concentrations that will confer them their different and specific properties. When faced with this diversity, we will instinctively try to define small and manageable water groups. Classification is the method used to confront the world that surrounds us [7].

To determine whether a substance will be found dissolved in natural waters, two factors need to be known: the abundance of the element in the Earth's crust, which in general diminishes as the atomic number increases, and the number of protons present in its nucleus. In addition, we should not forget that atoms whose atomic number is even are more abundant than those with an odd atomic number. This is because heavier elements are synthesized in the interior of stars from lighter elements, and for atomic numbers lower than 26, i.e that of iron, synthesis involves the capture of alpha particles, or helium nuclei, which have two protons. Elements of even atomic number are more abundant as they form part of the main synthesis pathway [8].

In Table 1, we detail the distributions of elements comprising the ions that serve to classify waters. These data, taken from Dickerson [8], indicate the abundance of elements expressed as the number of atoms per 100,000, for the universe, the Earth, the Earth's crust and in ocean waters. When no value is indicated, abundance is below 0.1 atoms per 100,000.

Table 1. Distributions of elements of the universe

Element	Atomic Nº	Universe	Earth	Crust	Ocean
C	6	8	99	55	1.4
F	9	-	3.8	77	-
Na	11	0.1	640	2554	290
Mg	12	2.1	12500	1784	34
S	16	0.9	1400	33	17
Cl	17	-	45	11	340
Ca	20	0.1	460	1878	6
Fe	26	1.4	18870	1858	-

Adapted from [8].

Since early times, analysis and classification systems were used by hydrologists to sort and name the different natural mineral waters they could use for therapeutic purposes. Table 2 provides the designations of natural mineral water types included by different Spanish authors in their books, over the last three hundred and twenty four years.

These designations are in disuse today, and an attempt has been made to unify them to give rise to a standardized classification system for waters. This has been possible for mineral waters because of the European Union legislation regarding bottled waters.

Table 2. Designations of natural mineral water types, by different Spanish authors, that are in disuse today

Author	Date	Waters
Alfonso Limón Montero [9]	1697	Salty, aluminous, bituminous, cuprous
Pedro Gomez de Bedoya [10]	1764	Nitrous, aluminous, bituminous, antimonial, mercurial.
Pedro Maria Rubio [11]	1853	Azootic, crenated, cuprous
Antonio Casares [12]	1866	Crenated
Anastasio García López [13]	1889	Nitrogenated, silicated, crenated, manganesian
Hipólito Rodriguez Pinilla [14]	1920	Azoadas or nitrogenated

CONCEPT

Bottled Natural Mineral Waters

The most correct definition of natural mineral water appears in the Directive 2009/54/EC that we transcribe [15, 16]:

> The term natural mineral water is legally defined and can only be used when the water complies with the specific source, compositional and labelling requirements of the following legislation: Directive 2009/54/EC (OJ L 164, p 45, 26/06/2009) of the European Parliament and of the Council, of 18 June 2009, on the exploitation and marketing of natural mineral waters and Directive 2003/40/EC (OJ L 126, p 34, 22/05/2003), of 16 May 2003, establishing the list, concentration limits and labelling requirements for the constituents of natural mineral waters and the conditions for using ozone-enriched air for the treatment of natural mineral waters and spring waters.

'Natural mineral water' refers to microbiologically wholesome water, originating in an underground water table or deposit and emerging from a spring tapped at one or more natural or bore exits.

Natural mineral water can be clearly distinguished from ordinary drinking water by:

(a) its nature, which is characterized by its mineral content, trace elements or other constituents and, where appropriate, by certain effects and;

(b) its original purity, both characteristics having been preserved intact because of the underground origin of such water, which has been protected from all risk of pollution.

The abovementioned characteristics, which may give rise to natural mineral water favourable properties for health, need to be assessed considering several parameters (geological and hydrological; physical, chemical and physico-chemical; microbiological; pharmacological, physiological and clinical) according to specific criteria and scientific methods [16].

Natural Mineral Waters Used in Health Resort Medicine

The Directive 2009/54/EC does not apply to natural mineral waters used at source for curative purposes in thermal or hydromineral establishments.

Therefore, the mineral and thermal waters used for baths or drinking in medical Spas must also be considered as natural mineral waters [16].

Natural mineral waters are defined as those of subterranean origin with a constant composition and, because of their special characteristics, have been officially confirmed as therapeutic agents and declared of public utility by the pertinent organisms [17].

In Italy, mineral waters are those that, based on their special therapeutic or hygienic properties, are used both as components of drinks and for curative purposes [18].

Classification of Bottled Natural Mineral Waters

Appendix III of Directive 2009/54/EC provides the label indications authorized for this type of natural mineral waters based on physical-chemical analysis data and if necessary on pharmacological, physiological and clinical analyses conducted using scientifically recognised methods. These label indications constitute a classification system according to fixed residue and ionic contents [16, 19], shown in Tables 3 and 4.

Fixed Residue Content

Table 3. Classes defined according to fixed residue content of minerals at 180 °C (bottled natural mineral waters)

Criterion **Mineral salt content calculated as a fixed residue**	**Label indications**
Not greater than 50 mg/L	Very low mineral content
Not greater than 500 mg/L	Low mineral content
Greater than 500 mg/L and not greater than 1500 mg/L	Intermediate mineral content
Greater than 1500 mg/L	High mineral content

Adapted from [16].

Ionic Content

Table 4. Classes defined according to ionic content (bottled natural mineral waters)

Ion	Criterion	Label indications
Cl^-	> 200 mg/L	Contains chloride
SO_4^{2-}	> 200 mg/L	Contains sulphate
HCO_3^-	> 600 mg/L	Contains bicarbonate
F^-	> 1 mg/L	Contains fluoride
Na^+	> 200 mg/L	Contains sodium
Ca^{2+}	> 150 mg/L	Contains calcium
Mg^{2+}	> 50 mg/L	Contains magnesium
Fe^{2+}	> 1 mg/L	Contains iron

Adapted from [16].

In addition, waters are considered acidulous if they contain more than 250 mg/L of free CO_2 [16].

Classification of Natural Mineral Waters Used in Health Resort Medicine

Bearing in mind that natural mineral waters are used in Health Resort Medicine, these can be classified according to: their temperature at their emergence point, fixed residue content at 110 °C, ionic content, presence of other compounds and the other classifications (hardness, molar concentration and BS ISO 21426:2018).

Temperature

To classify water according to its source temperature, this may be considered in relation to the physiological temperature of the organism. Hence, waters can be classified as hypothermal when their temperature is less than 35 °C, mesothermal when between 35 and 37 °C, and hyperthermal when over 37 °C [20].

In France, four categories of mineral waters are considered: hyperthermal from a temperature of 50 ºC, mesothermal from 49 to 35 ºC, hypothermal from 34 to 15 ºC and cold when below 15 ºC [21].

In Italy, mineral waters are defined as cold when their emergence temperature is lower than 20 ºC, and warm or thermal when above 20 ºC. The latter are then classified into: hypothermal for temperatures of 20 to 30 ºC, homothermal 31 to 40 ºC, and hyperthermal higher than 40 ºC [18, 22, 23].

In the United States of America, a general statement may be made about the relationship between temperature and sensation for a body bath as follows: very cold from 1 to 13 ºC, cold from 13 to 18 ºC, cool from 18 to 27 ºC, tepid from 27 to 33.5 ºC, neutral from 33.5 to 35.5 ºC, warm from 35.5 to 36.5 ºC, hot from 36.5 to 40 ºC and very hot from 40 to 46 ºC [24].

In Germany, mineral waters are defined as subthermale from 28 to 34 ºC, indifferent between 35 and 36 ºC and hyperthermal above 37 ºC [25].

Overall Mineralisation

In Spain [20], natural mineral waters have been classified by their fixed residue contents at 110 °C into:

- Oligomineral: less than 100 mg/L;
- Very weak mineralisation: 100 - 250 mg/L;
- Weak mineralisation: 250 - 500 mg/L;
- Medium mineralisation: 500 - 1000 mg/L;
- Strong mineralisation: greater than 1000 mg/L.

In France [21], five categories have been established according to the intensity of mineralisation:

- Very weak mineralisation: less than 50 mg/L;
- Weak mineralisation: 50 - 500 mg/L;
- Medium mineralisation: 500 - 1000 mg/L;
- Very mineralised: 1000 - 1500 mg/L;
- Strongly mineralised: greater than 1000 mg/L.

In Italy [18], three categories have been distinguished according to fixed residue content at 180 ºC:

- Oligomineral: less than 200 mg/L;
- Medium mineral: 200 - 1000 mg/L;
- Mineral: greater than 1 g/L.

Ionic Content

When natural mineral waters contain more than 1000 mg/L of fixed residue, they are classified according to their anion and cation contents as bicarbonate, chloride, sulphate, sodium, calcium or magnesium when the corresponding ion represents 20% of the anion or cation contents expressed in equivalents (Table 5) [25, 26].

The equivalent weight of a monoatomic ion is calculated as its atomic weight divided by its valence, and of a polyatomic ion, as the sum of the atomic weights of its constituents divided by its valence. The equivalent weight of an oxidant or reductant is defined as the ratio between its molecular weight and the number of electrons lost or gained in the process, i.e., equivalent weights vary according to the reaction. The concentration in milliequivalents of an ion is calculated by dividing its concentration in milligrams by its equivalent weight [5, 27].

Table 5. Classes defined according to ionic content (natural mineral waters used in Health Resort Medicine)

Ion	Criterion	Classification
Cl^-	> 20 % mEq	Chloride
SO_4^{2-}	> 20 % mEq	Sulphate
HCO_3^-	> 20 % mEq	Bicarbonate
Na^+	> 20 % mEq	Sodium
Ca^{2+}	> 20 % mEq	Calcium
Mg^{2+}	> 20 % mEq	Magnesium

Adapted from [20].

Interestingly, this classification system used in many countries is based on the concept that the different waters are electrically neutral solutions of ions such that the sums of the anions and cations expressed in mEq/L need to be balanced [28, 29].

Other authors use this ionic content-based classification system with a different threshold: the concentration of a given ion should be only greater than 12 mEq/L to give name to a water [26].

When the fixed residue content at 110 ºC is lower than 1000 mg/L, waters are known as oligomineral and only the predominant ions are indicated under the same criterion as described above [20].

As water may exist with the anions chloride, bicarbonate and sulphate, and the cations sodium, calcium and magnesium in concentrations above 20% of mEq, there may be several combinations of waters referred to as mixed with groups associated with one anion and subgroups associated with the cations (Table 6) [26].

Table 6. Examples according to ionic content (natural mineral waters used in Health Resort Medicine)

Anion	Cation	Source
HCO_3^-	Na^+	Challes les Eaux (FRA), Chateauneuf les Bains (FRA), Chaves (PRT), Las Trincheras (VEN), Le Boulou (FRA), Mondariz-Gandara (ESP), Saint Laurent les Bains (FRA), Verin-Cabreiroa (ESP), Vichy-Celetins (FRA), Vidago (PRT)
	Ca^{2+}	Sarein (IRN)
	$Na^+ Ca^{2+}$	Bussang (FRA), Royat (FRA), Pedras Salgadas (PRT)
	$Na^+ Mg^{2+}$	La Fortuna-Arenal Paraiso (CRI)
	$Ca^{2+} Mg^{2+}$	Borjomi (GEO), Melgaço (PRT), Krapinske Toplice (HRV)
	$Na^+ Ca^{2+} Mg^{2+}$	Cervantes-San Camilo (ESP), Mondariz-Molares (ESP), Spa (BEL)
Cl^-	Na^+	Aedipsos (GRC), Archena (ESP), Bad Ischl (AUT), Bad Kösen (DEU), Bad Salzungen (DEU), Baden Baden (DEU), Balaruc les Bains (FRA), Besançon la Mouillère (FRA), Beppu (JPN), Bourbon Lancy (FRA), Comarruga (ESP), Cucos (PRT), Domuyo (ARG), Druskininkai (LTU), Elguea (CUB), Elgorriaga (ESP), Fuente Santa (ESP), Klaipeda (LTU), La Hermida (ESP), La Toja (ESP), Lons le Saunier (FRA), Loutraki (GRC), Maizières (FRA), Montecatini-Regina (ITA), Montecatini-Tettuccio (ITA), Monticelli (ITA), Olmedo (ESP), Puente Viesgo (ESP), Reichenhall (DEU), Salies de Béarn (FRA), Salins les Bains (FRA), Salsomaggiore (ITA), San Juan de la Fuensanta (ESP), Salzuflen (DEU), Sochi-Matsesta (RUS), Techirghiol (ROM), Wiesbaden (DEU)

Table 6. (Continued)

Anion	Cation	Source
Cl^- (Continued)	Na^+ Ca^{2+}	Abano (ITA), Lanjarón-Capuchina (ESP)
	Na^+ Mg^{2+}	Frades de Vimeiro (PRT), Pozo de la Salud (ESP)
SO_4^{2-}	Na^+	Evaux les Bains (FRA)
	Ca^{2+}	Ariño (ESP), Bagnères de Bigorre (FRA), Bath (GBR), Camoins les Bains (FRA), Copahue-Chancho (ARG), Copahue-Laguna Verde (ARG), Fucoli (ITA), Les Fumades (FRA), Monte Real (PRT), San Diego de los Baños (CUB)
	Ca^{2+} Mg^{2+}	Alicun de las Torres (ESP), Boario-Antica (ITA), Contrexéville (FRA), Cransac (FRA), Curia (PRT), Encausse les Thermes (FRA), Fuentepodrida (ESP), Graena (ESP), Gravalos (ESP), Lierganes-Fuente Nueva (ESP), Trillo-Carlos III (ESP), Villavieja de Nules (ESP), Vittel (FRA)
	Na^+ Ca^{2+} Mg^{2+}	Miers Alvignac (FRA)
Cl^- HCO_3^-	Na^+	La Bourboule (FRA), Le Mont Dore (FRA), Piedade (PRT), Prats (ESP), Saint Nectaire (FRA), Saratoga Spa (USA), Vichy Catalan (ESP), Wiessee (DEU)
	Na^+ Ca^{2+}	Bourbon L`Archambault (FRA), Lanjarón-Salado (ESP), Lanjarón-Salud II (ESP), Nauheim (DEU), Tus (ESP)
	Ca^{2+} Mg^{2+}	Santa Rosa de Cabal (COL)
	Na^+ Ca^{2+} Mg^{2+}	Azuaje (ESP), Caxambu-Beleza (BRA), Chatelguyon (FRA)
HCO_3^- SO_4^{2-}	Na^+	Jermuk (ARM)
	Ca^{2+}	Bolu Karacasu (TUR), Nenndorf (DEU)
	Na^+ Ca^{2+}	Piestany (SVK), Valbuena (ESP)

Anion	Cation	Source
HCO_3^- SO_4^{2-} (Continued)	Ca^{2+} Mg^{2+}	Cofrentes-Hervideros (ESP), Rocallaura (ESP), Chianciano-Santa (ITA), Chianciano-Sillene (ITA)
	Na^+ Ca^{2+} Mg^{2+}	Cervantes- Pozo Mina (ESP), Marienbad (CZE)
Cl^- SO_4^{2-}	Na^+	Arnedillo (ESP), Brides les Bains (FRA), Chiclana-Fuente Amarga (ESP), Digne (FRA), Manzanera-El Paraiso (ESP), Paracuellos de Jiloca (ESP), Termales Nevado del Ruiz (COL), Uriage (FRA), Vallfogona-Sondeo (ESP), Villa Elisa (ARG)
	Na^+ Ca^{2+}	Alceda (ESP), Alhama de Murcia (ESP), Allevard les Bains (FRA), Baden Bei Wien (AUT), Budapest-Szechenyi (HUN), Cestona-Natividad (ESP), Cestona-San Ignacio (ESP), Dax (FRA), Dea sea area-Roman Spring (ISR), Fitero (ESP), Frantiskovy Lazne (CZE), Karlovy Vary (CZE), Kissingen (DEU), Mondorf (LUX), Pechelbronn (FRA), Saint Gervais les Bains (FRA), Vallfogona-Font Pudenda (ESP), Zujar (ESP)
	Ca^{2+} Mg^{2+}	Las Palmeras (ESP)
	Na^+ Ca^{2+} Mg^{2+}	Caldas da Rainha (PRT), Lierganes-Fuente Santa (ESP), Rochefort (FRA)

Adapted from [18, 20, 25, 30-36].

ISO3 Country Codes: Argentina (ARG), Armenia (ARM), Austria (AUT), Belgium (BEL), Brazil (BRA), Bulgaria (BGR), Colombia (COL), Costa Rica (CRI), Croatia (HRV), Cuba (CUB), Czech Republic (CZE), France (FRA), Georgia (GEO), Germany (DEU), Greece (GRC), Hungary (HUN), Iran (IRN), Israel (ISR), Italy (ITA), Japan (JPN), Lithuania (LTU), Luxembourg (LUX), Morocco (MAR), Poland (POL), Portugal (PRT), Romania (ROM), Russia (RUS), Slovak Republic (SVK), Slovak Republic (SVK), Spain (ESP), Turkey (TUR), Ukraine (UKR), United Kingdom (GBR), United States (USA), Venezuela (VEN).

Chlorides

Chlorine is found at low concentrations of 0.011% in the Earth's crust and chloride ions present in waters arise from evaporite rocks or those of marine origin. The chloride ion is always present in waters and its concentration depends on the corresponding underlying host rock making this range extremely wide [37].

Sulphates

Sulphates occur in most natural waters as the result of the dissolution of rocks, such as gypsum, or the oxidation of sulphides. The sulphate ion is very stable and resistant to reduction [37].

Bicarbonates

Bicarbonates are easily soluble in water such that this ion is present in most natural waters. The bicarbonate ion reacts as a base to form H_2CO_3 and OH^- through the reaction:

$$HCO_3^- + H_2O \rightleftharpoons H_2CO_3 + OH^-$$

It can also act as an acid and ionize water according to the reaction:

$$HCO_3^- + H_2O \rightleftharpoons H_3O^+ + CO_3^{2-}$$

The first of these two reactions is the predominant one and, so, in aqueous solution the water becomes alkaline [29].

According to hydrogen concentration (pH), CO_3^{2-}, HCO_3^- and CO_2 levels will be balanced. The percentage of each one according to pH is shown in Figure 1.

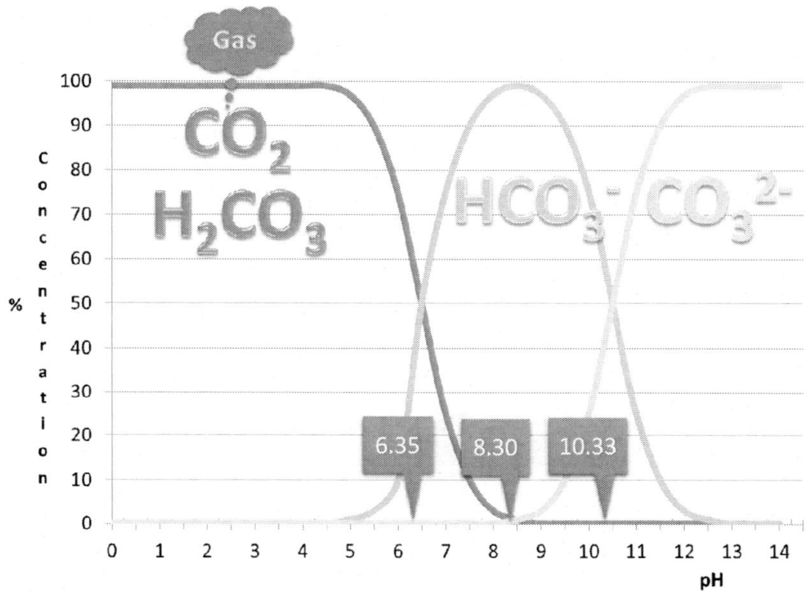

Figure 1. Carbonic, bicarbonate and carbonate ratio as a function of pH.

Sodium

Sodium is one of the most widely distributed elements and represents 2.36% of the Earth's crust. It is therefore present in greater or smaller proportion in all types of waters as all sodium compounds are soluble in water with the exception of pyroantimonate, fluosilicate, and some complex uranium and magnesium salts. Sodium is released by the meterorization of silicates, such as albite, the dissolution of sedimentary rocks of marine origin, and the evaporite deposits in which it is found like chloride, halite, and nitrate [29].

Calcium

The calcium ion is always present in water, is derived from igneous, silicate, sedimentary, and metamorphic rocks, since calcium does not exist free in nature. Its solubility decreases with increasing temperature, this behaviour is in harmony with the fact that the hydroxide dissolves in water with release of heat [29, 37].

Magnesium

Magnesium does not occur in a free state in nature, although in combination it is widely distributed in many minerals and rocks. Magnesium arises from the dissolution of carbonate rocks, such as dolomite and epsonite, and also from the weathering of iron magnesium silicates. It is generally found in water in much smaller quantities than calcium [29, 37].

Specific Compounds

Waters can also be classified according to the presence of a given concentration of other specific compounds (Table 7).

Table 7. Specific compounds (natural mineral waters used in Health Resort Medicine)

Compound	Spain	Italy	Germany	Classification
Fe^{2+}	> 5 mg/L	> 1 mg/L	> 20 mg/kg	Ferruginous
$H_2S + HS^-$	> 1 mg/L	> 10 mg/L	> 1 mg/kg	Sulphur
CO_2	> 250 mg/L	> 700 mg/L	1000 mg/kg	Carbogaseous or acidulous
Rn	> 67.3 Bq/L	20 Mache	18 nCi/L	Radioactive

Adapted from [18, 20, 25].

Ferruginous

Natural mineral waters described as ferruginous are those with a bivalent iron concentration greater than 1 mg/L. In Spain, this limit is > 5 mg/L [20].

Considering that iron is the fifth element of the Earth's crust, accounting for 5% in weight, most terrestrial waters contain iron although it can appear as traces. However, when its levels exceed the indicated minimum, this confers therapeutic properties determining its consideration as a specific mineralising element [38].

Ferruginous waters are those whose pH approaches neutrality and are hypothermal, colourless, odourless, and transparent upon their emergence. As they emerge, they become turbid when in contact with the air, as bivalent iron oxidizes to insoluble ferric oxide [37]:

$$4Fe^{2+} + 4H_2O + O_2 \rightarrow 2Fe_2O_3\downarrow + 8H^+$$

Ferric oxide forms characteristic reddish solid residues that appear in this type of spring, especially in volcanic zones. Examples, in Spain, are the zones of Olot and Campo de Calatrava [26].

Ferruginous waters with low concentrations of ferrous oxide are colourless but as concentrations increase, they may take on a greenish hue [29].

Examples of ferruginous waters: Blagoevgrad (BGR), Caxambu-Beleza (BRA), Cofrentes-Hervideros (ESP), Copahue-Chancho (ARG), Copahue-Pileta Ferruginosa (ARG), Fuente del Trampal (ESP), Incio (ESP), Kissingen (DEU), Lanjarón-Capuchina (ESP), Lanjarón-Salado (ESP), Marienbad (CZE), Mondariz-Molares (ESP), Mondariz-Gándara (ESP), Polczyn (POL), Spa (BEL).

Sulphur

Natural mineral waters are classed as sulphur waters when they contain more than 1 mg/L of reduced sulphur, i.e., with a valence of -2. Sulphur has as its main valences -2, +3, +4, and +6, and according to its oxidation state can give rise to oxides and sulphides. When sulphur is found in oxidation grade -2, it may be present in waters as a non-dissociated molecule H_2S, or hydrogen sulphide, as an HS^- ion, or bisulphide, and rarely as S^{2-}, or sulphide.

The presence of one or other of these forms is dependent on pH, there being no sulphides at pH values below 10 and a predominance of bisulphide above pH 9 (Figure 2).

Hydrogen sulphide is an inflammable poisonous gas and its characteristic rotten egg smell is perceivable in air at concentrations of 0.002 mg/L. One gram of H_2S dissolves in 187 mL of water at 10 ºC and in 314 mL at 30 ºC [39].

When dissolved in water, H_2S gives rise as main products to hydronium and bisulphide ions:

$$H_2S + H_2O \rightleftharpoons H_3O^+ + HS^-$$

Bisulphide ions in water give rise to a small proportion of sulphide ions:

$$HS^- + H_2O \rightleftharpoons H_3O + S^{2-}$$

When this dissolution is exposed to air, dissolved oxygen oxidizes sulphide, precipitating sulphur:

$$2S^{2-} + 4H^+ + O_2 \rightarrow 2H_2O + 2S\downarrow$$

This sulphur in the form of a colloid may be found in natural mineral waters and their bioglea [26].

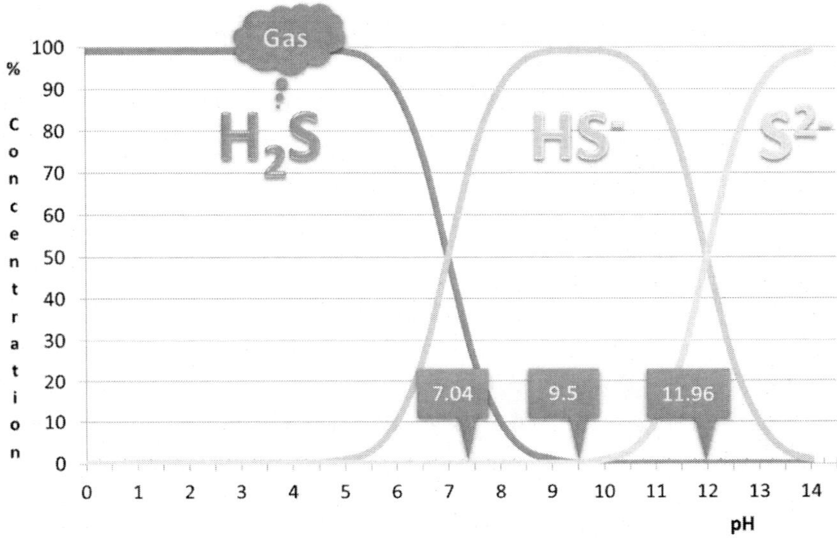

Figure 2. Sulfhydric, bisulphide and sulphide ratio as a function of pH (adapted from [40]).

Examples of sulphur waters: Aix-les-Bains (FRA), Araxa (BRA), Archena (ESP), Bad Deutsch Altenburg (AUT), Bad Ischl (AUT), Baden bei Wien (AUT), Bagnères de Bigorre (FRA), Beppu (JPN), Blagoevgrad (BGR), Caldas da Rainha (PRT), Caldas de Vizela (PRT), Chiclana-Fuente Amarga (ESP), Copahue-Pileta Ferruginosa (ARG), Cró (PRT), Fuentepodrida (ESP), Gravalos (ESP), Guitiriz (ESP), Héviz (HUN), Kırşehir (TUR), Küstendil (BGR), Lugo (ESP), Montemayor (ESP), Moulay Yacoub (MAR), Nenndorf (DEU), Paracuellos de Jiloca (ESP), Piestany (SVK), Poços de Caldas (BRA), Pyatigorsk (RUS), Retortillo (ESP), Río Hondo (ARG), Sao Jorge (PRT), Sao Pedro (BRA), Sao Pedro do Sul (PRT), San Diego de los Baños (CUB), Sirmione (ITA), Slavyansk (UKR), Tbilisi (GEO), Unhais da Serra (PRT), Uriage (FRA), Zujar (ESP).

Carbogaseous or Acidulous

Natural mineral waters are considered carbogaseous and acidulous if they contain more than 250 mg/L of free carbon dioxide [20].

Carbon dioxide is a non-flammable, odourless colourless gas. It is soluble in 880 ml/L of water at 20 °C and 760 mm Hg of pressure [39].

With water, carbon dioxide forms carbonic acid through the reversible reaction:

$$CO_2 + H_2O \rightleftharpoons H_2CO_3$$

Carbonic acid shows the properties of a weak acid although it has not been isolated as such. Carbonic acid gives these waters an astringent taste and a pH always lower than 8.3 that may reach 4 when present at high concentrations. They are usually hypothermal, given that the solubility of CO_2 in water diminishes as temperature rises, as the gas is more easily released [17].

Spring waters rich in CO_2 should be considered of deep origin and sometimes magmatic. This occurs in Campo de Calatrava (ESP), which is a Quaternary basalt eruptive zone where carbogaseous springs are common, some with high flow and from which large quantities of gas are released through intense bubbling. Examples of this are the hot springs, or "hervideros", of Fuensanta and Emperador (ESP), the latter located on the actual margins of the river Guadiana [41-43].

The waters from many springs in Galicia are also rich in CO_2, including those of Verín (ESP) and Mondariz (ESP). All of these springs are related to large fractures or faults that cut the granite massif and are marked by frequent natural mineral springs. These continue into Portugal where carbogaseous waters are also frequent e.g., the springs of Pedras Salgadas, Melgaço and Vidago, whose waters contain 2.276, 2.027 and 1.580 mg/L of CO_2 respectively.

Examples of carbogaseous waters: Bolu Karacasu (TUR), Borjomi (GEO), Caxambu-Beleza (BRA), Caxambu-Don Pedro (BRA), Cervantes-San Camilo (ESP), Cofrentes-Hervideros (ESP), Frantiskovy Lazne (CZE), Jermuk (ARM), Karlovy Vary (CZE), Lanjarón-Capilla (ESP), Lanjarón-Salud II (ESP), Marienbad (CZE), Melgaço (PRT), Mondariz-Gandara (ESP), Nauheim (DEU), Pedras Salgadas (PRT), Prats (ESP), Saint Nectaire (FRA), Vichy Catalan (ESP), Royat (FRA), Saint Laurent les Bains (FRA), Spa (BEL), Verin-Cabreiroa (ESP), Vichy-Celestines (FRA), Vidago (PRT) [18, 20, 25, 32-34].

Radioactive

Radioactive waters are those emitting ionising radiation due essentially to the presence of radon [17].

Radon is considered a noble gas because of its electronic structure. In its gaseous form it is colourless, odourless, and insipid. Its most abundant and stable natural isotope is 222Rn, which has a half-life of only 3.82 days. The decay of radon, whereby an alpha particle is emitted over a distance of 4.12 cm produces 218Po. Successive alpha and beta emissions give rise to stable 208Pb [44].

Radon is soluble in water, 230 cm^3/L at 20 °C, and highly absorbed by various surfaces [39].

Its half-life is the time period needed for radioactivity to drop to half its value at any instant. When 10 times its half-life has elapsed, activity is reduced to 0.1% its value at the moment when this time started to be counted [44].

At least 18 further isotopes with mass numbers of 202 to 224 have been prepared via several nuclear reactions. All these isotopes are radioactive over short half-lives [44].

Examples of radioactive waters: Abano Terme (ITA), Alange (ESP), Araxa (BRA), Arnedillo (ESP), Bad Steben (DEU), Baden Baden (DEU), Baños de Molgas (ESP), Boí-Tartera (ESP), Caldas de Oviedo (ESP), Caldelas de Tuy (ESP), Héviz (HUN), Jachymov (CZE), Joachimstal Grubenwasser (CZE), Lacco Ameno (ITA), La Bourboule (FRA), La Hermida (ESP), Lindoia (BRA), Loutraki (GRC), Lugo (ESP), Luso (PRT), Masutomi (JPN), Merano (ITA), Misasa Hot Spring (JAP), Monfortinho (PRT), Montecatini (ITA), Pyatigorsk (RUS), Retortillo (ESP), Royat (FRA), San Gregorio de Brozas (ESP), Titus (ESP), Tskaltubo (GEO), Vidago (PRT), Villavieja (ESP) [18, 20, 25, 32-34].

Other Classifications

Hardness

Initially, water hardness was a measure of water's capacity to precipitate soap. Soap is precipitated through the calcium and magnesium ions present. The total hardness of waters is due to the presence of calcium and magnesium ions expressed as the mg/L of $CaCO_3$ present [28].

The Girard classification [45] distinguishes five water hardness categories:

- Very soft: 0 - 100 mg/L $CaCO_3$;
- Soft: 100 - 200 mg/L $CaCO_3$;
- Hard: 200 - 300 mg/L $CaCO_3$;
- Very hard: 300 - 400 mg/L $CaCO_3$;
- Extremely hard: more than 400 mg/L $CaCO_3$.

Molar Concentration

Colligative properties are those that depend on the number of molecules or ions present and not on their nature, among them is the cryoscopic descent. It is the drop in the freezing point of a dilute solution that is proportional to the molar concentration of the solute [44].

When one mole of a substance is dissolved in 1000 g of pure water, this will reduce the freezing point of water by 1.85 ºC. Given the freezing point depression for our blood plasma is -0.56 ºC, natural waters may be classified into:

- Hypotonic: freezing point depression lower than -0.55 °C;
- Isotonic: freezing point depression from -0.55 ° to -0.58 °C;
- Hypertonic: freezing point depression greater than -0.58 °C.

BS ISO 21426:2018

The norm UNE-ISO 21426 applicable to Tourism and related services, which is identical to the International Norm ISO 21426:2018 [46], includes an informative appendix containing a guide to characterise mineral waters with therapeutic properties (minimum values). Table 8 may be used as a guide to the characterization of waters when there is no corresponding legislation ISO [46].

Table 8. ISO 21426:2018 Mineral waters with therapeutic properties

Compound	mg/L	Minerals waters with therapeutic properties
Ca^{2+}	500	Calcium
Mg^{2+}	150	Magnesium
Fe^{2+}	20	Bivalent iron
Li^{+}	2	Lithium
SO_4^{2-}	1200	Sulphate
HCO_3^-	1300	Bicarbonate
I^-	1	Iodide
F^-	1	Fluor
(HS^-, H_2S, HS_x^-)	1	Hydrogen sulphide
CO_2	1000	Carbon dioxide
Rn	666 Bq/L	Radon
Cl^-	8.5 g	Saline water

Adapted from [46].

Conclusion

Natural mineral waters have been classified, from the point of view of Medical Hydrology, to guide the reader on their possible beneficial effects for the organism [36, 47-49].

References

[1] Stillinger FH. Water revisited. *Science.* 1980;209(4455):451-7.
[2] Hannay N. *Treatise on solid state chemistry.* New York: Plenum Press; 1976.
[3] Reid R, Prausnitz J, Sherwood T. *The properties of gases and liquids.* New York: McGraw-Hill; 1977.
[4] Rodríguez Mellado J, Marín Galvín R. *Fisicoquímica de aguas.* [*Waters physicochemistry*]. Madrid: Díaz de Santos; 1999.
[5] Spice J, Alcaide García A. *Enlace químico y estructura.* [*Chemical bond and structure*]. Madrid: Alhambra; 1967.
[6] Wenclawiak B. *Analysis with supercritical fluids.* Berlin: Springer-Verlag; 1992.
[7] Heywood V. *Plant taxonomy.* London: Edward Arnold; 1967.
[8] Dickerson R. Chemical Evolution and the Origin of Life. *Sci Am.* 1978;239(3):70-87.
[9] Limón Montero A. *Espejo cristalino de las aguas de España, hermoseado, y guarnecido con el marco de variedad de fuentes y baños. Cuyas virtudes, excelencias, y propiedades se examinan, disputan y acomodan à la salud, provecho y conveniencias de la vida humana.* [*Crystal mirror of the waters of Spain, beautified, and decorated with the variety frame of fountains and baths. Whose virtues, excellences, and properties are examined, disputed, and accommodated to the health, benefit, and conveniences of human life*]. Madrid: IGME; 1979.

[10] Gómez de Bedoya y Paredes P. *Historia universal de las fuentes minerales de España.* [*Universal history of the mineral springs of Spain*]. Santiago: Tip. de Ignacio Aguayo. [Santiago: Typography of Ignacio Aguayo]; 1765.

[11] Rubio P. *Tratado completo de las fuentes minerales de España.* [*Complete treatise of the mineral springs of Spain*]. Madrid: Tip. de R. R. de Rivera. [Madrid: Typography of Ignacio Aguayo]; 1853.

[12] Casares y Rodríguez A, Calleja A. *Tratado práctico de análisis química de las aguas minerales y potables.* [*Practical treatise on chemical analysis of mineral and drinking waters*]. Madrid: Librería de D. Ángel Calleja. [Madrid: Bookshop of D. Ángel Calleja]; 1866.

[13] García López A. *Hidrología médica.* [*Medical Hydrology*]. Madrid: Pinto; 1889.

[14] Rodríguez Pinilla, H. *Medicaciones hidrológicas.* [*Hydrological medications*]. Madrid: Saturnino Calleja; 1920.

[15] Directive 2003/40/EC of 16 May 2003 establishing the list, concentration limits and labelling requirements for the constituents of natural mineral waters and the conditions for using ozone-enriched air for the treatment of natural mineral waters and spring waters. *OJEU.* 2003; line 126, page 34. Available at: https://www.legislation.gov.uk/eudr/2003/40/pdfs/eudr_20030040_adopted_en.pdf. Accessed on May 30, 2021.

[16] Directive 2009/54/EC of the European Parliament and of the Council of 18 June 2009 on the exploitation and marketing of natural mineral waters. *OJEU.* 2009; line 164, page 45. Available at: https://www.legislation.gov.uk/eudr/2009/54/contents. Accessed on May 30, 2021.

[17] Armijo M, San Martín J. *Curas balnearias y climáticas.* [*Balneo and climatic cures*]. Madrid: Editorial Complutense; 1994.

[18] Messina B, Grossi F. *Elementi di idrologia medica.* [*Elements of Medical Hydrology*]. Roma: Universo. [Rome: Universe]; 1984.

[19] Maraver F, Michán A. Es igual el agua del grifo que el agua envasada? No, sin duda, no. [Is tap water the same as mineral water? No, certainly, it is not]. *Med Clin* (*Barc*). 2010;134(1):40-2.

[20] Maraver F, Vazquez I, Armijo F. *Vademécum III de aguas mineromedicinales españolas*. [*Vademecum III of Spanish mineral-medicinal waters*]. Madrid: Editorial Complutense; 2020.
[21] Dubourg K, Fouquey J, Labarthe S. Produits hydrothermaux. [Hydrothermal products]. In: Queneau P, Roques Ch, coord. La médecine thermale. *Données scientifique*. [*Thermal medicine. Scientific data*]. Montrouge: John Libbey Eurotex; 2018:15-22.
[22] Agostini G. *Manuale de Medicina Termale*. [*Manual of Thermal Medicine*]. Torino: Archimedica. [Turin: Archimedica]; 2000.
[23] Nappi G. *Medicina e clinica termale*. [*Medicine and Spa clinic*]. Pavia: Selecta Medica; 2001.
[24] Behrend HJ. Hydrotherapy. In: Lych S, ed. *Medical Hydrology*. Baltimore: Wawerly Press; 1963:239-53.
[25] Amelung W, Hildebrandt G. *Balneologie und medizinische Klimatologie*. [*Balneology and Medical Climatology*]. Berlin: Springer; 1985.
[26] Armijo M. *Compendio de Hidrología médica*. [*Compendium of Medical Hydrology*]. Barcelona: Edit. Cientifico-Médica. [Barcelona: Publisher Scientific-Medical]; 1968.
[27] Armijo F. Expresión de los resultados del análisis de las aguas minero medicinales. [Expression of the results of the analysis of medicinal mineral waters]. In: Armijo M, San Martin J, eds. *Curas Balnearias y Climáticas*. [*Balneo and climatic cures*]. Madrid: Editorial Complutense; 1994:131-40.
[28] Rice EW, Baird RB, Eaton AD, eds. *Standard methods for the examination of water and wastewater*. 23rd edition. Washington, DC: American Public Health Association, American Water Works Association, Water Environment Federation; *2017*.
[29] Curtman L. *Análisis químico cualitativo; basado en las leyes de equilibrio y en la teoría de la ionización*. [*Qualitative chemical analysis; based on the laws of equilibrium and the theory of ionisation*]. Barcelona: Editorial Marín SA; 1959.
[30] Acciauiuoli LMC. Le *Portugal Hydromineral*. [*Hydromineral Portugal*]. Lisboa: Direcção Geral de Minas e dos Servicos

Geológicos. [Lisbon: General Directorate of Mines and Geological Services]; 1952.

[31] Araujo ARTS, Sarraguça MC, Ribeiro MP, Coutinho P. Physicochemical fingerprinting of thermal waters of Beira Interior region of Portugal. *Environ Geochem Health.* 2017;39(3):483-96.

[32] Direcção-Geral de Geologia e Minas. [Directorate-General for Geology and Mines]. *Termas e Águas Engarrafadas em Portugal.* [*Thermal Spas and Bottled Waters in Portugal*]. Lisboa: Grafispaço Lda. [Lisbon: Grafispaço Limited]; 1992.

[33] LaMoreaux PE, Tanner JT, eds. *Springs and Bottled waters of the world*. Berlin: Springer; 2001.

[34] Société Française d'Hydrologie et Climatologie médicale. [French Society of Hydrology and Medical Climatology]. *Précis de Pharmacologie et de Thérapeuthique Hydrominérale.* [*Precise of Pharmacology and Hydromineral Therapeutics*]. Paris: L'Expansion scientifique françaises; 1964.

[35] Teixeira F. O termalismo na Região Centro. [Thermalism in the Center Region]. *Bol Soc Esp Hidrol Med.* 2015;30(2):135-70.

[36] Teixeira FJ, Gomes CSF. Natural Mineral Water Used in Health Resort Medicine. In: Gomes C, Rautureau M, eds. *Minerals latu sensu and Human Health*. Cham: Springer; 2021:557-605.

[37] Catalán J. *Química del agua*. [*Chemistry of water*]. Madrid: Bellisco; 1990.

[38] Lutgens F, Tarbuck E. *Essentials of Geology*. Upper Saddle River, New Jersey: Prentice Hall; 2000.

[39] Budavari S, Windholz M. *The Merck Index.* Rahway, New Jersey: Merck; 1983.

[40] Carbajo JM, Maraver F. Sulphurous Mineral Waters: New Applications for Health. *Evid Based Complement Alternat Med.* 2017;2017:8034084.

[41] Armijo F. Viajes de agua IV. *Las aguas en los territorios del Quijote.* [*Waters in the territories of Quijote*]. 1st edition. Madrid: ACCI, Asociación Cultural y Científica Iberoamericana. [Madrid: ACCI, Ibero-american Cultural and Scientific Association]; 2016.

[42] Hernández-Pacheco F. *La tectónica peninsular y su relación con las aguas mineromedicinales.* [*The peninsular tectonics and its relationship with minero-medicinal waters*]. Madrid: Real Academia de Farmacia. [Madrid: Royal Academy of Pharmacy]; 1949.

[43] Poblete M, Beato S, Marino J. Landforms in the Campo de Calatrava Volcanic Field (Ciudad Real, Central Spain). *Journal of Maps.* 2016;12(sup1):271-279.

[44] Glasstone S. *Textbook of Physical Chemistry*. London: Macmillan; 1974.

[45] Girard R. *Essai de classification des eaux naturelles pour le transport et la distribution.* [*Classification trial of natural waters for transport and distribution*]. Paris: Tribune du CEBEDEAU. [Paris: Tribune of CEBEDEAU]; 1973.

[46] ISO21426:2018. *Tourism and related services. Medical spas. Service requirements.* November 2018. Available at: https://www.iso.org/ standard/70912.html. Accessed on May 30, 2021.

[47] Ferreira-Pêgo C, Babio N, Maraver F, Vitoria I, Salas J. Water mineralization and its importance for health. *Alim Nutri Salud.* 2016;23(1):4-18.

[48] Françon F, Traverse PM. Classification of therapeutic mineral waters. In: Lych S, ed. *Medical Hydrology*. Baltimore: Wawerly Press; 1963:390-98.

[49] Teixeira FJ, Gomes CSF. Mineral Water: Essential to Life, Health, and Wellness. In: Gomes C, Rautureau M, eds. *Minerals latu sensu and Human Health.* Cham: Springer; 2021:517-56.

In: Mineral Water
Editors: Maria João Martins

ISBN: 978-1-68507-458-6

Chapter 2

Clinical and Immunological Effects of Inhaled Thermal Waters in Chronic Obstructive Pulmonary Disease

Luís Taborda-Barata[1,2,3,*], MD, PhD
and Marco Contoli[4], MD, PhD

[1]NuESP-Planetary Health Study Group, Faculty of Health Sciences, University of Beira Interior, Covilhã, Portugal
[2]CICS-Health Sciences Research Centre, University of Beira Interior, Covilhã, Portugal
[3]Department of Allergy and Clinical Immunology, Cova da Beira University Hospital Centre, Covilhã, Portugal
[4]Department of Morphology, Surgery and Experimental Medicine, University of Ferrara, Italy

[*] Corresponding Author's E-mail: tabordabarata@fcsaude.ubi.pt.

ABSTRACT

Chronic Obstructive Pulmonary Disease (COPD) is a chronic respiratory pathology with a high global burden of disease worldwide. It involves persistent airflow limitation and other changes that are associated with an inflammatory component, to which neutrophils and mediators that chemoatttract them, as well as other mediators and oxidative bursts, contribute. The inhalation of thermal waters has been used, mainly empirically, for many centuries in patients with chronic respiratory diseases. However, the effectiveness of such treatments in COPD patients, in terms of modulation of inflammatory parameters and clinical improvement, is limited to very few studies. Further studies, involving a higher number of well-characterised COPD patients, with different severities and clinical phenotypes, are sought to support the use in COPD patients and to identify patients who would benefit the most from this therapeutic approach.

Keywords: chronic obstructive pulmonary disease, thermal water

INTRODUCTION

Chronic Obstructive Pulmonary Disease (COPD) is a chronic respiratory illness definitely contributing towards the global burden of diseases worldwide. It involves persistent airflow limitation and other changes that are associated with an inflammatory component. In this chapter, we will focus on clinical research involving thermal, natural mineral water treatments for COPD. In order to better understand the potential mechanisms of such treatments, we will also have to address some, but not all, of the clinical and inflammatory features of COPD that are more relevant to understanding such studies.

Finally, we will comment on the implications of such thermal water-based clinical studies and will outline the main future perspectives and knowledge gaps that will need to be addressed.

General Aspects about Chronic Obstructive Pulmonary Disease

As defined by GOLD (Global Initiative for Chronic Obstructive Lung Disease), COPD is "a common, preventable and treatable disease that is characterised by persistent respiratory symptoms and airflow limitation that is due to airway and/or alveolar abnormalities usually caused by significant exposure to noxious particles or gases and influenced by host factors including abnormal lung development." [1].

It is also important to highlight that the chronic, persistent airflow limitation which is observed in COPD is caused by a varying mixture of small airways disease (e.g., obstructive bronchiolitis) and parenchymal destruction (emphysema) [1].

COPD is currently the fourth most relevant cause of morbidity and mortality worldwide, and is expected to increase in importance even further in the coming years [1-4]. It should also be highlighted that COPD is associated with substantial and increasing economic and social costs, given the fact that it involves frequent exacerbations, hospitalizations, multimorbidity and low quality of life, particularly in more advanced cases [1]. In fact, COPD is frequently accompanied by significant concurrent morbidities (e.g., cardiovascular, diabetes, lung cancer, etc.), with a proportion of patients also having features of Asthma-COPD overlap (ACO), and such features also contribute to making COPD more difficult to manage [5, 6].

COPD is caused by significant, chronic exposure to noxious particles or gases, although it may also be influenced by a genetic component. Worldwide, cigarette smoking is the most common risk factor for developing the disease, particularly in developed countries [1]. In contrast, in low- and middle-income countries, other risk factors are quite relevant, particularly exposure to biomass particulate pollution, as occurs with wood smoke inhalation while cooking foods or when heating homes [1, 7-10]. Finally, various types of occupational exposure involving fumes, chemical agents, organic and inorganic dusts and other factors are also risk factors for COPD [11, 12] and may even condition worse morbidity [13].

Diagnosis and Clinical Assessment of Chronic Obstructive Pulmonary Disease

Lung function assessment is a *sine qua non condition* for COPD diagnosis. Besides spirometry, we will here briefly focus on other measurements that can be used in daily clinical practice to assess COPD patients.

Lung Function Tests

Lung function tests most frequently involve spirometry, although more complex techniques, namely plethysmography or other, can also be used. Among other aspects, spirometry allows detailed analysis of parameters of bronchial obstruction, namely its main location, as well as intensity [14]. Some of the most relevant parameters, such as forced expiratory volume in 1 second (FEV_1), forced vital capacity (FVC) and the ratio between these two parameters (FEV_1/FVC or Tiffeneau's index) are essential for confirmation of airflow obstruction and its severity [14]. In general, a FEV_1/FVC ratio of less than 0.70, even after short-acting adrenergic β-agonist bronchial dilation confirms the diagnosis of COPD [1]. Furthermore, it is possible to classify COPD into various stages of severity (GOLD 1 to 4), based on FEV_1 values, with the lowest values indicating very severe COPD [1].

Questionnaires for Symptoms and Quality of Life

Various validated questionnaires can be used for sub-classifying COPD, allocating patients to the degree of risk, or assessing quality of life, symptoms, and activity restriction due to the disease.

Borg Dyspnoea Score

The *Borg Dyspnoea Score* (BDS) is based on a category scale that specifically measures self-perception of the degree of dyspnoea affecting patients during exercise [15, 16]. It ranges between 6 and 20 units, directly depending on perceived intensity of exercise-associated dyspnoea. The higher the score, the more intensely is dyspnoea perceived. There is a later, *modified Borg dyspnoea scale*, which is a category-ratio scale ranging between 0 (nothing at all) and 10 units (maximal), aiming at more specifically recording symptomatic breathlessness, but the principle is the same [17].

COPD Assessment Test

The *COPD Assessment Test* (CAT) is a questionnaire which is an 8-item unidimensional measure of health status impairment, particularly in terms of symptoms, in COPD [18]. Each of the 8 items is scored from 0 to 5, with 0 being "Not affected" and 5 "Very affected". The total score thus ranges from 0 to 40, and the higher its score is the more affected the patient is [18, 19]. In this context, a score < 10 is equivalent to a "low COPD impact", 11-20 implies "medium COPD impact", 21-30 means "high COPD impact" and ≥ 30 indicates "very high COPD impact".

St George's Respiratory Questionnaire

The *St George's Respiratory Questionnaire* (SGRQ) is a more complex standardised, self-completed, broad 76-item questionnaire, divided into three sections (symptoms – 24 items, activity – 16 items, and psychosocial impacts – 36 items), focusing on various domains of patient activity and perceived "well-being" or quality of life in airways disease [20]. This questionnaire is largely used in Randomised Controlled Trials (RCTs); however, because of its complexity it is not routinely used in daily clinical practice. A score is calculated for each section but a total score is also obtained. A higher score means worse quality of life. It is designed to allow comparison of health parameters between patient populations and also to quantify treatment- or other intervention-associated respiratory health changes.

Exercise Tolerance Tests

The 6-Minute Walk Test

The 6-minute walk test measures the distance, in metres, which is walked during a 6-minute period [21, 22]. It is easy to administer, well tolerated and fairly accurately predicts morbidity and mortality from heart or lung disease. Its main indications include measuring outcomes before and after a therapeutic intervention, although it can also be used to assess disease progression [21, 22].

Tests for Analysis of Lung Inflammation

Assessment of lung inflammation is not used in daily clinical practice but can provide valuable information in COPD patients.

Induced Sputum

Induced sputum is a method which involves inhalation of either increasing concentrations (3-5%) of an aerosol of hypertonic saline [23] or inhalation of the same concentration for progressively longer periods [24]. In any case, inhalation occurs via an ultrasonic nebuliser, for defined periods, up to a total of 30 minutes, with some pauses in between, and then collecting sputum that is thus produced [23-25]. The induced sputum that is obtained needs to be processed and can then be stored for subsequent analysis of cells and mediators.

Exhaled Breath Condensate

Exhaled Breath Condensate (EBC) is a recent and non-invasive method performed during quiet breathing, for detection of a wide variety of metabolic, proteomic, lipidomic and genomic biomarkers which mostly stem from the lower airways [26]. EBC seems to adequately reflect the airway epithelial function, and this is quite useful for the study of respiratory diseases, such as COPD [27].

Clinical Concepts about Chronic Obstructive Pulmonary Disease

General Aspects

The most common manifestations of COPD are progressive dyspnoea, chronic cough and/or sputum production, which may be associated with or even precede the development of spirometry-confirmed airflow limitation [1]. In addition, COPD patients often have a history of recurrent lower respiratory tract infections, which are associated with COPD exacerbations [28], and may contribute towards a vicious cycle leading to progressive lung function decline [29].

However, there are clearly different clinical phenotypes of COPD, with some patients having predominantly small airways disease, whereas others mainly have pathological emphysema, with increased alveolar space and destruction. These and other aspects may contribute to different clinical manifestations. In addition, other heterogeneous aspects observed in different COPD patients include age of onset, rate of progression, frequency of exacerbations and the association with other comorbidities, such as chronic cardiovascular diseases and metabolic syndrome. Although various studies have classified COPD patients into different clinical phenotypes based on cluster analysis or application of algorithms to clinical and radiological characteristics [30], it has been difficult to reliably identify such phenotypes in different populations and, furthermore, no solid relationship with common underlying inflammatory disease mechanisms or endotypes has been established [31-33]. In contrast, some cellular, inflammatory endotypes have been characterised [32] and we will comment upon these aspects further on.

Independently of such aspects, COPD is generally characterised by an irreversible persistent decline of airflow associated with an enhanced chronic inflammatory response and emphysematous changes [34].

Pathophysiology of Chronic Obstructive Pulmonary Disease

Cellular Aspects of Inflammation

COPD is a chronic inflammatory disease, with inflammation being predominantly localized to peripheral airways and lung parenchyma [32, 35]. However, COPD-associated inflammation seems not to affect just the lung but also appears to include a systemic component which, in fact, may explain some of the comorbidities [36].

Inflammation in COPD involves the influx by infiltrating cells of both innate and adaptive components of the immune system, particularly neutrophils and macrophages in the airway lumen as well as macrophages, T lymphocytes and B lymphocytes in the airway wall and parenchyma [35, 37-39]. Of all these cells, neutrophils are possibly the most common effector cells with a role in inflammation underlying COPD.

In fact, increased numbers of neutrophils have long been known to be the predominant feature of intraluminal airway inflammation in the disease [40, 41], although other cellular inflammatory types may also occur in COPD, namely with an influx of eosinophils in the eosinophil-rich COPD endotype [32]. Nevertheless, neutrophils are most frequently key inflammatory cells in the pathogenesis of COPD, with sputum and blood neutrophilia being a characteristic feature of most COPD patients, although with varying degrees. Furthermore, neutrophils are not only a possible biomarker of COPD, albeit not a very specific one, but have also been reported as a marker of its severity and symptoms [42-44]. These aspects can be translated into practical issues. In this context, in terms of potential impact of neutrophilia in COPD, an observational study found that patients with higher sputum neutrophil percentages had a higher dyspnoea score across different severities of COPD [45]. In addition, higher numbers of sputum neutrophils have been shown to correlate with accelerated decline of FEV_1 [46, 47].

It should be again stated that COPD is not just an inflammatory disease with bronchial obstruction. The airway obstruction in COPD is usually progressive with accelerated decline in lung function over many years, although longitudinal studies have shown that only about 50% of patients with COPD have accelerated decline in lung function [48]. Progressive obstruction in COPD can be due to the fact that the underlying inflammatory component is associated with progressively severe lung structural, pathological and functional changes, namely basal, goblet and mucous cell hyperplasia, increased mucus production and plugging, as well as airway fibrosis [49, 50] and airways remodelling [51, 52]. Fibrosis and collapse of peripheral airways due to loss of elasticity in the lung parenchyma, which leads to air trapping, are the predominant causes of airways obstruction in small airway narrowing [53]. However, concurrent, reversible, cholinergic contraction of small airways may also play a part, and mucus hypersecretion also contributes to airway obstruction, namely by formation of mucous plugs [51, 54], indicating a chronic bronchitis component in a high proportion of patients [55].

It is also important to realize that although inflammatory cells, such as neutrophils and macrophages, have a key role in antibacterial defences [56], they may also induce and maintain inflammation in COPD, particularly neutrophils, due to the release of oxidants, inflammatory mediators and destructive proteases [35, 57]. In fact, neutrophil-derived proteases, such as neutrophil elastase, may contribute to COPD by increasing the release of inflammatory cell-attracting chemokines from epithelial cells [58], by triggering extracellular matrix elastin breakdown [59], besides impairing the antimicrobial interleukin (IL)-22/IL-22 receptor signaling pathway and by decreasing the expression of antimicrobial effectors, such as β-defensin-2 [60]. Finally, neutrophils can also release web-like extracellular structures, known as neutrophil extracellular traps (NETs) [61], that retain microbicidal and cytotoxic proteins, and which are an important mechanism in innate immunity against pathogens, but that may also contribute to the damage of the host tissue [61, 62]. It should be highlighted that there is a significant increase in NET formation in sputum of patients with stable COPD [63], where these structures may be involved not only in antimicrobial but also pathological effects [61].

In this context, various studies have endeavoured to define COPD-related biomarkers, many of which reflect underlying inflammatory parameters, and may, in some cases, eventually predict COPD exacerbations [64]. The main problem with biomarkers in COPD is their low specificity and their longitudinal changes depending upon disease progression.

Nevertheless, a wide variety of biomarkers have been studied and these include neutrophils and neutrophil-related enzymes, cytokines and chemokines (such as IL-8), eosinophils and eosinophil-related enzymes and biomarkers, arachidonic acid-derived inflammatory mediators, biomarkers of oxidative stress, as well as multiple other molecules, namely those reflecting extracellular matrix proteins and epithelial cell-derived molecules [3, 65-67].

We will next only address some of the soluble mediators that have been studied in clinical trials of thermal water treatments of COPD patients (leukotrienes [LTs], pH in EBC, and oxidative stress-related mediators) as well as other parameters that are relevant to the involved context, such as production of endogenous hydrogen sulphide (H_2S).

Mediators of Inflammation

Arachidonic Acid Derivatives

Arachidonic acid is the main source of several families of lipid mediators, including prostaglandins (PGs), thromboxanes (TXs), LTs, and lipoxins, via the cyclooxygenase (COX) and lipoxygenase (LOX) pathways [68]. In addition, isoprostanes, derived from arachidonic acid via peroxidation, are both biomarkers and mediators of oxidative stress [69]. On the other hand, LTs, such as LTB_4, and cysteinyl-leukotrienes, such as LTC_4, LTD_4 and LTE_4, are produced by activated macrophages, neutrophils, eosinophils and epithelial cells and all seem to be relevant to the pathogenesis of COPD [70].

LTB_4, in particular, seems to have direct or indirect inflammatory and clinical implications in COPD. In fact, it has previously been shown that LTB_4 levels were increased in induced sputum of COPD patients undergoing an exacerbation, in comparison with stable patients [71]. In addition, in longitudinal studies, LTB_4 was also a good factor predicting exacerbations [64]. Furthermore, LTB_4 may contribute to the COPD inflammation-associated neutrophil influx into the lung [72], since it is one of the most potent chemotactic agents for these cells [70].

Oxidative Stress

Oxidative stress is a fundamental component of airway inflammation in COPD [73, 74). In particular, reactive oxygen species (ROS), such as superoxide anion ($O_2^{-\bullet}$) and hydrogen peroxide (H_2O_2), can be produced, under stress, in excessive amounts not only by resident epithelial and vascular cells in the lung but also by infiltrating inflammatory cells [73-76]. This excessive production may thus exceed pulmonary anti-oxidant defence mechanisms, such as glutathione and thioredoxin redox systems, or catalase and superoxide dismutase enzymatic systems [77]. Those molecules can induce further relevant oxidative processes in various cell types. In addition, ROS are also associated with multiple other effects in the lung, namely remodelling of the extracellular matrix, protease-antiprotease imbalance, reduction of surfactant production, slowing down the airway epithelial repair process or changes in cellular respiration [74-76]. In addition, ROS also affect immune responses in the lung, namely by interfering with proliferation, activation and function of cells, such as macrophages [73-76].

Finally, it should be highlighted that excessive production of ROS in COPD may be associated with increased inflammation, and contribute towards disease development or severity, namely regarding exacerbations [73, 78, 79].

Endogenous Hydrogen Sulphide

In the human lung, H_2S is produced by epithelial, vascular, and smooth muscle cells, and is mainly synthesised from L-cysteine via cytoplasmic and mitochondrial cystathionine-β-synthase and cystathionine-γ-lyase enzymes [80, 81]. Other sources of endogenous H_2S also exist [80, 82] and it should also be borne in mind that H_2S can also be produced by gastrointestinal and pulmonary tract microbiomes [83, 84]. After being synthesised, H_2S can either act on its biological targets or be stored as a bound sulfane sulphur pool [84, 85] as well as an acid-labile sulphur pool [83, 86]. In the presence of oxygen, H_2S undergoes oxidation in mitochondria and also methylation in the cytoplasm [80, 87]. Free H_2S can also be scavenged by methemoglobin and metal- or disulphide bond-carrying molecules, and excreted in biological fluids, namely urine and flatuses, as well as exhaled in breath [80, 81].

In terms of function, H_2S can act as a cellular oxygen sensor [88] and may contribute towards body homeostasis [82]. Indeed, the decrease in H_2S oxidation under hypoxic conditions has been associated with the production of significant amounts of H_2S by airway epithelial cells (AECs) [89].

In COPD, various aspects regarding endogenous H_2S have to be taken into account and we will focus on studies involving larger samples of patients.

First of all, there seems to be an association between levels of H_2S and the inflammatory profile of COPD patients. For example, in a study carried out in 2009/2010 by Zhang and collaborators, involving 77 COPD patients [60 male, 67.09±8.29 years old (mean±standard deviation, SD)], subdivided into "eosinophilic" and "non-eosinophilic" groups, there was a negative correlation between exhaled levels of H_2S and sputum eosinophilia, suggesting that increased levels of exhaled H_2S may predict a non-eosinophilic phenotype in these patients [90].

In fact, this finding appeared to have clinical implications, since "eosinophilic" COPD patients had lower levels of exhaled H_2S than "non-eosinophilic" ones, and this was associated with longer disease course, lower quality of life scores, worse lung function (although they had a better response to bronchodilators) and health status, and more frequent exacerbations [90]. Association of serum H_2S levels with non-neutrophilic profiles was also observed in another study performed in 2005 by Chen and collaborators enrolling 64 COPD patients [27 undergoing an exacerbation (AECOPD, 16 male), 76.7±1.3 years old (mean±standard error of the mean, SEM); 37 with stable COPD (29 male), 65.6±1.6 years old] and 13 healthy individuals (6 male, 58.7±2.3 years old) [91]. This study showed that serum H_2S levels had a negative correlation with sputum neutrophils, and a positive association with sputum lymphocytes and macrophages in all patients with COPD. However, these results have to be interpreted carefully, since other studies have shown an association between higher levels of sputum H_2S and neutrophils, as we will see further on [92].

Secondly, H_2S availability may also be related to the stage of airway obstruction in COPD since its levels seem to be significantly decreased in the more advanced GOLD stage 3 than in the milder stage 1, as seen in the study by Chen *et al.* [91].

Thirdly, different levels of H_2S may vary between stable phases and exacerbations of COPD. For instance, in the study by Chen *et al.,* serum levels of H_2S were higher in stable COPD patients than in AECOPD patients [91]. This was also seen in another study performed by Saito *et al.*, in 2012/2013, involving 29 AECOPD patients [18 male, 74.7±9.06 years old (mean±SD)], 64 patients with stable COPD (33 male, 69.1±8.6 years old), 14 healthy smokers (6 male, 54.4±7.31 years old) and 21 healthy non-smokers (13 male, 49.2±9.24 years old), in which serum H_2S levels were significantly lower in AECOPD than in stable COPD patients and healthy smokers and non-smokers [92]. However, it should be highlighted that the same study also showed that sputum H_2S levels were significantly higher in AECOPD than in stable COPD patients and healthy smokers and non-smokers [92], suggesting that there may be target organ-specific changes in H_2S production in COPD exacerbations. In addition, it should be stressed that this same study allowed calculation of a sputum-to-serum H_20 ratio in COPD, which was, by inference, higher in exacerbations and which, importantly, was positively correlated with SGRQ, sputum neutrophils, and IL-6 as well as IL-8 levels in sputum, and inversely correlated with lung function parameters [92].

Overall, despite some of the abovementioned contradictions, all studies indicated significant changes of H_2S and H_2S synthesis-involved enzyme levels in COPD subjects. These alterations in H_2S metabolism seem to contribute, at least in part, to exacerbations and worsening of this respiratory disease state, thereby affecting general lung function.

pH in Exhaled Breath Condensate

EBC is essentially composed of water and aerosolised droplets from the airway lining fluid, as well water-soluble volatile compounds, all of which contribute towards determining the pH of EBC [93]. It should be highlighted that EBC pH may reflect acidity present in the airways in a robust and reproducible way [94]. Furthermore, EBC pH may be a biomarker of COPD severity at least in ex-smokers [95].

At least in part due to the inflammatory component of the disease as well as infections that may change pH homeostasis in the airways [96], EBC pH has been shown to be lower in patients with COPD than in healthy subjects [95, 97]. Furthermore, hypopharyngeal gastric acid reflux, which is very common in patients with COPD may also play a part in lower airways pH in these patients, although a causal link has not been firmly established [98].

Figure 1 shows a conceptual outline of various aspects concerning COPD and the corresponding effects of inhaled crenotherapy.

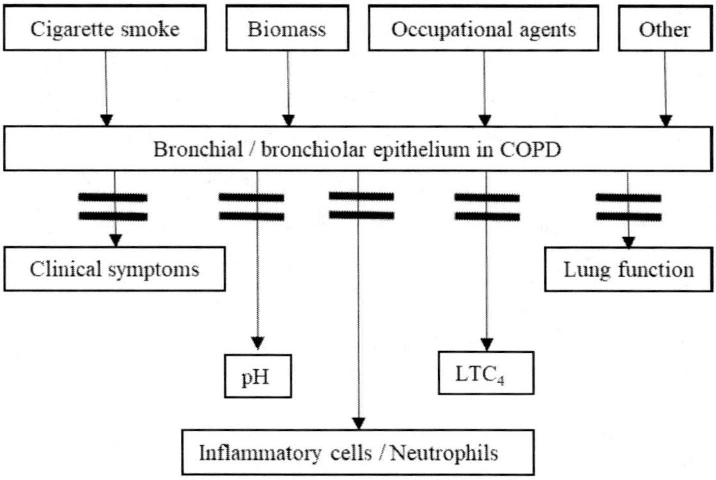

Figure 1. Conceptual outline of various COPD parameters and demonstrated treatment efficacy by inhaled crenotherapy for the disease. ═ Blocked by thermal water treatments.

Clinical and Anti-Inflammatory Effects of Sulphurous Thermal Natural Mineral Waters in Chronic Obstructive Pulmonary Disease

Various studies have taken place, over time, involving different treatment approaches in patients with COPD. Many of these approaches were implemented in different countries [99-131], involving patients with different COPD definitions and including treatment options such as sauna, balneotherapy and mud therapy, climate therapy or speleotherapy (treatment in natural caves). In addition, most of them have been non-controlled studies, with small patient samples and frequently not focused on respiratory crenotherapy (or such information was not adequately displayed). We will, therefore, not focus on these studies.

Respiratory, inhalational crenotherapy involves the inhalation of thermal water. Although it is not regarded as a therapeutic option for

COPD patients in international guidelines [1], inhalation of thermal water has been used since ancient times to treat patients suffering from chronic disorders, including respiratory symptoms. Various aspects regarding this therapeutic approach have been previously discussed by several authors over time [132-140]. It is plausible that benefits of inhalation of thermal water as treatment of chronic respiratory disorders may be partially due to putative mucolytic, anti-inflammatory, immunomodulatory, antioxidant and vasodilatory and vascular trophic properties [140-143]. For further detailed information please read the chapter regarding *Thermal Waters in Otorhinolaryngology*.

Assumptions that thermal waters have anti-inflammatory properties are mostly based on *in vivo* studies using sulphurous and non-sulphurous waters, performed in patients with rhinitis/rhinosinusitis/upper respiratory tract diseases, with collection of samples for analysis of nasal cytology, but also on *in vitro* studies (for the respective references please see the next two paragraphs).

In vivo treatment with sulphurous thermal waters resulted in a reduction of polymorphonuclear cells in nasal cytology of patients with nonallergic chronic rhinosinusitis/chronic inflammation of the upper respiratory airways [144, 145]. Similar results were observed with non-sulphurous thermal waters in chronic rhinosinusitis/allergic rhinitis/upper respiratory tract inflammations [146-148]. In addition, an improvement of symptoms, along with a decrease in serum immunoglobulin (Ig) E and an increase in serum IgA, was observed in patients with perennial allergic rhinitis after treatment with iodine bromide thermal water [149].

An *in vitro* study using cultures of T lymphocytes exposed to sulphurous thermal water showed a decrease in mitogen-induced proliferative responses [141]. Furthermore, these results were reproduced in other *in vitro* study in which exogenous H_2S highly significantly reduced mitogen-induced proliferative responses and IL-2 production in T lymphocytes, and, simultaneously, increased caspase-independent cell death [150]. Together, these results suggest that sulphurous thermal waters and H_2S may potentially decrease inflammation at least in part through the reduction of the functional properties of effector T-lymphocytes, namely in target organs.

H_2S is, as we have discussed before, a potent reducing agent that is present at high levels in sulphurous thermal waters and in lower concentrations in salt-bromide-iodine thermal waters. Treatment of bronchial epithelial cell lines with sulphurous thermal water before rhinovirus infection resulted in increased concentrations of the endogenous intracellular reducing agent glutathione (GSH) and in the inhibition of a rhinovirus induced intracellular oxidative burst [151].

A non-controlled study carried out by Nappi and collaborators (2001 and 2003) at Tabiano Spa, in Italy, involved the treatment of 37 COPD patients [25 male, 12 female, 59.6±8.7 years old (mean±SD)] for 12 days with inhalation and nebulisation with sulphur-salt-calcium-magnesic thermal water (from the Arvé spring of the Tabiano Spa) [152]. Patients were assessed before (baseline) and after treatment (day 12) only in terms of induced sputum and IgG and IgA antibodies against *Chlamydia pneumoniae* but not in clinical terms. This study showed that inhaled crenotherapy with sulphurous thermal water was associated with a decrease in *C. pneumoniae*-specific IgG and IgA antibodies, which may be pertinent since this pathogen commonly infects COPD patients [153, 154], although it may only be relevant in a subgroup of COPD patients who are frequent exacerbators [154]. However, the study by Nappi *et al.* [152] did not clearly state whether COPD patients improved clinically with the thermal treatment and this does not allow inferences regarding the relevance of changes in *C. pneumoniae*-specific IgG and IgA antibodies, namely whether that reflects a reduction in bacterial burden.

Contoli and collaborators (2013) recruited 40 patients [29 male, 11 female, 69.9±1.0 years old (mean±SEM)] suffering from moderate to severe COPD (stages 2 and 3, according to GOLD criteria [1]) for a 12-day randomised placebo-controlled double-blind study in order to evaluate the effects of the inhalation of sulphurous thermal water on airway oxidative stress as well as on patients' clinical outcomes [155]. Patients continued to use their maintenance treatment, and were randomised to receive home-delivered treatments involving inhalation and aerosol treatments, either with sulphurous thermal water (Acqua Breta, Terme di Riolo; Ravenna, Italy) or with control isotonic saline solution, both of which had been previously bottled and delivered to patients' homes. The treatment schedule reproduced the standard treatments performed at the Spa, and consisted of once daily inhalation of either sulphurous thermal water or isotonic saline, as follows: (a) 500 mL warm inhalation, and, after 20 minutes, (b) 5 mL conventional aerosolisation. Patients were observed at three time points: before the onset of treatment (baseline), the day after the conclusion of the 12-day treatment (day 13), and one month after the end of the inhalation treatment, as follow-up. Patients who underwent active treatment with sulphurous thermal water had a significant reduction in COPD symptoms and improvement of health status, as detected by a reduction in the CAT score, although not accompanied by improvement in lung function, when compared with baseline. Furthermore, clinical improvement was still observed one month after cessation of thermal water treatment. In contrast, patients who had been allocated to saline treatment did not show any significant clinical improvement. Finally, the significant improvement in CAT score in patients treated with sulphurous thermal water showed a clear trend for a significant, positive correlation with a reduction in oxidative stress parameters, as detected by a decrease in superoxide radical ($O_2^{-\bullet}$) production in EBC. Thus, this study [155] showed that a course of sulphurous thermal water treatment may improve symptoms of the disease in patients with moderate to severe COPD, and this may be associated with reduced oxidative stress in the airways.

The relevance of an oxidant/antioxidant imbalance to the pathogenesis of COPD is well-established, as previously mentioned [74]. Thus, therapeutic strategies targeting oxidative stress may be beneficial as an additional option in the treatment of COPD patients. In fact, potentially, such interventions may even increase corticosteroid sensitivity in COPD, as predicted from *in vitro* studies in mice and in human peripheral blood mononuclear cells from COPD patients [156-160].

Another randomised but not placebo-controlled study was carried out by Lopalco and collaborators (2004) and involved 63 patients (mean age 70 years old) with what the authors called "chronic bronchopneumopathy"

[161]. The study took place at "Pompeo" Spa Center, in Ferentino, Italy. All patients underwent mechanical pulmonary ventilation associated with sulphurous thermal water aerosol treatments, for 12 days. However, before the onset of treatments, patients were randomly allocated to two groups: one group (n=33) was treated with inhaled corticosteroids (flunisolide), whereas the other group (n=30) was not given any corticosteroids. Patients were studied in terms of symptoms and lung function (spirometry), before (baseline) and immediately after treatment. All patients reported an improvement in symptoms, such as dyspnoea and cough. In addition, there was a significant improvement in FEV_1 in both groups. This study showed that sulphurous thermal water inhaled crenotherapy may show clinical efficacy in patients with chronic bronchopneumopathies (most likely including some patients with COPD), independently of patients being medicated or not with inhaled corticosteroids.

Clinical and Anti-Inflammatory Effects of Salt-Bromide-Iodine Natural Mineral Thermal Waters in Chronic Obstructive Pulmonary Disease

A few other studies studied the effects of salt-bromide-iodine thermal waters in COPD patients.

In this context, a randomised placebo-controlled single-blind study carried out by Pellegrini and collaborators (2003) involved 39 patients [35 male; 4 female; aged 44 to 76 years; 64±2 years old (mean±SEM)] mostly with mild to moderate COPD [162]. Patients were matched in terms of smoking habits (pack-years) and those on inhaled or oral steroids during the previous month were excluded from the study. Unfortunately, no information was given regarding how many patients were current smokers. Patients were randomly allocated to either active treatment (aerosol nebulisation at 37 °C, for 20 minutes, once daily, for 12 days) with salt-bromide-iodine thermal water from Terme Euganee area [Abano-

Montegrotto, Veneto, Italy (n=20; 19 male; 1 female)] or control treatment using sterile normal saline solution (n=19; 16 male, 3 female). Patients were studied before (baseline) and immediately after treatment, in terms of symptoms (BDS) and health-related quality of life (using the Italian version of the SGRQ), physical exercise capacity, lung function and induced sputum. In contrast with patients on isotonic saline, those who underwent thermal water inhalation treatment had a small but significant reduction in sputum neutrophilic inflammation and a short-term improvement in quality of life, particularly in terms of SGRQ (activity and impact of disease domains). However, there was no short-term effect on exercise capacity (measured by 6-minute walk test) or on lung function parameters. This was the first controlled study [164] to examine the effect of a standard course of inhaled salt-bromide-iodine thermal water treatment on respiratory function and airway inflammation in COPD and suggests that this intervention may have a mild anti-inflammatory effect in COPD patients that is associated with some partial clinical improvement.

Another randomised placebo-controlled and single-blind cross-over study using the same thermal water was performed by the same Italian group (2010). Its aim was to determine whether treatment with this type of thermal natural mineral water could modify inflammatory aspects of airway lining fluid in patients with mild or moderate COPD (mostly GOLD stages 1-3 [1]) [163]. Thirteen COPD patients [10 male, 3 female; 69±3 years old (mean±SEM)] who were current or ex-smokers with at least a 5 pack-year smoking history, were allocated either to active treatment with salt-bromide-iodine thermal water or isotonic saline, delivered by aerosol, once daily, for 20 minutes, for a total period of 12 days, and then switched to the other treatment, after a 4-week washout period. The cross-over design allowed reaching conclusions even with a low number of patients. In addition, patients on inhaled or oral steroids during the previous month were excluded from the study but 5 of the 13 patients were current smokers. Patients were studied at the Spa before (baseline) and immediately after treatment, in terms of lung function (spirometry) and inflammatory parameters in EBC. There were no significant clinical changes with thermal water treatment in comparison with isotonic saline in terms of dyspnoea score (only a non-significant trend towards reduction of this score was found) or lung function. It should be highlighted that this study had a small patient sample and was not designed to analyse potential clinical effects of such treatments. In addition, LTB_4 concentration in EBC did not significantly change after any of the treatments. Nevertheless, a significant increase in EBC non-deaerated pH measurements was described after thermal water inhalation. Overall, this study suggested that 2-week inhalation treatment with salt-bromide-iodine thermal water may modify components of the biological substrate of COPD.

CONCLUSION

In summary, in spite of generally effective drug-based treatments for most cases of chronic rhinitis, bronchial asthma, and COPD, some patients still show a sub-optimal response to such treatments. Furthermore, over time, long-term high-dose therapy may be associated with the development of some adverse effects. Thus, additional Spa thermal water treatments, involving both sulphurous and non-sulphurous thermal waters, may be complementary non-pharmacological therapeutic tools in subjects whose symptoms are not adequately controlled with the usual drugs. With supplementary thermal water treatment, it may be possible to regain symptom control in COPD and eventually reduce baseline drug therapy. Another aspect which must be borne in mind is that with thermal water treatments at Spas, additional psychological components may also contribute towards clinical improvement. These components include leisure time, opportunity for relaxation, being aware of regular clinical monitoring, and various cultural aspects, all of which may play a part in Spa treatment-associated final results, namely in COPD [164].

However, further randomised placebo-controlled double-blind studies are needed to firmly assess clinical, antioxidant and anti-inflammatory efficacy of thermal water treatments in COPD patients. These studies should ideally involve larger samples of patients, in order to be able to adequately detect minimal clinically relevant differences in outcomes, between active and control saline treatments. Furthermore, these studies should also broaden the scope of biomarkers included for detection in oxidative- and inflammation-related parameters as well as others. In addition, studies should also include different COPD phenotypes, endotypes and/or disease symptom / exacerbation risk groups (A, B, C and D) [1], in order to better understand which type(s) of patients may best benefit from thermal water treatments.

References

[1] GOLD. *Global Strategy for the Diagnosis, Management and Prevention of COPD Report.* 2020. Available at: https://goldcopd.org/wp-content/uploads/2019/11/GOLD-2020-REPORT-ver1.0wms.pdf. Accessed on January 8, 2020.

[2] Lozano R, Naghavi M, Foreman K, Lim S, Shibuya K, Aboyans V, Abraham J, Adair T, Aggarwal R, Ahn SY, Alvarado M, Anderson HR, Anderson LM, Andrews KG, Atkinson C, Baddour LM, Barker-Collo S, Bartels DH, Bell ML, Benjamin EJ, Bennett D, Bhalla K, Bikbov B, Bin Abdulhak A, Birbeck G, Blyth F, Bolliger I, Boufous S, Bucello C, Burch M, Burney P, Carapetis J, Chen H, Chou D, Chugh SS, Coffeng LE, Colan SD, Colquhoun S, Colson KE, Condon J, Connor MD, Cooper LT, Corriere M, Cortinovis M, de Vaccaro KC, Couser W, Cowie BC, Criqui MH, Cross M, Dabhadkar KC, Dahodwala N, De Leo D, Degenhardt L, Delossantos A, Denenberg J, Des Jarlais DC, Dharmaratne SD, Dorsey ER, Driscoll T, Duber H, Ebel B, Erwin PJ, Espindola P, Ezzati M, Feigin V, Flaxman AD, Forouzanfar MH, Fowkes FG, Franklin R, Fransen M, Freeman MK, Gabriel SE, Gakidou E, Gaspari F, Gillum RF, Gonzalez-Medina D, Halasa YA, Haring D, Harrison JE, Havmoeller R, Hay RJ, Hoen B, Hotez PJ, Hoy D, Jacobsen KH, James SL, Jasrasaria R, Jayaraman S, Johns N,

Karthikeyan G, Kassebaum N, Keren A, Khoo JP, Knowlton LM, Kobusingye O, Koranteng A, Krishnamurthi R, Lipnick M, Lipshultz SE, Ohno SL, Mabweijano J, MacIntyre MF, Mallinger L, March L, Marks GB, Marks R, Matsumori A, Matzopoulos R, Mayosi BM, McAnulty JH, McDermott MM, McGrath J, Mensah GA, Merriman TR, Michaud C, Miller M, Miller TR, Mock C, Mocumbi AO, Mokdad AA, Moran A, Mulholland K, Nair MN, Naldi L, Narayan KM, Nasseri K, Norman P, O'Donnell M, Omer SB, Ortblad K, Osborne R, Ozgediz D, Pahari B, Pandian JD, Rivero AP, Padilla RP, Perez-Ruiz F, Perico N, Phillips D, Pierce K, Pope CA 3rd, Porrini E, Pourmalek F, Raju M, Ranganathan D, Rehm JT, Rein DB, Remuzzi G, Rivara FP, Roberts T, De León FR, Rosenfeld LC, Rushton L, Sacco RL, Salomon JA, Sampson U, Sanman E, Schwebel DC, Segui-Gomez M, Shepard DS, Singh D, Singleton J, Sliwa K, Smith E, Steer A, Taylor JA, Thomas B, Tleyjeh IM, Towbin JA, Truelsen T, Undurraga EA, Venketasubramanian N, Vijayakumar L, Vos T, Wagner GR, Wang M, Wang W, Watt K, Weinstock MA, Weintraub R, Wilkinson JD, Woolf AD, Wulf S, Yeh PH, Yip P, Zabetian A, Zheng ZJ, Lopez AD, Murray CJ, AlMazroa MA, Memish ZA. Global and regional mortality from 235 causes of death for 20 age groups in 1990 and 2010: a systematic analysis for the Global Burden of Disease Study 2010. *Lancet.* 2012;380(9859):2095-128. Erratum in: *Lancet.* 2013;381 (9867):628.

[3] López-Campos JL, Tan W, Soriano JB. Global burden of COPD. *Respirology.* 2016;21(1):14-23.

[4] ALA - American Lung Association Epidemiology and Statistics Unit. *Trends in COPD (Chronic Bronchitis and Emphysema): morbidity and mortality.* 2013. Available at: https://www.lung.org/getmedia/4f74781e-481f-4f10-9255-8dfc9dc56974/copd-trend-report.pdf. Accessed on December 16, 2019.

[5] Negewo NA, McDonald VM, Gibson PG. Comorbidity in chronic obstructive pulmonary disease. *Respir Investig.* 2015;53(6):249-58.

[6] Westerik JA, Metting EI, van Boven JF, Tiersma W, Kocks JW, Schermer TR. Associations between chronic comorbidity and exacerbation risk in primary care patients with COPD. *Respir Res.* 2017;18(1):31.

[7] Salvi SS, Barnes PJ. Chronic obstructive pulmonary disease in non-smokers. *Lancet.* 2009;374(9691):733-43.

[8] Salvi SS, Brashier BB, Londhe J, Pyasi K, Vincent V, Kajale SS, Tambe S, Mandani K, Nair A, Mak SM, Madas S, Juvekar S, Donnelly LE, Barnes PJ. Phenotypic comparison between smoking and non-smoking chronic obstructive pulmonary disease. *Respir Res.* 2020;21(1):50.

[9] Sana A, Somda SMA, Meda N, Bouland C. Chronic obstructive pulmonary disease associated with biomass fuel use in women: a systematic review and meta-analysis. *BMJ Open Respir Res.* 2018;5(1):e000246.

[10] Assad NA, Balmes J, Mehta S, Cheema U, Sood A. Chronic obstructive pulmonary disease secondary to household air pollution. *Semin Respir Crit Care Med.* 2015;36(3):408-21.

[11] Eisner MD, Anthonisen N, Coultas D, Kuenzli N, Perez-Padilla R, Postma D, Romieu I, Silverman EK, Balmes JR; Committee on Nonsmoking COPD, Environmental and Occupational Health Assembly. An official American Thoracic Society public policy statement: Novel risk factors and the global burden of chronic obstructive pulmonary disease. *Am J Respir Crit Care Med.* 2010;182(5):693-718.

[12] De Matteis S, Jarvis D, Darnton A, Hutchings S, Sadhra S, Fishwick D, Rushton L, Cullinan P. The occupations at increased risk of COPD: analysis of lifetime job-histories in the population-based UK Biobank Cohort. *Eur Respir J.* 2019;54(1):1900186.

[13] Paulin LM, Diette GB, Blanc PD, Putcha N, Eisner MD, Kanner RE, Belli AJ, Christenson S, Tashkin DP, Han M, Barr RG, Hansel NN; SPIROMICS Research Group. Occupational exposures are associated with worse morbidity in patients with chronic obstructive

pulmonary disease. *Am J Respir Crit Care Med.* 2015; 191(5):557-65.

[14] Graham BL, Steenbruggen I, Miller MR, Barjaktarevic IZ, Cooper BG, Hall GL, Hallstrand TS, Kaminsky DA, McCarthy K, McCormack MC, Oropez CE, Rosenfeld M, Stanojevic S, Swanney MP, Thompson BR. Standardization of Spirometry 2019 Update. An Official American Thoracic Society and European Respiratory Society Technical Statement. *Am J Respir Crit Care Med.* 2019;200(8):e70-e88.

[15] Borg GA. Psychophysical bases of perceived exertion. *Med Sci Sports Exerc.* 1982;14(5):377-81.

[16] Mador MJ, Kufel TJ. Reproducibility of visual analog scale measurements of dyspnea in patients with chronic obstructive pulmonary disease. *Am Rev Respir Dis.* 1992;146(1):82-7.

[17] Johnson MJ, Close L, Gillon SC, Molassiotis A, Lee PH, Farquhar MC; Breathlessness Research Interest Group (BRIG). Use of the modified Borg scale and numerical rating scale to measure chronic breathlessness: a pooled data analysis. *Eur Respir J.* 2016; 47(6): 1861-4.

[18] Jones PW, Harding G, Berry P, Wiklund I, Chen WH, Kline Leidy N. Development and first validation of the COPD Assessment Test. *Eur Respir J.* 2009;34(3):648-54.

[19] Jones PW, Brusselle G, Dal Negro RW, Ferrer M, Kardos P, Levy ML, Perez T, Soler Cataluña JJ, van der Molen T, Adamek L, Banik N. Properties of the COPD assessment test in a cross-sectional European study. *Eur Respir J.* 2011;38(1):29-35.

[20] Jones PW, Quirk FH, Baveystock CM. The St George's Respiratory Questionnaire. *Respir Med.* 1991;85(Suppl B):25-31; discussion 33-7.

[21] ATS Committee on Proficiency Standards for Clinical Pulmonary Function Laboratories. ATS statement: guidelines for the six-minute walk test. *Am J Respir Crit Care Med.* 2002;166(1):111-7.

[22] Enright PL. The six-minute walk test. *Respir Care.* 2003; 48(8):783-5.

[23] Pin I, Gibson PG, Kolendowicz R, Girgis-Gabardo A, Denburg JA, Hargreave FE, Dolovich J. Use of induced sputum cell counts to investigate airway inflammation in asthma. *Thorax*. 1992;47(1):25-9.

[24] Iredale MJ, Wanklyn SA, Phillips IP, Krausz T, Ind PW. Non-invasive assessment of bronchial inflammation in asthma: no correlation between eosinophilia of induced sputum and bronchial responsiveness to inhaled hypertonic saline. *Clin Exp Allergy*. 1994;24(10):940-5.

[25] Tsoumakidou M, Tzanakis N, Siafakas NM. Induced sputum in the investigation of airway inflammation of COPD. *Respir Med.* 2003;97(8):863-71.

[26] Hao W, Li M, Zhang C, Zhang Y, Wang P. Inflammatory mediators in exhaled breath condensate and peripheral blood of healthy donors and stable COPD patients. *Immunopharmacol Immunotoxicol.* 2019;41(2):224-30.

[27] Konstantinidi EM, Lappas AS, Tzortzi AS, Behrakis PK. Exhaled Breath Condensate: Technical and Diagnostic Aspects. *Scientific World Journal.* 2015;2015:435160.

[28] Miravitlles M, Anzueto A. Role of infection in exacerbations of chronic obstructive pulmonary disease. *Curr Opin Pulm Med.* 2015;21(3):278-83.

[29] Hogea SP, Tudorache E, Fildan AP, Fira-Mladinescu O, Marc M, Oancea C. Risk factors of chronic obstructive pulmonary disease exacerbations. *Clin Respir J.* 2020;14(3):183-197.

[30] Burgel PR, Paillasseur JL, Janssens W, Piquet J, Ter Riet G, Garcia-Aymerich J, Cosio B, Bakke P, Puhan MA, Langhammer A, Alfageme I, Almagro P, Ancochea J, Celli BR, Casanova C, de-Torres JP, Decramer M, Echazarreta A, Esteban C, Gomez Punter RM, Han MK, Johannessen A, Kaiser B, Lamprecht B, Lange P, Leivseth L, Marin JM, Martin F, Martinez-Camblor P, Miravitlles M, Oga T, Sofia Ramírez A, Sin DD, Sobradillo P, Soler-Cataluña JJ, Turner AM, Verdu Rivera FJ, Soriano JB, Roche N; Initiatives BPCO, EABPCO, Leuven and 3CIA study groups. A simple

algorithm for the identification of clinical COPD phenotypes. *Eur Respir J.* 2017;50(5):1701034.

[31] Burgel PR, Paillasseur JL, Caillaud D, Tillie-Leblond I, Chanez P, Escamilla R, Court-Fortune I, Perez T, Carré P, Roche N; Initiatives BPCO Scientific Committee. Clinical COPD phenotypes: a novel approach using principal component and cluster analyses. *Eur Respir J.* 2010;36(3):531-9.

[32] Barnes PJ. Inflammatory endotypes in COPD. *Allergy.* 2019;74(7): 1249-56.

[33] Castaldi PJ, Dy J, Ross J, Chang Y, Washko GR, Curran-Everett D, Williams A, Lynch DA, Make BJ, Crapo JD, Bowler RP, Regan EA, Hokanson JE, Kinney GL, Han MK, Soler X, Ramsdell JW, Barr RG, Foreman M, van Beek E, Casaburi R, Criner GJ, Lutz SM, Rennard SI, Santorico S, Sciurba FC, DeMeo DL, Hersh CP, Silverman EK, Cho MH. Cluster analysis in the COPDGene study identifies subtypes of smokers with distinct patterns of airway disease and emphysema. *Thorax.* 2014;69(5):415-22.

[34] World Health Organization. *COPD–Fact Sheets*. 2018. Available at: http://www.who.int/mediacentre/factsheets/fs315/en/. Accessed on January 8, 2020.

[35] Barnes PJ. Inflammatory mechanisms in patients with chronic obstructive pulmonary disease. *J Allergy Clin Immunol.* 2016; 138(1):16-27.

[36] Sinden NJ, Stockley RA. Systemic inflammation and comorbidity in COPD: a result of 'overspill' of inflammatory mediators from the lungs? Review of the evidence. *Thorax.* 2010;65(10):930-6.

[37] Barnes PJ. Cellular and molecular mechanisms of chronic obstructive pulmonary disease. *Clin Chest Med.* 2014;35(1):71-86.

[38] Bagdonas E, Raudoniute J, Bruzauskaite I, Aldonyte R. Novel aspects of pathogenesis and regeneration mechanisms in COPD. *Int J Chron Obstruct Pulmon Dis.* 2015;10:995-1013.

[39] Eapen MS, McAlinden K, Tan D, Weston S, Ward C, Muller HK, Walters EH, Sohal SS. Profiling cellular and inflammatory changes

in the airway wall of mild to moderate COPD. *Respirology.* 2017;22(6):1125-32.
[40] Thompson AB, Daughton D, Robbins RA, Ghafouri MA, Oehlerking M, Rennard SI. Intraluminal airway inflammation in chronic bronchitis. Characterization and correlation with clinical parameters. *Am Rev Respir Dis.* 1989;140(6):1527-37.
[41] Baraldo S, Turato G, Badin C, Bazzan E, Beghé B, Zuin R, Calabrese F, Casoni G, Maestrelli P, Papi A, Fabbri LM, Saetta M. Neutrophilic infiltration within the airway smooth muscle in patients with COPD. *Thorax.* 2004;59(4):308-12.
[42] Singh D, Edwards L, Tal-Singer R, Rennard S. Sputum neutrophils as a biomarker in COPD: findings from the ECLIPSE study. *Respir Res.* 2010;11(1):77.
[43] Mendy A, Forno E, Niyonsenga T, Gasana J. Blood biomarkers as predictors of long-term mortality in COPD. *Clin Respir J.* 2018;12(5):1891-1899.
[44] Meijer M, Rijkers GT, van Overveld FJ. Neutrophils and emerging targets for treatment in chronic obstructive pulmonary disease. *Expert Rev Clin Immunol.* 2013;9(11):1055-68.
[45] Bartoli ML, Costa F, Malagrinò L, Nieri D, Antonelli S, Decusatis G, Simone CD, Santerini S, Cianchetti S, Latorre M, Vagaggini B, Paggiaro P. Sputum inflammatory cells in COPD patients classified according to GOLD 2011 guidelines. *Eur Respir J.* 2016;47(3): 978-80.
[46] Stănescu D, Sanna A, Veriter C, Kostianev S, Calcagni PG, Fabbri LM, Maestrelli P. Airways obstruction, chronic expectoration, and rapid decline of FEV1 in smokers are associated with increased levels of sputum neutrophils. *Thorax.* 1996;51(3):267-71.
[47] Donaldson GC, Seemungal TA, Patel IS, Bhowmik A, Wilkinson TM, Hurst JR, Maccallum PK, Wedzicha JA. Airway and systemic inflammation and decline in lung function in patients with COPD. *Chest.* 2005;128(4):1995-2004.
[48] Lange P, Celli B, Agustí A, Boje Jensen G, Divo M, Faner R, Guerra S, Marott JL, Martinez FD, Martinez-Camblor P, Meek P, Owen

CA, Petersen H, Pinto-Plata V, Schnohr P, Sood A, Soriano JB, Tesfaigzi Y, Vestbo J. Lung-Function Trajectories Leading to Chronic Obstructive Pulmonary Disease. *N Engl J Med.* 2015; 373(2):111-22.

[49] Crystal RG. Airway basal cells. The "smoking gun" of chronic obstructive pulmonary disease. *Am J Respir Crit Care Med.* 2014;190(12):1355-62.

[50] Shaykhiev R, Crystal RG. Early events in the pathogenesis of chronic obstructive pulmonary disease. Smoking-induced reprogramming of airway epithelial basal progenitor cells. *Ann Am Thorac Soc.* 2014;11 Suppl 5(Suppl 5):S252-8.

[51] Hogg JC, Chu F, Utokaparch S, Woods R, Elliott WM, Buzatu L, Cherniack RM, Rogers RM, Sciurba FC, Coxson HO, Paré PD. The nature of small-airway obstruction in chronic obstructive pulmonary disease. *N Engl J Med.* 2004;350(26):2645-53.

[52] Hirota N, Martin JG. Mechanisms of airway remodeling. *Chest.* 2013;144(3):1026-32.

[53] McDonough JE, Yuan R, Suzuki M, Seyednejad N, Elliott WM, Sanchez PG, Wright AC, Gefter WB, Litzky L, Coxson HO, Paré PD, Sin DD, Pierce RA, Woods JC, McWilliams AM, Mayo JR, Lam SC, Cooper JD, Hogg JC. Small-airway obstruction and emphysema in chronic obstructive pulmonary disease. *N Engl J Med.* 2011;365(17):1567-75.

[54] Higham A, Quinn AM, Cançado JED, Singh D. The pathology of small airways disease in COPD: historical aspects and future directions. *Respir Res.* 2019;20(1):49.

[55] Lahousse L, Seys LJM, Joos GF, Franco OH, Stricker BH, Brusselle GG. Epidemiology and impact of chronic bronchitis in chronic obstructive pulmonary disease. *Eur Respir J.* 2017;50(2):1602470.

[56] Francis SM, Tan ME, Fung PR, Shaw JG, Semmler AB, Nataatmadja M, Bowman RV, Fong KM, Yang IA. Peripheral compartment innate immune response to Haemophilus influenzae and Streptococcus pneumoniae in chronic obstructive pulmonary disease patients. *Innate Immun.* 2013;19(4):428-37.

[57] Noda N, Matsumoto K, Fukuyama S, Asai Y, Kitajima H, Seki N, Matsunaga Y, Kan-O K, Moriwaki A, Morimoto K, Inoue H, Nakanishi Y. Cigarette smoke impairs phagocytosis of apoptotic neutrophils by alveolar macrophages via inhibition of the histone deacetylase/Rac/CD9 pathways. *Int Immunol.* 2013;25(11):643-50.

[58] Victoni T, Gicquel T, Bodin A, Daude M, Tenor H, Valença S, Devillier P, Porto LC, Lagente V, Boichot E. Roflumilast n-oxide associated with PGE2 prevents the neutrophil elastase-induced production of chemokines by epithelial cells. *Int Immunopharmacol. 2016*;30:1-8.

[59] Bihlet AR, Karsdal MA, Sand JM, Leeming DJ, Roberts M, White W, Bowler R. Biomarkers of extracellular matrix turnover are associated with emphysema and eosinophilic-bronchitis in COPD. *Respir Res.* 2017;18(1):22.

[60] Guillon A, Jouan Y, Brea D, Gueugnon F, Dalloneau E, Baranek T, Henry C, Morello E, Renauld JC, Pichavant M, Gosset P, Courty Y, Diot P, Si-Tahar M. Neutrophil proteases alter the interleukin-22-receptor-dependent lung antimicrobial defence. *Eur Respir J.* 2015;46(3):771-82.

[61] Obermayer A, Stoiber W, Krautgartner WD, Klappacher M, Kofler B, Steinbacher P, Vitkov L, Grabcanovic-Musija F, Studnicka M. New aspects on the structure of neutrophil extracellular traps from chronic obstructive pulmonary disease and *in vitro* generation. *PLoS One.* 2014;9(5):e97784.

[62] Brinkmann V, Reichard U, Goosmann C, Fauler B, Uhlemann Y, Weiss DS, Weinrauch Y, Zychlinsky A. Neutrophil extracellular traps kill bacteria. *Science.* 2004;303(5663):1532-5.

[63] Pedersen F, Marwitz S, Holz O, Kirsten A, Bahmer T, Waschki B, Magnussen H, Rabe KF, Goldmann T, Uddin M, Watz H. Neutrophil extracellular trap formation and extracellular DNA in sputum of stable COPD patients. *Respir Med.* 2015;109(10):1360-2.

[64] Tufvesson E, Ekberg M, Bjermer L. Inflammatory biomarkers in sputum predict COPD exacerbations. *Lung.* 2013;191(4):413-6.

[65] Paone G, Leone V, Conti V, De Marchis L, Ialleni E, Graziani C, Salducci M, Ramaccia M, Munafò G. Blood and sputum biomarkers in COPD and asthma: a review. *Eur Rev Med Pharmacol Sci. 2016*;20(4):698-708.

[66] Aggarwal T, Wadhwa R, Thapliyal N, Sharma K, Rani V, Maurya PK. Oxidative, inflammatory, genetic, and epigenetic biomarkers associated with chronic obstructive pulmonary disorder. *J Cell Physiol.* 2019;234(3):2067-82.

[67] Stockley RA, Halpin DMG, Celli BR, Singh D. Chronic Obstructive Pulmonary Disease biomarkers and their interpretation. *Am J Respir Crit Care Med*. 2019;199(10):1195-1204.

[68] Haeggström JZ, Funk CD. Lipoxygenase and leukotriene pathways: biochemistry, biology, and roles in disease. *Chem Rev.* 2011;111(10):5866-98.

[69] Milne GL, Dai Q, Roberts LJ 2nd. The isoprostanes-25 years later. *Biochim Biophys Acta.* 2015;1851(4):433-45.

[70] Wan M, Tang X, Stsiapanava A, Haeggström JZ. *Biosynthesis of leukotriene B_4. Semin Immunol.* 2017;33:3-15.

[71] Drozdovszky O, Barta I, Antus B. Sputum eicosanoid profiling in exacerbations of chronic obstructive pulmonary disease. *Respiration.* 2014;87(5):408-15.

[72] Corhay JL, Henket M, Nguyen D, Duysinx B, Sele J, Louis R. Leukotriene B4 contributes to exhaled breath condensate and sputum neutrophil chemotaxis in COPD. *Chest.* 2009;136(4):1047-54.

[73] de Groot LES, van der Veen TA, Martinez FO, Hamann J, Lutter R, Melgert BN. Oxidative stress and macrophages: driving forces behind exacerbations of asthma and chronic obstructive pulmonary disease? *Am J Physiol Lung Cell Mol Physiol.* 2019;316(2):L369-L384.

[74] Psarras S, Caramori G, Contoli M, Papadopoulos N, Papi A. Oxidants in asthma and in chronic obstructive pulmonary disease (COPD). *Curr Pharm Des.* 2005;11(16):2053-62.

[75] Hancock JT, Desikan R, Neill SJ. Role of reactive oxygen species in cell signalling pathways. *Biochem Soc Trans.* 2001;29(Pt 2):345-50.

[76] Faux SP, Tai T, Thorne D, Xu Y, Breheny D, Gaca M. The role of oxidative stress in the biological responses of lung epithelial cells to cigarette smoke. *Biomarkers.* 2009;14(Suppl 1):90-6.

[77] Rahman I, Biswas SK, Kode A. Oxidant and antioxidant balance in the airways and airway diseases. *Eur J Pharmacol.* 2006;533(1-3):222-39.

[78] MacNee W. Oxidative stress and lung inflammation in airways disease. *Eur J Pharmacol.* 2001;429(1-3):195-207.

[79] Aggarwal T, Wadhwa R, Rohil V, Maurya PK. Biomarkers of oxidative stress and protein-protein interaction in chronic obstructive pulmonary disease. *Arch Physiol Biochem.* 2018;124(3):226-231.

[80] Bazhanov N, Ansar M, Ivanciuc T, Garofalo RP, Casola A. Hydrogen Sulfide: A Novel Player in Airway Development, Pathophysiology of Respiratory Diseases, and Antiviral Defenses. *Am J Respir Cell Mol Biol.* 2017;57(4):403-410.

[81] Wallace JL, Wang R. Hydrogen sulfide-based therapeutics: exploiting a unique but ubiquitous gasotransmitter. *Nat Rev Drug Discov.* 2015;14(5):329-45.

[82] Viegas J, Esteves AF, Cardoso EM, Arosa FA, Vitale M, Taborda-Barata L. Biological Effects of Thermal Water-Associated Hydrogen Sulfide on Human Airways and Associated Immune Cells: Implications for Respiratory Diseases. *Front Public Health.* 2019;7:128.

[83] Kolluru GK, Shen X, Bir SC, Kevil CG. Hydrogen sulfide chemical biology: pathophysiological roles and detection. *Nitric Oxide.* 2013;35:5-20.

[84] Pouokam E, Althaus M. Epithelial Electrolyte Transport Physiology and the Gasotransmitter Hydrogen Sulfide. *Oxid Med Cell Longev.* 2016;2016:4723416.

[85] Wang R. Physiological implications of hydrogen sulfide: a whiff exploration that blossomed. *Physiol Rev.* 2012;92(2):791-896.

[86] Predmore BL, Lefer DJ, Gojon G. Hydrogen sulfide in biochemistry and medicine. *Antioxid Redox Signal.* 2012; 17(1):119-40.

[87] Mishanina TV, Libiad M, Banerjee R. Biogenesis of reactive sulfur species for signaling by hydrogen sulfide oxidation pathways. *Nat Chem Biol.* 2015;11(7):457-64.

[88] Olson KR, Dombkowski RA, Russell MJ, Doellman MM, Head SK, Whitfield NL, Madden JA. Hydrogen sulfide as an oxygen sensor/transducer in vertebrate hypoxic vasoconstriction and hypoxic vasodilation. *J Exp Biol.* 2006;209(Pt 20):4011-23.

[89] Krause NC, Kutsche HS, Santangelo F, DeLeon ER, Dittrich NP, Olson KR, Althaus M. Hydrogen sulfide contributes to hypoxic inhibition of airway transepithelial sodium absorption. *Am J Physiol Regul Integr Comp Physiol.* 2016;311(3):R607-17.

[90] Zhang J, Wang X, Chen Y, Yao W. Exhaled Hydrogen Sulfide Predicts Airway Inflammation Phenotype in COPD. *Respir Care.* 2015;60(2):251-8.

[91] Chen YH, Yao WZ, Geng B, Ding YL, Lu M, Zhao MW, Tang CS. Endogenous hydrogen sulfide in patients with COPD. *Chest.* 2005;128(5):3205-11.

[92] Saito J, Mackay AJ, Rossios C, Gibeon D, Macedo P, Sinharay R, Bhavsar PK, Wedzicha JA, Chung KF. Sputum-to-serum hydrogen sulfide ratio in COPD. *Thorax.* 2014;69(10):903-9.

[93] Davis MD, Hunt J. Exhaled breath condensate pH assays. *Immunol Allergy Clin North Am.* 2012;32(3):377-86.

[94] Vaughan J, Ngamtrakulpanit L, Pajewski TN, Turner R, Nguyen TA, Smith A, Urban P, Hom S, Gaston B, Hunt J. Exhaled breath condensate pH is a robust and reproducible assay of airway acidity. *Eur Respir J.* 2003;22(6):889-94.

[95] Papaioannou AI, Loukides S, Minas M, Kontogianni K, Bakakos P, Gourgoulianis KI, Alchanatis M, Papiris S, Kostikas K. Exhaled breath condensate pH as a biomarker of COPD severity in ex-smokers. *Respir Res.* 2011;12(1):67.

[96] Kostikas K, Papatheodorou G, Ganas K, Psathakis K, Panagou P, Loukides S. pH in expired breath condensate of patients with

inflammatory airway diseases. *Am J Respir Crit Care Med.* 2002;165(10):1364-70.

[97] Borrill Z, Starkey C, Vestbo J, Singh D. Reproducibility of exhaled breath condensate pH in chronic obstructive pulmonary disease. *Eur Respir J.* 2005;25(2):269-74.

[98] Broers C, Tack J, Pauwels A. Review article: gastro-oesophageal reflux disease in asthma and chronic obstructive pulmonary disease. *Aliment Pharmacol Ther.* 2018;47(2):176-91.

[99] Turmann R. [Emphysematous bronchitis and its treatment in a health resort]. *Dtsch Med J.* 1963;14:57-62.

[100] Mielke U. Die balneotherapie der chronischen bronchitis. [Balneotherapy of chronic bronchitis]. *Dtsch Med J.* 1966;17(16): 484-5.

[101] Kolesár J, Antal M. Hladina hemolytického úćinku komplementu pocas liecby v Kúpel'ock Nimnica u chronických bronchitikov. [Level of the hemolytic effect of the complement during treatment of chronic bronchitis in the spa Nimnica]. *Fysiatr Revmatol Vestn.* 1968;46(3):137-42.

[102] Maczyński B. Sprawność termoregulacji u doroslych chorych na dychawice oskrzelowa i przewlekly niezyt oskrzeli po klimatycznym leczeniu na wybrzezu Baltyku. [Thermoregulating efficiency in adult patients with bronchial asthma and chronic bronchitis after climatic treatment on the Baltic coast]. *Przegl Lek.* 1970;26(2):313-6.

[103] Antal M, Kolesár J. Zmeny fagocytárnej schopnosti leukocytov u chronických bronchitikov pocas liecby v kúpel'och Nimnica. [Variations in the phagocytic ability of leukocytes in patients with chronic bronchitis during a treatment course at the Nimnice health resort]. *Fysiatr Revmatol Vestn.* 1970;48(3):133-8.

[104] Reinert M, Trendelenburg F, Horbach L, Jordan A, von Blohn H, Schön U. Die Lungenfunktion bei chronischer Bronchitis und allergischem Asthma bronchiale. Untersuchungen vor und nach Heilverfahren. [Pulmonary function in chronic bronchitis and

allergic bronchial asthma. Studies before and after therapy]. *Munch Med Wochenschr.* 1972;114(11):484-7.

[105] Schmidt OP. Physikalisch-balneologische Therapie beim chronischen bronchitischen Syndrom. [Physical and balneological therapy in the chronic bronchitis syndrome (author's transl)]. *Munch Med Wochenschr.* 1973;115(34):1457-9.

[106] Kossmann S. Badania plwociny jako miernik skuteczności balneoterapii w przewlekłých niezytach oskrzeli u górników. [Studies of sputum as a measure of the effectiveness of balneotherapy in chronic bronchitis in miners]. *Pol Tyg Lek.* 1974;29(41):1757-9.

[107] Kossmann S, Wysocki J, Fraczek M. Zmiany zawartości immunoglobulin w plwocinie i w surowicy podczas balneoterapii przewlekłych niezytów oskrzeli wikłajacych pylice. [Changes in the immunoglobulin content of sputum and serum in the course of balneotherapy in chronic bronchitis complicating coal workers's pneumoconiosis]. *Pol Tyg Lek.* 1974;29(26):1105-7.

[108] Kossmann S, Pilarek M, Bednarski W. Zmiany aktywości proteolitycznej plwociny w czasie leczenia balneologicznego przewlekłych niezytów oskrzeli u górników. [Changes in plasma proteolytic activity during balneological treatment of chronic bronchitis in miners]. *Pol Tyg Lek.* 1974;29(5):172-4.

[109] Bednarski W, Kossmann S, Pilarek M. Zmiany aktywności histaminazy w surowicy i w plwocinie w czasie balneoterapii przewlekłych niezytów oskrzeli u górników. [Changes in the serum and sputum histaminase activity during balneotherapy for chronic bronchitis in miners]. *Pol Tyg Lek.* 1976;31(6):221-2.

[110] Dobes L, Kubík A. Vliv komplexní lázenské lécby v Lázních Jeseníku na základní spirometrické hodnoty u pacientů trpících chronickou bronchitidou. [Influence of complex balneotherapy on the basic spirometric values in patients with chronic bronchitis]. *Fysiatr Revmatol Vestn.* 1977;55(1):22-6.

[111] Eliseev VA. Lechenie termal'nymi radonovymi vodami bol'nykh khronicheskim bronkhitom. [Treatment of chronic bronchitis

patients with thermal radon waters]. *Vopr Kurortol Fizioter Lech Fiz Kult.* 1986;(4):57-9.

[112] Simonenko TS, Povazhnaia EL. Kliniko-funktsional'noe obosnovanie SMT-griazelecheniia bol'nykh khronicheskim obstruktivnym bronkhitom. [Clinico-functional basis for sinusoidal modulated current-mud therapy of patients with chronic obstructive bronchitis]. *Vopr Kurortol Fizioter Lech Fiz Kult.* 1987;(6):54-5.

[113] Povazhnaia EL, Simonenko TS, Davydova OB. Peloidoterapiia bol'nykh khronicheskim obstruktivnym bronkhitom v usloviiakh srednegornogo kurorta. [The pelotherapy of patients with chronic obstructive bronchitis at a central highlands health resort]. *Vopr Kurortol Fizioter Lech Fiz Kult.* 1990;(6):17-21.

[114] Krasik IaD, Zorina SS, Lebedev AS, Makarova AA, Ivchenko MM, Zalkind AE, Musienko GI, Fomkina AI. Otsenka éffektivnosti i obosnovanie metodov lecheniia bol'nykh khronicheskim obstruktivnym bronkhitom na kurorte Evpatoriia. [An assessment of the efficacy and a validation of the methods of treating patients with chronic obstructive bronchitis at the Yevpatoriya health resort]. *Ter Arkh.* 1990;62(3):46-9.

[115] van Hengstum M, Festen J, Corstens F. Measurement of tracheobronchial clearance after sauna in subjects with chronic bronchitis. *Thorax.* 1991;46(10):732-3.

[116] Petrovska Ia, Petrov A. Promeni v niakoi kliniko-funktsionalni i imunologichni pokazateli pri bolni s khronichna obstruktivna belodrobna bolest--alergichna forma, sled kompleksno klimatolechenie v kurorta Sandanski. [Changes in the clinico-functional and immunological indices of patients with chronic obstructive lung disease, the allergic form, following combined climatotherapy at Sandanski health resort]. *Vutr Boles.* 1991;30(1):41-4.

[117] Rychkova MA, Aĭrapetova NS, Davydova OB, Krivtsova IE, Doronina IuV, Derevnina NA. Kontrastnye vanny v reabilitatsii bol'nykh khronicheskim bronkhitom. [Contrast baths in the

rehabilitation of patients with chronic bronchitis]. *Vopr Kurortol Fizioter Lech Fiz Kult.* 1994;(3):3-6.

[118] Anisimkina AN, Aĭrapetova NS, Davydova OB, Doronina IuV, Derevnina NA, Gontar' EV. Primenenie khloridnykh natrievykh vann u bol'nykh khronicheskim bronkhitom. [The use of sodium chloride baths in patients with chronic bronchitis]. *Vopr Kurortol Fizioter Lech Fiz Kult.* 1996;(3):14-8.

[119] Nakahiro K, Murata A, Kaneko Y, Takasaki Y. [Effects of bathing on lung mechanics in patients with severe COPD]. *Nihon Kokyuki Gakkai Zasshi.* 1998;36(2):150-6.

[120] Ivanov EM, Shakirova OV, Zhuravskaia NS. Ul'trafioletovoe obluchenie krovi i peloidoterapiia (traditsionnye i ukorochennye kursy) bol'nykh khronicheskim bronkhitom. [Ultraviolet irradiation of blood and peloid therapy (standard- and short-course) of patients with chronic bronchitis]. *Vopr Kurortol Fizioter Lech Fiz Kult.* 2001;(4):13-7.

[121] Ivanov EM, Shakirova OV, Zhuravskaia NS. Peloidoterapiia v kompleksnom vosstanovitel'nom lechenii bol'nykh khronicheskim bronkhitom. [Pelotherapy in combined aftertreatment of patients with chronic bronchitis]. *Vopr Kurortol Fizioter Lech Fiz Kult.* 2002;(4):18-21.

[122] Balaban IE, Ponomarenko GN. Peloidointerferentsterapiia bol'nykh khronicheskim obstruktivnym bronkhitom na kurorte. [Peloid interference therapy of patients with chronic obstructive bronchitis in health resort]. *Vopr Kurortol Fizioter Lech Fiz Kult.* 2002;(6):11-4.

[123] Golich LG, Ponomarenko GN. Lechebnye éffecty uglekislykh mineral'nykh vann u bol'nykh khronicheskoĭ obstruktivnoĭ bolezn'iu legkikh. [Therapeutic effects of carbon dioxide mineral baths in patients with chronic obstructive lung disease]. *Vopr Kurortol Fizioter Lech Fiz Kult*. 2003;(1):32-6.

[124] Aĭrapetova NS, Polikanova EB, Davydova OB, Gosn LD, Kulikova OV, Ksenofontova IV, Nikoda NV, Rassulova MA, Nitchenko OV, Siziakova LA, Doronina IuV, Derevnina NA. [Turpentine baths in

rehabilitation of patients with chronic obstructive pulmonary disease]. *Vopr Kurortol Fizioter Lech Fiz Kult.* 2007;(4):17-22.

[125] Rassulova MA. [Sylvinite speleochamber and general chloride sodium baths in medical rehabilitation of patients with chronic obstructive pulmonary disease]. *Vopr Kurortol Fizioter Lech Fiz Kult.* 2008;(2):20-3.

[126] Zunnunov ZR, Ubaĭdullaev AM, Nurov IKh. [Application of ammotherapy for the remedial treatment of patients with chronic obstructive pulmonary disease in the rehabilitative phase]. *Vopr Kurortol Fizioter Lech Fiz Kult. 2009*;(2):22-5.

[127] Zunnunov ZR. [The clinical efficiency and safety of iodide-bromine balneotherapy in patients with coronary heart disease concurrent with chronic obstructive pulmonary disease]. *Ter Arkh.* 2010;82(1):24-7.

[128] Zaripova TN, Antipova II, Smirnova IN, Khon VB. [Mathematical prognostication of the efficacy of peloidotherapy in the patients with chronic bronchitis and obstructive pulmonary disease]. *Vopr Kurortol Fizioter Lech Fiz Kult.* 2012;(1):9-13.

[129] Aĭrapetova NS, Uianaeva MA, Pershin SB. [The approaches to realization of the therapeutic action of gas-air carbonate baths and lysozyme inhalation during their combined application for the treatment of patients presenting with chronic obstructive pulmonary disease]. *Vopr Kurortol Fizioter Lech Fiz Kult.* 2013;(2):8-13.

[130] Uyanaeva AI, Airapetova NS, Badalov NG, Tupitsina YY, L'vova NV, Nitchenko OV, Uyanaeva MA, Ksenofontova IV. [The role of physiobalneotherapy in the prevention of weather-dependent exacerbations in the patients presenting with chronic obstructive pulmonary disease]. *Vopr Kurortol Fizioter Lech Fiz Kult.* 2015;92(6):17-22.

[131] Kendrova L, Takác P, Kubincová A, Mikuláková W, Nechvátal P. Effect of spa treatment and speleotherapy in the treatment of chronic obstructive pulmonary disease – a pilot study. *Clinical Social Work and Health Intervention.* 2016;7:7-15. Available at: https://www.

clinicalsocialwork.eu/wp-content/uploads/2016/06/01-kendrova-takac-kubincova.pdf. Accessed on December 16, 2019.

[132] Cornet HA. Bäderbehandlung bei chronischer Bronchitis. [Inhalation and balneologic therapy in chronic bronchitis]. *Arch Phys Ther* (Leipz). 1954;6(2):120-5.

[133] Delore P, Megard M, Marin A. Bilan de la crénotherapie et de la climatothérapie dans let états de bronchite chronique. [Assets and liabilities of crenotherapy and climatotherapy in chronic bronchitis]. *J Med Lyon.* 1956;37(875):477-90.

[134] Otto JH. Bronchitis, Asthma und Emphysem und ihre Behandlung an der Nordsee. [Bronchitis, asthma & emphysema & their treatment at North Sea health resorts]. *Allerg Asthma* (Leipz). 1957;3(3):144-51.

[135] Dionigi R. [On the behavior of the excrescence in chronic bronchitis treated with sulfurea crenotherapy]. *Arch Med Interna.* 1960; 12:53-7.

[136] Passa J. S'enescence et possibilit'es de la cr'enoth'erapie sulfureuse en pathologie respiratoire. [Senescence and possibilities of sulfurous crenotherapy in respiratory pathology]. *Gaz Med Fr.* 1964;17: 1741-2.

[137] Jean R. Le traitement thermal dans la bronchite chronique. [Thermal treatment in chronic bronchitis]. *Presse Therm Clim.* 1971;108(2):51-4.

[138] Piegaia G, Re A. Le broncoinstillazioni come tecnica preparatoria della crenoterapia sulfurea nella bronchite cronica. [Bronchial instillations as a preparatory technic in sulfur crenotherapy in chronic bronchitis]. *Minerva Ecol Idroclimatol Fis Sanit.* 1976;16(3-4):141-3.

[139] Melillo G, Nappi G, Valenti M. L'inaloterapia termale nel trattamento delle broncopneumopatie croniche. Risultati del progetto NAIADE. Rassegna di Patologia dell'Aparato Respiratorio. [Thermal inhalotherapy in the treatment of chronic bronchopneumopathies. Results of the NAIADE project. Review of

Pathology of the Respiratory System]. *Ital Rev Resp Dis*. 2002;17:37-42.

[140] Petraccia L, Masciullo SG, Grassi M, Pace A, Lucchetta MC, Valenzi VI, Avino P, Fraioli A. Possibilità crenoterapiche e climatoterapiche nelle malattie ostruttive polmonari corniche. [Spa and climate therapy in chronic obstructive pulmonary diseases]. *Clin Ter*. 2005;156(1-2):23-31.

[141] Valitutti S, Castellino F, Musiani P. Effect of sulfurous (thermal) water on T lymphocyte proliferative response. *Ann Allergy*. 1990;65(6):463-8.

[142] Braga PC, Ceci C, Marabini L, Nappi G. The antioxidant activity of sulphurous thermal water protects against oxidative DNA damage: a comet assay investigation. *Drug Res (Stuttg)*. 2013;63(4):198-202.

[143] Braga PC, Sambataro G, Dal Sasso M, Culici M, Alfieri M, Nappi G. Antioxidant effect of sulphurous thermal water on human neutrophil bursts: chemiluminescence evaluation. *Respiration*. 2008;75(2):193-201.

[144] Cristalli G, Abramo A, Pollastrini L. Trattamento delle flogosi croniche delle vie aeree superiori con crenoterapia inalatoria solfureo-solfato-bicarbonato-carbonica-alcalinoterrosa: studio della citologia nasale. [Treatment of chronic inflammation of the upper respiratory airways by inhalation thermal therapy with sulfur-sulfate-bicarbonate-carbonate-alkaline earth mineral water: a study of nasal cytology]. *Acta Otorhinolaryngol Ital*. 1996;16(6 Suppl 55):91-4.

[145] Ottaviano G, Marioni G, Staffieri C, Giacomelli L, Marchese-Ragona R, Bertolin A, Staffieri A. Effects of sulfurous, salty, bromic, iodic thermal water nasal irrigations in nonallergic chronic rhinosinusitis: a prospective, randomized, double-blind, clinical, and cytological study. *Am J Otolaryngol*. 2011;32(3):235-9.

[146] Passali D, De Corso E, Platzgummer S, Streitberger C, Lo Cunsolo S, Nappi G, Passali GC, Bellussi L. Spa therapy of upper respiratory tract inflammations. *Eur Arch Otorhinolaryngol*. 2013;270(2):565-70.

[147] Cantone E, Marino A, Ferranti I, Castagna G, Maione N, Di Rubbo V, Iengo M. Nasal cytological assessment after crenotherapy in the treatment of chronic rhinosinusitis in the elderly. *Int J Immunopathol Pharmacol.* 2014;27(4):683-7.

[148] Passali D, Gabelli G, Passali GC, Magnato R, Platzgummer S, Salerni L, Lo Cunsolo S, Joos A, Bellussi LM. Radioactive Merano SPA Treatment for Allergic Rhinitis Therapy. *Int J Otolaryngol.* 2016;2016:2801913.

[149] Barbieri M, Salami A, Mora F, Casazza A, Sovatzis A, Teglia R, Cordone MP, Mora R. Comportamento delle IGE e IGA sieriche in pazienti con rinite allergica trattata con acque salsobromoiodiche. [Behavior of serum IgE and IgA in patients with allergic rhinitis treated with iodine bromide thermal water]. *Acta Otorhinolaryngol Ital.* 2002;22(4):215-9.

[150] Mirandola P, Gobbi G, Sponzilli I, Pambianco M, Malinverno C, Cacchioli A, De Panfilis G, Vitale M. Exogenous hydrogen sulfide induces functional inhibition and cell death of cytotoxic lymphocytes subsets. *J Cell Physiol.* 2007;213(3):826-33.

[151] Papi A, Contoli M, Gasparini P, Bristot L, Edwards MR, Chicca M, Leis M, Ciaccia A, Caramori G, Johnston SL, Pinamonti S. Role of xanthine oxidase activation and reduced glutathione depletion in rhinovirus induction of inflammation in respiratory epithelial cells. *J Biol Chem.* 2008;283(42):28595-606.

[152] Nappi G, De Luca S, Guinzoni-Confortini M, Strinati F, Masciocchi M. [Short term effects of inhalation with sulphureous water on Chlamydia pneumoniae bodies in patients affected by COPD]. *Medicina e Clinica Termale.* 2003;55:535-45.

[153] Von Hertzen L, Alakärppä H, Koskinen R, Liippo K, Surcel HM, Leinonen M, Saikku P. Chlamydia pneumoniae infection in patients with chronic obstructive pulmonary disease. *Epidemiol Infect.* 1997;118(2):155-64.

[154] Paplinska-Goryca, Magdalena, Renata Rubinsztajn, Patrycja Nejman-Gryz, Tadeusz Przybylowski, Rafael Krenke, Ryszarda Chazan. The association between Chlamydia pneumonia chronic

infection and inflammation in COPD patients. *Eur Resp J.* 2017;50:PA4096.

[155] Contoli M, Gnesini G, Forini G, Marku B, Pauletti A, Padovani A, Casolari P, Taurino L, Ferraro A, Chicca M, Ciaccia A, Papi A, Pinamonti S. Reducing agents decrease the oxidative burst and improve clinical outcomes in COPD patients: a randomised controlled trial on the effects of sulphurous thermal water inhalation. *ScientificWorldJournal.* 2013;2013:927835.

[156] Ito K, Lim S, Caramori G, Chung KF, Barnes PJ, Adcock IM. Cigarette smoking reduces histone deacetylase 2 expression, enhances cytokine expression, and inhibits glucocorticoid actions in alveolar macrophages. *FASEB J.* 2001;15(6):1110-2.

[157] Ito K, Chung KF, Adcock IM. Update on glucocorticoid action and resistance. *J Allergy Clin Immunol.* 2006;117(3):522-43.

[158] Marwick JA, Caramori G, Stevenson CS, Casolari P, Jazrawi E, Barnes PJ, Ito K, Adcock IM, Kirkham PA, Papi A. Inhibition of PI3Kdelta restores glucocorticoid function in smoking-induced airway inflammation in mice. *Am J Respir Crit Care Med.* 2009;179(7):542-8.

[159] Sun Y, Wang K, Li MX, He W, Chang JR, Liao CC, Lin F, Qi YF, Wang R, Chen YH. Metabolic changes of H2S in smokers and patients of COPD which might involve in inflammation, oxidative stress and steroid sensitivity. *Sci Rep.* 2015;5:14971.

[160] Mitani A, Azam A, Vuppusetty C, Ito K, Mercado N, Barnes PJ. Quercetin restores corticosteroid sensitivity in cells from patients with chronic obstructive pulmonary disease. *Exp Lung Res.* 2017;43(9-10):417-425.

[161] Lopalco M, Proia AR, Fraioli A, Serio A, Cammarella I, Petraccia L, Grassi M. Effetto terapeutico dell'associazione ventilazione polmonare e aerosol-inalazione con acqua minerale solfurea nelle broncopneumopatie cronico-ostruttive (BPCO). [Therapeutic effect of the association between pulmonary ventilation and aerosol-inhalation with sulphureous mineral water in the chronic bronchopneumopathies]. *Clin Ter.* 2004;155(4):115-20.

[162] Pellegrini M, Fanin D, Nowicki Y, Guarnieri G, Bordin A, Faggian D, Plebani M, Saetta M, Maestrelli P. Effect of inhalation of thermal water on airway inflammation in chronic obstructive pulmonary disease. *Respir Med.* 2005;99(6):748-54.

[163] Guarnieri G, Ferrazzoni S, Scarpa MC, Lalli A, Maestrelli P. Effects of inhalation of thermal water on exhaled breath condensate in chronic obstructive pulmonary disease. *Respiration.* 2010;79(3):216-21.

[164] Gutenbrunner C, Bender T, Cantista P, Karagülle Z. A proposal for a worldwide definition of health resort medicine, balneology, medical hydrology and climatology. *Int J Biometeorol.* 2010; 54(5):495-507.

In: Mineral Water
Editors: Maria João Martins
ISBN: 978-1-68507-458-6

Chapter 3

THERMAL WATERS IN OTORHINOLARYNGOLOGY

João Filipe Simões[1,*], MD, Helena Castro[2], MD, Maria João Martins[3,4], PhD and António Miguéis[5], MD, PhD

[1]Otorhinolaryngology Department, Centre Hospitalier de Mouscron, Réseau Santé Louvain, Mouscron, Belgium
[2]Termas de São Jorge, Santa Maria da Feira, Portugal
[3]Department of Biomedicine, Biochemistry Unit, Faculty of Medicine, University of Porto, Porto, Portugal
[4]i3S-Instituto de Investigação e Inovação em Saúde, University of Porto, Porto, Portugal
[5]Otorhinolaryngology University Clinic, Faculty of Medicine, University of Coimbra, Coimbra, Portugal

* Corresponding Author's E-mail: jofsim@gmail.com.

Abstract

This chapter aims to present and discuss the benefits of Spa therapy in the pathology within the Otorhinolaryngology (ORL) field. A literature search, from January 2000 until the 31st of January 2021, was performed in MedLine, Up-to-Date, Cochrane and clinicaltrials.gov databases. A total of 29 articles were selected (counting 4 reviews). Sixteen studies refer to sinonasal diseases, 5 to ear diseases and 4 include pharyngeal and laryngeal conditions; 11 studies describe cures with sulphurous thermal waters. Nowadays, although more well-designed studies are needed to clarify specific issues and further unravel the mechanisms of action of distinct thermal waters in the ORL field, there is a large set of scientific evidence supporting the use of Spa therapy in ORL diseases. Thermal water treatments in ORL are well-accepted and tolerated, presenting a high safety level. Spa therapy deserves relevant application in the ORL field, in prevention, treatment and rehabilitation.

Keywords: nasal endoscopic surgery, otitis media with effusion, rhinitis, rhinosinusitis, sinusitis, thermal water, upper respiratory tract disease

Introduction

Therapy with thermal waters is considered one of the most basic medical methodologies. The external and/or internal use of thermal waters in the medical area, for health promotion and disease cure, is as old as humanity. History reveals that the aforementioned use of thermal waters started as a belief in gods, being then linked to hygiene and appropriate health state. For centuries, thermal waters use reflected, exclusively, an evidence-based approach, lacking the experimental scientific methodology that validates modern medical procedures and treatments. Recently, in the last years, relying on precise mechanisms (although not completely characterised neither their full extent known), thermal waters use has been stablished as important and/or effective preventive, rehabilitative and curative non-pharmacological therapeutic options, as well as co-adjuvant in the pharmacological treatment, for several diseases. Readers are suggested to read other chapters in this book for acknowledgement of thermal waters' impact upon rheumatic, pulmonary, dermatologic and metabolic alterations/diet-induced pathological conditions. Ear, nose and throat diseases are very prevalent in the modern society, affecting all age groups. Surgeries and/or drugs may not always achieve their management and symptomatic control (no drug is universally efficacious) or, sometimes, a medical contra-indication for surgery and/or pharmacological treatment could exist. Therefore, adequate research that adds evidence regarding non-surgical and/or non-pharmacological therapeutic interventions should be collected and adequately disclosed aiming to improve and spread scientific medical knowledge as well as to support and encourage their implementation. Although the use of thermal waters in upper respiratory airways and ears diseases is a traditional longstanding practice to improve head and neck mucosa status (being the oldest therapy in medical history for upper airways disorders), it is not unanimously acknowledged [1-9].

Topics in this chapter were organized not only by anatomic treated region but also by chemical type of thermal waters used. Thermal waters can be applied in the ear, nose and throat regions by different ways, namely through irrigations, nebulisations/inhalations, sprays and/or aerosols as well as Eustachian tube (direct and indirect) applications. Here, we disclose that patients with (chronic) upper respiratory tract diseases and middle ear disorders may benefit from treatments with thermal waters and we suggest and discuss what is missing to further strength and spread the use of thermal waters in Otorhinolaryngology (ORL). A summary of the mechanisms behind thermal waters impact in ORL is presented.

METHODS

To write this chapter, a literature search in MedLine, Up-to-Date, Cochrane and clinicaltrials.gov databases was performed, including articles published from January 2000 until the 31st of January 2021, conducted by specific keywords. Considering the principal clinical indications for thermal treatment in ear, nose and throat diseases, the search included disease-associated terms, namely rhinitis, sinusitis, otitis, pharyngitis or laryngitis, combined with several terms/designations used in different countries and associated with thermal medicine, specifically balneotherapy, crenotherapy, Spa therapy or thermal water. A total of 29 articles was selected.

RESULTS AND DISCUSSION

The main clinical use found for thermal treatments in prevention, treatment and/or recovery in ORL was in chronic rhinosinusitis (CRS), with or without nasal polyposis, rhinitis, after nasal endoscopic surgery, otitis media with effusion (OME), and auditory tubal dysfunction (and subsequent rhinogenic deafness). No thermal treatments were specifically found in pharyngeal or laryngeal diseases separately, but always (and less frequently) along with other ORL conditions. Among the 29 articles selected, 16 studies involved patients with sinonasal conditions [5, 7, 10-23], 5 assessed thermal waters upon ear diseases [4, 24-27] and 4 evaluated patients with pharyngeal and laryngeal conditions (among others in ORL) [8, 28-30]. The other 4 publications reviewed the literature [31-34]. Sulphurous thermal waters were the most often found in ORL treatments (11 publications included in this chapter) [4, 11, 12, 16, 18, 20, 24-26, 28, 29]. Table 1 briefly discriminates the type of thermal waters tested in each ORL condition along with a summary of the results obtained in the 25 experimental publications just cited (data from the reviews by Olina *et al.*, Hermelingmeier *et al.*, Keller *et al.* and Casale *et al.* [31-34] were not included).

Table 1. Thermal waters: applications and benefits in Otorhinolaryngology

Thermal water	Application	Effect	Ref.
Salso-bromo-iodine Salt-bromide-iodine	• Nonseasonal rhinitis • Recurrent rhinosinusitis or CRS (with/out I degree nasal polyposis) • CRS (with/out I degree nasal polyposis) • After endoscopic surgery (for chronic sinonasal polyposis, with inflammatory conditions) • Monolateral or bilateral OME • Chronic upper respiratory tract infections (tonsillitis, pharyngitis, rhinitis, sinusitis, otitis, common cold and bronchitis)	• Improvement of symptoms and objective examination • Improvement of mucociliary transport time • Improvement of rhinomanometric data • Improvement of nasal mucosal recovery • Decreased nasal mucus content • Decrease of nasal IgA • Modulation of circulating cytokine and immunoglobulin profiles (↓IL-2, IL-4, IFNγ, IgE;↑IL-1β, IL-6, IL-8, IL-17, IL-21, TNF-α, IgA) • Lower upper respiratory tract infections frequency • Improvement of audiometric and tympanogram data	[15] [16] [17] [18] [19] [20]
Bicarbonate-calcium-magnesium	• Allergic rhinitis	• Improvement of symptom scores (TSS and VAS)	[22]
Sulphurous	• Chronic sinonasal disease • CRS (without visible polyps) • Nonallergic CRS • After nasal functional endoscopic surgery (for CRS) • Monolateral or bilateral OME • Chronic inflammatory upper respiratory tract and middle ear disturbances associated with rhinogenic deafness	• Improvement of nasal mucociliary clearance: increase of nasal respiratory flow, reduction of nasal resistance and mucociliary transport time • Improvement of mucosal recovery • Improvement of audiometric data • Decreased hearing loss • Modulation of circulating immunoglobulin profile (↓IgE; ↑IgA)	[1] [2] [3] [4] [5] [6] [7] [8] [9] [10] [11]

Table 1. (Continued)

Thermal water	Application	Effect	Ref.
Sulphurous (Continued)	• OME[1] + tubal dysfunction • OME with deafness (as a consequence of chronic upper airways inflammatory status) • Laryngitis, pharyngitis, rhinitis and rhinosinusitis • Recurrent upper respiratory tract infections[2]	• Improvement of endoscopic data/ethmoid biopsy (↓eosinophils; ↓ mastocytes; ↓cellular inflammatory influx) • Modulation of nasal cytology (↓bacteria; ↓ ↑neutrophils;↑plasma cells; ↑ciliated cells) • Decreased number of primary airways infections • Lower consumption of antibiotics • Amelioration of symptoms (cough, nasal itch, and expectoration, for example) • Decrease of frequency, duration, severity and social impact of diseases[2] • Improvement of symptom score (VAS) • Improvement of quality of life • Full disease recovery[1]	
Chloride-sodium	• Seasonal allergic rhinitis and intermittent asthma (without respiratory tract abnormalities) • CRS (without nasal polyps) • CRS	• Improvement of symptoms (including TSS); reduction of the percentage of patients presenting symptoms • Improvement of SN5 and QoL scores • Improvement of inflammation (↓exhaled FeNO; ↓nasal TNF-α, calprotectin and hBD-2) • Improvement of nasal ciliary motility and neutrophil and spore counts	[12] [13] [14]
Carbon dioxide-enriched	• Allergic rhinitis	• Improvement of scores of each symptom and nasal chemokine levels (↓IL-3, IL-5, eotaxin) • Improvement of nasal inflammation (↓eosinophils)	[21]

Thermal water	Application	Effect	Ref.
Radioactive	• Chronic sinonasal inflammation (CRS, persistent allergic rhinitis, and vasomotor rhinitis with inferior turbinate hypertrophy; without obstructive polyposis) • Perennial allergic rhinitis (without nasal polyps)	• Improvement of nasal mucociliary transport time • Improvement of symptom score (SNOT) • Improvement of nasal cytology data (inflammatory cell infiltration profile; ↓eosinophils; ↑ciliated cells)	[23] [24]
Salty-earthy-alkaline	• Chronic rhinitis, pharyngitis or sinusitis	• Improvement of symptom and clinical scores (TSS and CES) • Modulation of genes involved in tissue repair, innate immune response, antioxidant defence and inflammation (↑CXCR4, SOD2, NF-KB1; ↓FLT1, TLR4)	[25]

CES: clinical evaluation score; CRS: chronic rhinosinusitis; CXCR4: C-X-C motif chemokine receptor 4; FeNO: exhaled nitric oxide; FLT1: Fms related receptor tyrosine kinase 1; hBD-2: human β-defensin 2; IFN: interferon; Ig: immunoglobulin; IL: interleukin; NF-KB1: nuclear factor kappa B subunit 1; OME: otitis media with effusion; QoL: quality of life; Ref: referefence; SOD2: superoxide dismutase 2; SN5: sino-nasal 5; SNOT: sino-nasal outcome test; TLR4: toll-like receptor 4; TNF: tumour necrosis factor; TSS, total symptom score; VAS: visual analogue scale.

Rhinology

General Aspects of Sinonasal Diseases

Prevalence of sinonasal diseases is continuously increasing, reaching epidemic proportions worldwide. They markedly deteriorate patient's quality of life (morbidity can be significant) and associate with relevant socioeconomic costs, in terms of therapy, friendship and socialisation, academic performance and labour productivity (the latter takes into account missed workdays, absenteeism and productivity loss). Curiously, nasal diseases may have a greater impact on social function than cardiovascular diseases [17, 19, 23, 35-37].

Rhinitis, a common heterogeneous chronic disease, affecting children and adults, is an inflammation of the nasal mucosa characterised by one or more nasal symptoms (like nasal discharge and blockage, sneezing and itching). Rhinitis phenotypes include allergic rhinitis [the most common form of non-infectious rhinitis and the most common form of atopic disease; previously subdivided into seasonal, perennial or occupational based on exposure time to allergens (now as intermittent or persistent)], nonallergic rhinitis [that includes the so-called idiopathic (previously vasomotor) rhinitis] and other rhinitis syndromes. Children with a parental background of atopic diseases present symptoms more frequently, and earlier, than those with nonallergic parental family history [19, 35]. Nonallergic rhinitis has a prevalence of 2.8% and 11.8% at the age of 4 and 18 years, respectively, and allergic rhinitis 3.4% and 27.3%, respectively. On adults, the adjusted prevalence rate is 9.6% and 29.8%, respectively. Allergic rhinitis, forming part of a systemic multicomplex inflammatory disorder, is frequently/highly associated with asthma and the risk of asthma-related hospitalisations (emergency department visits are amplified for patients with non-controlled rhinitis) [17, 19, 23, 35, 38]. Allergic rhinitis is considered an eosinophilic, immunoglobulin (Ig) E-mediated and T helper type (Th) 2 immune disease that can be divided into early and late responses. The former, that displays sneezing, itching, rhinorrhoea and congestion, occurs within minutes of allergen exposure and is primarily caused by the release of several pre-formed and newly synthesised mast cell products (for example histamine); the latter occurs from 4 to 8 hours after allergen exposure, is characterised by congestion, malaise, fatigue, irritability and neurocognitive deficits and includes the recruitment of additional inflammatory cells (neutrophils, eosinophils, basophils and mast and mononuclear cells) that sustain and perpetuate disease mechanisms. Eosinophils, that release an array of pro-inflammatory mediators, are the main cells in the late-phase response, correlating with symptom progression and disease severity [19, 35, 39]. Treatment involves a combination of actions (alleviating symptoms, limiting risk factors and preventing sensitisation), being pharmacological therapy based on histamine antagonists, topical intranasal steroids (the most used) and specific immune therapy [23].

Rhinitis and sinusitis frequently coincide and have been proposed as rhinosinusitis. Rhinosinusitis incidence has been gradually increasing, especially in its chronic and recurrent forms in which anatomical abnormalities, allergy, infections, and other systemic diseases perform a central role. CRS has an estimated incidence of 12.3% in the USA, 10.9% in Europe and 13% in China; besides being one of the most common chronic medical conditions worldwide, CRS is the most common cause of primary care physician consultations. CRS affects all age groups, being the elderly, children, heart patients, diabetics and immunocompromised patients suffering from chronic lower respiratory tract diseases at the highest risk. CRS is characterised by mucosal inflammation of the nose and paranasal sinuses that leads to nasal blockage and discharge, facial pressure/pain and loss of sense of smell (involving different inflammatory, antimicrobial and immune-regulatory mediators and cell types, suggestive of differences in the pathogenic processes in an age-dependent way). CRS can be divided into two broad clinical categories: CRS with and without nasal polyposis [21, 22, 34, 37, 40]. CRS can be treated with general or topical antibiotics and steroids, cromoglycate sodium, ipratropium bromide and sodium hyaluronate [8, 22, 33, 40]. Anti-inflammatory medication characterises the first-line treatment for both allergic rhinitis and CRS [33].

Assessments on the available treatments for the abovementioned sinonasal conditions have been published reporting low quality of several clinical studies and low quality evidence for their use as well as unsatisfactory/inadequate/not complete efficacy, adverse effects and contraindications. Poor compliance, sometimes associated with corticophobia (e.g., 64% of allergic rhinitis patients present steroid phobia), occurs when therapy must be pursued for long time. Quite often, patients desire other non-pharmacological treatment options [5, 8, 22, 33, 40].

Sulphurous Thermal Water

Staffieri & Abramo studied the effects of a 12-day course of nasal inhalations (at 38 ºC, for 10 min, to 20 cm from patient's face) with a sulphurous-arsenical-ferruginous thermal water (Levico Spa, Levico Terme, Trento, Italy), followed by nasal aerosol of the same Spa water (7 µm micelle, for 10 min), in 37 consecutive patients with chronic sinonasal disease (20 women, 17 men; mean age of 40 y). The Spa water intervention significantly increased total nasal respiratory flow but reduced total nasal resistance as well as mucociliary transport time. Additionally, nasal cytology disclosed significant changes after the thermal water treatment: bacteria and neutrophils decreased while plasma cells increased. No adverse effects were reported by patients. All together, these findings support the hypothesis of a pharmacological type of action of sulphurous-arsenical-ferruginous thermal water inhalations [11].

To confirm these stimulating preliminary results, Staffieri and co-workers, in a randomised controlled double-blind prospective study, investigated the effects of sulphurous-arsenical-ferruginous thermal water irrigation (Levico Spa, Levico Terme, Trento, Italy) in mucosal cicatrisation/recovery after nasal functional endoscopic surgery for CRS (University Hospital of Padova, Padova, Italy). Consecutive patients (37 male and 19 female; 18-65 y) were assigned to one of the two irrigation treatments (4 times per day, for 6 months) with 20 mL of either isotonic sodium chloride solution (control group; n=18 patients) or sulphurous-arsenical-ferruginous thermal water diluted to 10% with distilled water (treatment group; n=38 patients), being intraoperative and postoperative biopsies performed (at 1, 3 and 6 months after surgery). Thermal treatment induced a statistically significant reduction of eosinophils and mastocytes (cellular inflammatory influx) but the control treatment led to a mixed impact by increasing eosinophils and decreasing mastocytes levels. No modifications in the cellular population of lymphocytes, neutrophils, plasmocytes and histiocytes were seen for both treatments. Very few adverse events to thermal water were communicated: 2 patients felt nasal irritation and local burning and 1 patient developed a generalised cutaneous hypersensitivity reaction. These results suggest the use of this type of thermal water in irrigations after nasal endoscopic surgery for CRS in order to improve mucosal recovery [12].

Sulphurous thermal water (Tabiano Spa, Parma, Italy) was tested in a randomised double-blind study enrolling 80 CRS (without visible polyps) patients (45 men and 35 women; 26-58 y, mean age 46.4 y), at the ENT (Ear, Nose and Throat) Department of the University of Genoa (Genoa, Italy). All patients underwent a 12-day course of warm inhalations (for 10 min, at 38 °C, 20 cm from the face, once a day), followed by nasal irrigations (for 6 min, at corporeal temperature, once a day). Nasal decongestants and oral antihistamines, antibacterials and corticosteroids were allowed during the study. Sulphurous thermal water significantly decreased circulating IgE concentration levels and nasal mucociliary transport time values as well as significantly improved visual analogue scale (VAS) score results [overtime (baseline, 12 days and 3 months) and *versus* 0.9% sodium chloride solution]; no changes were observed in circulating IgG, IgA and IgM (overtime and with both treatments). Adverse effects were not experienced by patients. These data highlight thermal treatment efficacy and applicability in CRS treatment [16].

A randomised controlled double-blind prospective 1-month protocol (follow-up 2 months later), including 70 consecutive smokers with nonallergic CRS (18-65 y) carrying out 20 mL/day irrigations with sulphurous-arsenical-ferruginous thermal water [from Levico Spa (Levico Terme, Trento, Italy); pre-diluted to 10% with distilled water] or isotonic sodium chloride solution (each treatment group included 35 individuals: 11 men and 24 women), was performed by Ottaviano and colleagues. No topical nasal treatments, systemic steroids or antibiotics were used during the intervention. Spa thermal water irrigations revealed a strong beneficial impact upon nasal resistance (by lowering it, both at 1 and 3 months) and nasal cytology results (by increasing ciliated cells number, at 1 month) *versus* control group or baseline data. Endoscopic results were still improved at 3 months in thermal water group *versus* control group. However, overtime (at 1 and 3 months), the olfactory threshold was significantly greater in the control group than in the thermal water-treated group; *versus* baseline, it was significantly higher at 1 month in the control group. Unexpectedly, nasal neutrophil count increased with thermal water treatment. No local adverse effects in consequence of thermal water use were recorded in this intervention. These results show a potential pharmacological type of action of sulfurous-arsenical-ferruginous in smoking associated nonallergic CRS [20].

A previous randomised controlled double-blind prospective study by the same research team assessed the effects of a 1-month irrigation treatment with sulphurous-salty-bromic-iodic thermal water [from Sirmione Spa (Sirmione, Brescia, Italy); 5 mL 4 times/day] upon clinical (endoscopic and functional) and microbiological evidence as well as cytological profile in 66 consecutive nonallergic CRS adult and elderly patients (Padova University Hospital, Padova, Italy; 18-65 y). No topical nasal treatments, systemic steroids or antibiotics occurred during the study. Possible side effects pointed out after thermal water irrigation: mild nasal irritation and local burning sensation (6 cases) and episodes of limited epistaxis (5 cases). At baseline, *Staphylococcus aureus* was isolated in 5 patients in the thermal water group (n=35) and 4 in the isotonic sodium chloride solution group (control) (n=31). After the nasal irrigations, a) there was no sign of the bacteria in either group, b) a statistical significant clinical (endoscopic) improvement was seen in both groups, and c) no significant differences in the cytological results were encountered between groups. The only statistically significant difference between the 2 irrigation treatments was the reduction of total nasal resistance observed in the thermal water group while no change occurred in the control group (also 5 mL 4 times/day). The need of more studies is expressed [18].

Chloride-Sodium Thermal Water

The randomised controlled prospective study conducted by Del Giudice and co-workers in 34 children (6-14 y) with seasonal allergic rhinitis and intermittent asthma (without respiratory tract abnormalities) assessed the effects of nasal irrigations with a hyper-mineral chloride-sodium Ischia thermal water during the period of natural exposure to Parietaria pollen. Children were selected from both the Department of Pediatrics, Second University of Naples (Italy), and the Children's Hospital

"Anna Rizzoli" of Ischia, Naples (Italy), and treated for 3 consecutive months, 15 days per month, either with thermal water (n=18; aerosol by nasal adapter), at the Lacco Ameno Spa services (Italy), or with isotonic sodium chloride solution (n=16; micronised nasal douche), with follow-up assessment 2 weeks after the end of the treatment. On demand, they were also treated with cetirizine, no other treatment being allowed; intervention without significant side effects. A statistically significant reduction of the nasal symptoms (total symptom score, TSS) was observed in thermal water group *versus* control group, at the end of therapy. At baseline both groups had comparable levels of exhaled nitric oxide (FeNO, a marker that allows monitorization of airway inflammation). On thermal water-treated children, there was a statistically significant reduction of FeNO levels at the end of the treatment (that remained unaltered at the follow-up period) while in controls no statistically significant difference was found between baseline and follow-up period; after 3 months of treatment, thermal water-treated children had significantly lower FeNO values than the control children. A statistically significant correlation between TSS score and FeNO values happened. Data obtained by Del Giudice and co-workers highlight the relevance of inflammation in the development of allergic rhinitis and points out to a new possible effect of this thermal water: the reduction of airway inflammation [17].

Passarielo *et al.* explored the modulation of symptom (sino-nasal 5, SN5) and quality of life (QoL) scores as well as nasal mucosal markers of inflammation on 60 consecutive children [28 boys; 3.3±0.9 y (mean±standard deviation; SD)] with CRS, without nasal polyps, by sulphate-sodium-chloride thermal water (Ischia, Italy) inhalations by nasal aerosol (15 minutes/day, for 15 days). Fifty healthy children (28 boys; 3.4±1.0 y), not undergoing therapy, were included for comparison. A significant decrease of nasal tumour necrosis factor (TNF)-α, calprotectin, and human β-defensin-2 (hBD-2) levels (towards normal values) as well as of percentage of patients presenting reduction of sense of smell or symptoms of facial pain, nasal obstruction or nasal discharge was observed at the end of treatment, in addition to a significant improvement of SN5 and QoL scores. This set of beneficial impacts remained unaltered at follow-up (after 4 weeks) what, in conjunction with the good tolerability of the thermal intervention that was observed, points towards its use upon paediatric CRS [21].

Cantone and co-workers (ENT Unit of the Department of Neuroscience, Federico II University of Naples, Italy) determined, for the first time, the effects of Spa therapy with sodium-chloride-sulphate hyperthermal water in a two-arm interventional study with 84 elderly subjects with CRS (males < females; mean age 70.3±11 y). All volunteers were treated at the Thermae Oriente (Ischia, Italy): 49 patients with thermal water rich in mineral salts [individual steam hot-vapour inhalation for 10 min, at 38 °C, 20 cm from the face, followed by individual aerosol, with a nasal adapter, for 10 min, at 38 °C; for 12 consecutive days] and 35 patients with isotonic saline solution (according to the same protocol; groups were matched for sex and age, without significant differences in cytological and clinical parameters). Thermal water treatment, unlike sodium chloride treatment, induced a statistically significant improvement of symptoms as well as of ciliary motility and neutrophil and spore counts (as determined by nasal cytological assessment, at baseline and 1 month after the beginning of the treatment). Contrariwise, the count of mast cells, eosinophils, bacteria and biofilm did not significantly change in both groups. Patients reported having no aggressive reactions. This study suggests that in these patients sodium-chloride-sulphate hyperthermal water Spa therapy could be safely used as a primary treatment [22].

Salso-Bromo-Iodine Thermal Water

The effects of the iodine bromide water from Salsomaggiore Terms (Salsomaggiore, Italy) were assessed on 80 patients suffering from specific nonseasonal rhinitis (*Dermatophagoides Farinae* and *Dermatophagoides Pteronyssinus*). After the trial period, patients treated with the thermal water (by endonasal Acqua Sal spray, 7 times/day, for 30 days) presented a 100% improvement in their subjective perception of their symptomatology while patients in the control group (oily drops, 7 times/day, for 30 days) showed a 33% improvement. Circulating IgE decreased while IgA increased in the former group. Iodine bromide water presents an anti-inflammatory effect, besides its cleansing action [10].

Passali and co-workers enrolled 120 patients to characterise the efficacy of the modulation of recurrent rhinosinusitis or CRS (with/out I degree nasal polyposis) by salt-bromine-iodic thermal water (Salsomaggiore water) *versus* sodium chloride solution. Patients were randomised into 2 groups: a) 60 underwent vapour inhalation, aerosol and nasal douching treatment with thermal water (study group), for 14 days at the Salsomaggiore Spa, and b) 60 underwent nasal douching and aerosol treatment with saline (control group), twice/day, also for 14 days, but at the Rhinologic Centre of the ENT Clinic of Siena University (Siena, Italy). After treatment, a significant improvement of symptoms (nasal obstruction, rhinorrhoea and number of nocturnal arousals) was observed only in the former group. When existent in the control group, the improvement of those symptoms was not significant. Significant improvement of nasal mucosa congestion, nasal secretion and mucociliary transport time also happened in the study group. This randomised controlled protocol puts forward salt-bromine-iodic water treatment as a non-pharmacological therapeutic efficient tool in the treatment of chronic and recurrent rhinosinusitis [13].

In a similarly structured randomised controlled study in CRS (with/out I degree nasal polyposis), the Salsomaggiore thermal water was tested through a distinct administration method - nasal spray, 4 times/day, for 4 weeks (study group: n=30; control group: n=25). A significant improvement of symptoms (headache, rhinorrhoea and hyposmia), *versus* control group, was seen. Significant changes in objective examination (nasal mucosa appearance and crusts) and instrumental analysis (rhinomanometric and mucociliary transport time data) were detected between the 2 groups. Nasal cytology data (epithelial and goblet cells, neutrophils, eosinophils, bacteria) equally improved in both groups. Nasal Salsomaggiore thermal water spray shows a greater efficacy than saline in the resolution of CRS [14].

Later, the effects of the aforementioned salso-bromo-iodine thermal water (Salsomaggiore Terms) were also compared with those of standard topical treatment, in 30 consecutive patients scheduled for endoscopic surgery for chronic sinonasal polyposis, with inflammatory conditions. After surgery, patients were assigned (by alternative randomisation) to one of the two treatment groups: a) topical antibiotic ointments (mupirocin) and saline douching 3 times a day (comparison group; positive control group) and b) isotonic salso-bromo-iodine water-based product douching 3 times a day (study group), at the Department of Otolaryngology, University of Sassari (Sassari, Italy); 15 volunteers with no clinical signs of upper respiratory tract diseases formed the negative control. A solution of the salso-bromo-iodine thermal water (6%) in deionized water (94%), available as Acquasal® spray (Scharper Healthcare, Milan, Italy), was used by the study group. Cytology analysis after nasal brushings, 1 month subsequently to surgery, showed that in the pharmacologically-treated group mucus content was slightly lower than at baseline but epithelial cells had not recovered their junction sites while in the thermal water-treated group epithelial cells were intimately connected to each other and goblet cells had no mucus content. Secretory IgA levels in nasal brushings significantly decreased from preoperatively patients scheduled for surgery, to postoperatively patients in the positive control group, to postoperatively patients in the thermal water-based product-treated group and, finally, to the negative control group. The expression or not of adverse side effects is not mentioned in the publication. This randomised controlled prospective study shows that this type of thermal water may improve postoperative mucosal healing [15].

Carbon Dioxide-Enriched Thermal Water

In a controlled study of the CO_2-enriched thermal water at the Fonti di Rabbi Spa Centre (Trento, Italy), the scores of nasal obstruction, itching and sneezing were evaluated, in addition to chemokine levels quantification and cell population assessment in nasal lavage fluid, on 25 consecutive patients with allergic rhinitis. Both patients [13 men and 12 women; 18-65 y (45.3±2.4 y, mean±SD)] and healthy controls (n=25, 12 males and 13 females; age- and gender-matched subjects, 46.6±3.1 y) inhaled, in the same way, saline solution and the aforementioned thermal water (for 2 consecutive weeks, 6 days a week, once a day, per water). Nasal lavage samples were collected from all subjects, before the first inhalation and immediately after the last one. Statistically significant differences between controls and patients were observed before treatments (at baseline) in nasal obstruction, itching and sneezing score values as well as in chemokine levels [interleukin (IL)-3, IL-5 and eotaxin) and in percentage of eosinophils: lower values were always observed in the former group. The CO_2-enriched thermal water enabled a statistically significant improvement in patients which was not obtained with the saline solution (just a tendency) [19]. As in the previous publication, the occurrence or not of adverse side effects is not declared here. As well as with the study of the exhaled nitric oxide [17], this research underlines that CO_2-enriched thermal water inhalation ameliorates the inflammatory status besides the most common symptoms of allergic rhinitis [19].

Bicarbonate-Calcium-Magnesium Thermal Water

A bicarbonate-calcium-magnesium thermal water was tested in allergic rhinitis patients (mean age 40.9 y) at the Comano thermal centre (Trento, Italy). Thirty consecutive patients (13 men, 17 women) were treated daily, for 15 days, with inhalation of 1 L of thermal water, supplied by Asema inhaler, for 10 min, at 37-38 °C (diameter of inhaled drops was 8-12 μm). Interfering drugs were prohibited; as before, cetirizine syrup was allowed as SOS medication [7, 17]. The treatment significantly reduced nasal symptoms (itching, sneezing, rhinorrhoea, and obstruction) and significantly increased the patient's perception of nasal patency [evaluated by the TSS and VAS scores, respectively], being these outcomes partially long-lasting (after a 2-week follow-up). As in many other studies presented in this chapter, this thermal water treatment had a high tolerability, without the disclosure of significant adverse events. Unfortunately, this preliminary study did not include a control group. Nevertheless, these results are in accordance with previous significant data from a randomised placebo-controlled double-blind intervention with Comano thermal water in vasomotor rhinitis (significantly affected nasal symptoms, improved nasal blood supply and strengthened local nasal immune response). Again, previous data confirm the effective, beneficial and/or safe pattern of Comano thermal water on patients with sub-acute and/or chronic inflammation of upper airways caused by mucosal hyper-reactivity or with chronic pharyngitis [7].

Radioactive Thermal Water

In a comparative prospective study with a pre-post design, Passali and colaborators enrolled 33 consecutive patients of both genders (males 70%), older than 12 y of age, affected by chronic sinonasal inflammation (comprising CRS, persistent allergic rhinitis, and vasomotor rhinitis with inferior turbinate hypertrophy; without obstructive polyposis), in a 14-day course of double radioactive thermal water administration: by warm vapour inhalation (at 38 °C, 20 cm from patient's face, 8-10 μm micelles, 10 min/day) followed by aerosol (2-4 μm micelles, 10 min/day), at the Merano Therme (Merano, Italy). Adverse effects did not occur. Nasal respiratory flow and nasal resistance did not significantly change but pathological mucociliary transport times significantly reduced to physiological ones after treatment. Additionally, before treatment, nasal cytology analysis showed an inflammatory cell infiltration profile in 42% of patients; nasal cytology was normal in 2/3 of these patients after therapy. So, radioactive water SPA therapy could be an alternative option in chronic inflammatory diseases of the upper airways, nonresponsive to pharmacological interventions [5].

Later, in a randomised comparative prospective study, the same research group aimed to evaluate the clinical efficacy of nasal inhalation plus aerosol therapy (8-10 *μ*m micelles, at 38 ºC, 20 cm from the face, for 10 min/day; 2–4 *μ*m micelles for 10 min) of radioactive oligomineral thermal water for 14 days (at the Merano hot springs, as before) and to compare it with the clinical efficacy of mometasone furoate nasal spray for 14 days, in consecutive perennial allergic rhinitis (without nasal polyps) patients (n=54 and n=36, respectively; 14-80 y, including both genders). The radioactive thermal water treatment significantly improved subjective [sino-nasal outcome test (SNOT) score] and objective (mucociliary transport time) clinical data as well as non-significantly improved the cytological exam (number of ciliated cells), similarly to the results obtained with mometasone furoate nasal spray. Additionally, the radioactive thermal water treatment decreased eosinophil levels (tendency). It was well tolerated with no side effects being reported by patients. This thermal treatment could be considered a non-pharmacological therapeutic intervention in allergic patients, an alternative similar to the use of medium-strength corticosteroids [23].

Several Waters - Review Articles

Interestingly, in a recent review, in line with the data just presented, Casale *et al.* state that, regardless of studies heterogeneity in CRS in adult patients [in terms of saline solution characteristics, volume (dose), frequency per day and duration of treatment, administration methods, nasal device types and aims], administration of a hypertonic saline solution, with the addition of natural minerals and oligo-elements found in seawater and some thermal waters, once or twice-daily, *versus* isotonic solutions, associates with a pattern towards a larger clinical improvement, better endoscopic scores and enhanced nasal resistance [34]. On the other hand, from a previous review regarding the use of either isotonic or hypertonic solutions [Salsomaggiore thermal water [10] and sodium chloride solutions; and including seawater gel] on allergic rhinitis patients, overall, lower improvements were obtained when using hypertonic solutions. Nevertheless, 8 out of the 10 studies analysed used sodium chloride solutions [32] and, so, the effects of hypertonicity could be dependent on the type of salts and on the targeted disease [32, 41].

Final Remarks

There is a large set of beneficial data from the use of thermal waters at the sinonasal level [improvement of nasal ciliary motility and mucociliary clearance (as a result of an increase of nasal respiratory flow/improvement of rhinomanometric data and of a reduction of nasal mucus content, resistance and mucociliary transport time), improvement of symptoms and objective examination, reduction of the percentage of patients presenting symptoms (and, consequently, improvement of QoL, SN5, SNOT, TSS and VAS scores), improvement of nasal mucosal recovery, improvement of inflammation (reduction not only of exhaled FeNO but also of nasal eosinophils, eotaxin, IL-3, IL-5, TNF-α, calprotectin and hBD-2); Table 1], without the disclosure of relevant side effects. In what concerns the impact upon nasal and circulating immunoglobulins as well as cell types, bacteria, fungi and biofilm profiles from cytology and/or biopsy data some inconsistency was found, although improvements were quite frequent (Table 1) [5, 7, 10-23]. Supporting the relevance of those beneficial findings is the fact that very few of the abovementioned studies were conducted without a control group [5, 7, 11]. The discrepancy just mentioned is, most likely, due to particular features of the distinct experimental designs, namely a) time that elapsed from surgery up to the first sampling point prevented the characterisation of the treatment impact upon the initiation of the healing process [example [12, 15]]; b) type of thermal water and methodology chosen for its use [example [14, 20]], c) patients clinical condition (and its evolution), patients age, and treatment duration (and number of cycles as well) [example [22]], and d) parameters used for monitoring treatment clinical impact [example [18]].

However, to strength the knowledge about the impact of thermal water cures upon sinonasal diseases a) longer treatments, with control groups, should be performed [only two studies tested the thermal water for more than 1 month [12, 17]], b) follow-up periods should always be included in the study design, for as long as possible [it only occurred in 5 of the studies presented above, 3 months maximum [7, 16, 17, 20, 21]], c) different waters should be tested against each other while using placebo, isotonic and/or hypertonic sodium chloride solutions as control groups, aiming to find out the best mineral content (and concentration) for a given clinical condition, d) comparison as well as synergism with standard sinonasal disease pharmacological therapies should be assessed (as thermal cures, for specific patient populations, could be preferable and more easier to comply with, besides reducing drugs dosage and duration of drugs usage or strengthening drug effects), and e) patient sample size should reflect patient age range, providing statistical power to analyse the response to the cure of age subgroups within the patients sample [missing in [12, 18-20, 23]].

Otology

General Aspects of Otitis Media with Effusion

Otitis media is a very common condition, affecting approximately 11% of the globe's population each year - over 700 million people. The majority of these are children, accounting for more than half of all. Middle ear otitis is the main cause of rhinogenic deafness and effusion in childhood while chronic inflammatory conditions, namely sinusitis, rhinosinusitis and pharyngitis, are important aetiology factors of inflammation of the middle ear with effusion in adults. OME is defined as the presence of fluid in the middle ear, without signs or symptoms of acute ear infection. Middle ear effusion prevalence is 15-40% in healthy children up to 5 y. Furthermore, among children performing regular yearly check-ups, 50-60% of child care attendees and 25% of school-aged children were found to have a middle ear effusion. Below 10 y of age, approximately 80% of children have had an episode of OME, usually under 8 y of age, being bilateral in 80% of the cases. Most OME episodes resolve spontaneously within 3 months (supporting the management of children presenting OME who are not at risk with watchful waiting for 3 months), although 30% to 40% of children have repeated OME episodes, and 5% to 10% of episodes last ≥ 1 y. Typically, a simple episode of classic middle ear infection initially occurs but it tends to be recurrent and self-maintaining, what exacerbates the local chronic inflammation that leads to tympanic effusion. Various degrees of conductive hearing loss are present. Treatment is aimed to a) restore ventilation in the middle ear, b) resolve the chronic inflammatory status, and c) recover the hearing function. OME treatment combines vigilant waiting, pharmacological therapy and surgical intervention. Frequently, first-choice pharmacological cures include aerosol therapy with mucolytics, topical corticosteroids and nasal decongestants, even though with a) relatively uncertain efficacy, b) absence of precise quantification of benefits, and c) manifestation of problems/adverse effects with long-term treatments. There is no scientific evidence about the effectiveness of the use of antihistamines and/or decongestants in OME treatment. In fact, recommendations exist against using intranasal or systemic steroids as well as antihistamines and/or decongestants for treating OME. Less often, structural damage to the tympanic membrane, requiring surgical intervention for its correction, may occur as a consequence of OME [4, 27, 42-45].

Sulphurous Thermal Water

The effects of a slightly sulphurous-sulphated-bicarbonate-calcic thermal water were evaluated on 35 children with OME (n=25) and marked tubal dysfunction [girls & boys; 3-7 y (5.64±1.41 y, mean±SD)] at the thermal baths Bagni delle Galleraie (Radicondoli, Siena, Italy), in a collaboration with the Hygiene Institute from the University of Siena (Siena, Italy). The initial population possessed a mild hearing loss (around 27 dB), but only 71% accepted to undergo the thermal cures cycle. Out of the 35 children followed in the 1st year, 28 returned to Bagni delle Galleraie for the 2 following years as a preventive strategy (only 5 of them went through adenotonsillectomy surgery). After 3 stays at the Bagni delle Galleraie, children were no longer affected by OME and a lower number of infections of the primary airways was observed during the winter as well as less antibiotics were taken. The thermal intervention consisted of 3 sequential steps: micronised nasal wash with physiological solution, b) aerosol treatment with thermal water (2-5 μm particles), and c) Politzer insufflation. The existence of adverse effects was not described. Focused on infant school children, the authors argue for the relevance of an early diagnosis and therapy aiming to prevent any negative social development, with sulphurous thermal water cures playing a crucial role [25].

Costantino and co-workers evaluated the tolerability, effectiveness and impact upon the quality of life of sulphurous Spa therapy, on 27 individuals [28-88 y (62±2.2 y, mean±standard error of the mean),] with chronic inflammatory upper respiratory tract and middle ear disturbances responsible for the onset or persistence of rhinogenic deafness [linked to a light to mild hearing loss (31.1 dB at 500, 1000 and 2000 Hz; 45.0 dB at 4000 Hz)]. Patients did 12 individual humid-hot inhalation sessions (at 38 °C, for 10 min, vapour jet 20 cm from the face) followed by Politzer insufflation with sulphurous-sodium-chloride-bicarbonate-alkaline thermal water at the Rosapepe Spa (Contursi, Salerno, Italy). At the end of the treatment, *versus* baseline, patients showed a statistically significant a) increase in audiometric normoacoustic curves and decrease in pathological curves, b) decrease in auditory loss percentage, and c) hearing improvement at the frequencies required for daily activities (500, 1000 and 2000 Hz) [24]. As in the next study [4], good local and systemic tolerability to the Spa therapy was perceived during the study by Costantino *et al.* (with the occurrence of adverse effects not being observed during the protocol) what supports the use of Spa therapy in rhinogenic deafness. Nevertheless, it should be stated that no control group was included, with or without standard widely available treatments, which could also had shown improvements [24].

A controlled retrospective observational study conducted by Mirandola *et al.*, at an Italian medical Spa, looked at registered audiometric data obtained on children (5-9 y) affected by hearing impairment due to chronic upper airways inflammatory status resulting in OME with deafness. Fifty eight children (presenting a hearing loss ≤ 25dB) had been treated by 1 cycle of standard therapy [12 consecutive days of standard Politzer insufflation [24], with a sulphurous thermal water] per year for a total of 3 consecutive years (between the age of 5 to 7 y) while 37 children had been treated for 1 cycle of therapy per year for a total of 5 consecutive years (between the age of 5 to 9 y). Control children, selected by identical inclusion/exclusion criteria, were represented by 3 untreated age matched groups (5, 6, and 7 y). An almost always significantly decreased dB loss at 500, 1,000 and 2,000 Hz was found at the end of the 2nd cycle, which even improved in the 3rd cycle, *versus* controls. The recovery pattern was particularly important at 500 Hz where the hearing damage was greater. Hearing function improved significantly each year, at the end of each single therapeutic cycle. Almost no children presented significant hearing loss when up to 4 treatments were performed. Unfortunately, the Spa centre and the detailed characteristics of the thermal water were not specified in this study. Since adverse effects did not occur and a high efficacy was disclosed, middle ear insufflation treatment with sulphurous thermal waters is suggested as a consistent, long-term non-pharmacological therapeutic option in OME [4].

A randomised controlled protocol with 80 children suffering of monolateral or bilateral OME [44 boys, 36 girls; 4-12 y (average age around 7.2 y)] compared the effectiveness of a systemic steroid therapy *versus* a thermal therapy based on the Salimbani-Politzer insufflation technique with sulphurous water from Terme di Telese (Telese, Italy). Children were evaluated at baseline and 7 days after the beginning of the therapy as well as 7-10 and 30-35 days after the end of the therapy. The change either from a type B tympanogram to C or A and from C to A was considered a positive outcome while either the persistence of the same type of tympanogram or the shift from a type C tympanogram to B or from A to C or B was considered a negative outcome. Sulphurous water insufflation therapy associated with enhanced outcomes at each time point, with differences in improvement and healing sometimes reaching statistical relevance. The presence of an initial type B tympanogram was the most important prognostic marker, associated to a worst prognosis in both groups and in each subgroup of OME. Sulphurous water insufflation therapy acts as an appropriate non-pharmacological therapeutic option in paediatric OME treatment [26].

Salso-Bromo-Iodine Thermal Water

Beyond their sole application, thermal waters can be used in ORL mixed with other non-pharmacological compounds. A randomised controlled prospective pilot study, planned at the ENT Unit, Acireale Hospital (Catania, Italy), enrolled 80 children with OME (monolateral or bilateral) divided randomly and equally into two treatment groups: with either a salt-bromine-iodine thermal water solution with hyaluronic acid and grapefruit seed extract (Broncalt, Aurora Biofarma Srl, Milano) or isotonic saline (both administered by nasal nebulisation for 3 consecutive months, for 10 days/month, twice/day, with Rinowash micronised nasal douche). Therapy with the salso-bromo-iodine thermal water solution *versus* sodium chloride solution originated a better and statistically significant drift not only for tympanogram data [with greater improvement (type C tympanogram)] and healing (type A tympanogram)] but also for audiometric records (increased patients number with normal hearing and lower patients number with moderate hypoacusis). The manifestation of adverse effects is not addressed in the publication. The research team claims the effectiveness of this thermal therapy in the OME treatment [27].

Final Remarks

Taking into consideration data collected from the 5 abovementioned publications on ear pathology (key benefits being the improvement of audiometric data and tympanogram outcomes along with reduction of not only the number of primary airways infections and but also of antibiotic consumption as well as improvement of quality of life and full disease recovery; Table 1), OME and tubal dysfunction, and consequent rhinogenic deafness, emerge as good targets for Spa therapy [4, 24-27]. Interestingly, Spa therapy could be considered as a valid first-choice treatment option as it appears lacking adverse effects, is simple and, usually, cost-effective; so, it may even be preferred over pharmacological and surgical therapies. And, why not think about thermal water therapy (if available) as a helpful treatment option during the 3-month management waiting period, mentioned above in the "General aspects of Otitis Media with Effusion" section? It might improve quality of life in this period, assisting (speeding and/or anticipating) OME natural self-limiting mechanisms, and, at an earlier management point, contribute to prevent, delay and/or shorten future OME recurrences/relapses/crises (lowering complications and therapeutic expenses as well as personal, family and social burdens).

Still, at the moment, in order to stronger support the application of Spa therapy in the aforementioned ear pathological conditions, more (and better well-designed) clinical trials are needed: a) considering/including pneumatic otoscopy and acoustic impedance/tympanometry [the latter can be used in suspected OME when the diagnosis is uncertain after performing (or attempting) pneumatic otoscopy] as diagnostic tools within the inclusion criteria, to enhance research objectivity [[43]; for instance, used in [25] and [27] but lacking in [4] where, although being considered an indirect and subjective test [43], audiometry was performed], b) with extended treatment duration [treatments lasted 7 or 12 days in [24, 26]] and (longer) follow-up periods [inexistent in [24, 27]], c) comprising more patients and including more centres per trial as well as patients with higher hearing loss, not only amplifying the magnitude and statistical relevance of the results but also expanding patients age and clinical status ranges (by assessing cases that would need surgery for treatment) as well as disease aetiology factors, to enhance research strength [for example, in the study by Costantino *et al.*, from the clinical point of view, a quite modest improvement of hearing loss (4.3 dB) was obtained within patients that had light hearing loss (31.1 dB) [24]], d) testing thermal waters with other and distinct characteristics (and against each other), e) including adequate control groups [absent in [24] and [25]] to allow comparison of applicability and efficacy with standard pharmacological and surgical therapies, f) identifying the effects specific to each component of the solution used [when to thermal waters are added additives (other compounds or solutions)] and confirm and characterise their interaction [is there a synergism in the mechanisms of action? in [27] this is hypothesised but not established neither categorised by the use of suitable control groups], and g) further unravelling the biochemical, physiological and/or molecular mechanisms behind thermal waters protective effects. Detailed characterisation of the selected clinical situation considered in the thermal treatment study is also vital as is the inclusion of enlarged/diverse patient age ranges, as abovementioned [while taking into consideration the sample size to allow adequate statistical analysis per age subgroups when their formation is viable; 4 out of the 5 studies included children [4, 25-27]; 1 study included young and old adults, but the group was small to allow identification of underlying distinct aetiology factors [24]].

Laryngology, Pharyngology, and Upper Respiratory Tract Diseases

General Aspects of Laryngitis and Pharyngitis

(Chronic) upper respiratory tract infections [embracing (recurrent) nose, sinuses, throat, pharynx, larynx and/or trachea infections] are very frequent diseases, involving millions of people annually, with all ages being affected. They are among the most common diseases encountered in paediatric ages. Due to the decline of the immune response, affecting not only the clinical presentation but also the therapeutic approach, these infections are complex in the elderly. Antibacterial and antiviral drugs are only exceptionally suitable in their prevention since the benefit is modest and the risk of resistant bacteria emergence is high; likewise surgery efficacy is unclear [8, 29, 30, 46].

A yearly incidence of 3.47 cases per 1,000 subjects has been published for chronic laryngitis. Around 21% of the population will develop chronic laryngitis in their life. Proton pump inhibitors, nasal steroids and antihistamines are used (in decreasing percentage order) in its initial pharmacological treatment [47]. Pharyngitis, commonly encountered by family physicians, is an inflammation of the pharynx, caused not only by one of many different viruses and/or bacteria but also by reflux, rhinitis and postnasal drip, persistent cough and allergy. Group A streptococcal pharyngitis represents 15% to 30% of infections in children and 5% to 15% in adults. Penicillins are the first choice for treatment of streptococcal pharyngitis [46].

Sulphurous Thermal Water

Constantino *et al.*, in a study including 83 patients (45 men and 38 women, mean age around 53 y), with the diagnosis of laryngitis, pharyngitis, rhinitis and rhinosinusitis, tested a cycle of sulphurous mineral inhalant therapy (at 38 °C, at 20 cm from the face, for 10 min) followed by an aerosol treatment (for 10 min). An amelioration of most of the symptoms examined, namely cough, nasal itch and expectoration, was found in parallel to an excellent local and systemic tolerability [28].

Besides the already described myriad of beneficial known effects, thermal waters also have a positive immunomodulatory activity (at the systemic level) contributing to their therapeutic effects [29, 30]. Characterisation of the impact and efficacy of sulphurous thermal water inhalations in the treatment of paediatric recurrent upper respiratory tract infections [where cough (dry or productive) was one of the symptoms within the inclusion criteria] was accomplished by Salami and collaborators. This research team included 100 children [55 boys and 45 girls; 6-14 y (9 y on average)] in a 12-day course (consecutive days) warm vapour inhalations randomised double-blind comparative protocol, at the ENT Department of the University of Genoa (Genoa, Italy), using sulphurous-sulphate-calcium-magnesium thermal water (with one of the highest levels of sulphur in the world; Tabiano SPA Mineral Water, Tabiano, Parma, Italy; n=50) and physiological solution (n=50; both at 38 ºC, 20 cm from patient's face, for 10 min). Compared against the physiological solution, after the 12-day treatment and at the end of the follow-up of the study (3 months after the start), children treated with the sulphurous thermal water had a) lower and higher circulating IgE (significantly) and IgA levels, respectively, b) unchanged circulating IgG and IgM levels, c) significantly improved subjective assessment of symptoms (by VAS score), d) normal nasal mucociliary transport time, and e) significantly decreased frequency, duration, severity and social impact of recurrent upper respiratory tract occurrences. The thermal water treatment induced no side effects on children. It is claimed that the immunomodulant activity of the sulphurous thermal water used plays a pivotal role in its therapeutic effects [29].

Salt-Bromide-Iodine Thermal Water

In line, further deepening the knowledge upon immune system modulation by thermal water inhalation, Magrone *et al.* measured the impact of inhalatory therapy with salt-bromide-iodine thermal water at the Margherita di Savoia Spa (Margherita di Savoia, Barletta-Andria-Trani,

Italy) on young (24-58 y, mean age 48 y) and elderly (66-86 y, mean age 68 y) individuals with chronic upper respiratory tract infections (pharyngitis included, among other ORL diseases; n=51/group). The inhalatory treatment consisted of nebulised thermal water (2–10 μm microparticles) administered daily through a rhino-pharynx tubal unit (at 37°C), for 2 consecutive weeks, for 10 min (at 2-3° Baumè density). It reduced, with different patterns, the excessive secretion of Th1-related cytokines (IL-2 and interferon-γ) and Th2-related cytokine (IL-4) observed at baseline on both elderly and young patients. In both groups of patients, circulating IL-10 values were above normality at baseline and at 6 and 12 months after treatment. Circulating IL-17 levels increased following therapy in both groups of patients but those of IL-21 increased only on the elderly patients. Circulating IL-1β, IL-6, IL-8 and TNF-α values were lower than normal in the 2 patient groups at baseline but increased after the inhalatory protocol. For both groups of patients (more effectively in the young), a sharp reduction of the frequency of upper respiratory tract infections was recorded 1 year after the inhalatory intervention; this clinical amelioration is long-lasting enduring after 1 y from the initial treatment. Salt-bromide-iodine thermal water therapy attenuates the pro-inflammatory arm of the immune response [30].

Salty-Earthy-Alkaline Thermal Water

Neri and co-workers evaluated the impact of combined warm vapour inhalations and aerosol (by nasal adapter; 12 days in 2 weeks) with Cappelletta salty-earthy-alkaline thermal water (Acquasanta, Genoa, Italy) upon 183 consecutive adult and elderly patients [20-86 y, (60.6±15.2 y, mean±SD)] with chronic rhinitis, pharyngitis or sinusitis [29% from (naso) pharyngitis]. The elderly complied better to the inhalation+aerosol treatment. At the end of the treatment, patient percentage with symptoms slightly decreased among those with low intensity symptoms while strongly decreased among those with symptoms with an intermediate to strong intensity. TSS significantly decreased more than 50% at the end of the treatment, with symptoms remaining at considerably low levels at the 1-y-follow-up. Clinical evaluation score (CES) significantly decreased

57% with treatment. Age or pathology did not significantly modulate TSS and CES. At the end of treatment, rhinomanometric data were irregular: although inhalation resistance remained unaltered, exhalation resistance significantly changed only among patients with sinusitis (increased), what led to a significant change when considering the entire population. Related events or side effects were uncommon and not severe. In nasal epithelial cells, differential modulation of the expression level of several genes was observed: the increase of C-X-C motif chemokine receptor 4 (CXCR4; for the 3 pathologies), superoxide dismutase 2 (SOD2; only for pharyngitis) and nuclear factor kappa B subunit 1 (NF-KB1; only for sinusitis) as well as the decrease of Fms related receptor tyrosine kinase 1 (FLT1; only for sinusitis) and toll-like receptor 4 (TLR4; only for rhinitis) were significant treatment consequences. CXCR4 showed the highest change in absolute figures (and for the first time), which was not age-dependent although smoking status-dependent (lower in current smokers *versus* non-smokers). Additionally, no dependency on gender, exposure to noxious inhalable substances or to second-hand smoke, allergy or fruit and vegetables consumption was found. FLT1 significant change occurred only among non-smokers. Along with an improvement of the clinical condition, modulation of genes involved in tissue repair, innate immune response, antioxidant defence and inflammation by a thermal treatment is displayed [8]. These (local) results, like the previous ones (systemic), could open the way for new possible applications of this therapeutic strategy in other conditions characterised by inflammation.

Several Waters - Review Articles

Olina *et al.* reviewed that, in pharyngitis caused by nonbacterial inflammatory processes (induced by virus, mycoses, reflux of gastric juices, tobacco or alcohol abuse), inhalation, irrigation or aerosol-therapy with distinct thermal waters could be indicated both as alternative and preventive therapies [31]. A systematic review and meta-analysis by Keller *et al.* in the treatment of upper respiratory tract diseases with thermal waters presented no specific results for events in laryngeal or pharyngeal locations [33].

Final Remarks

No studies solely evaluating the impact of thermal water treatments upon pharyngeal or laryngeal diseases were retrieved from the literature search, showing a lower focus of the medical research specifically in these domains. Nevertheless, their aetiology is linked to the other upper respiratory tract conditions [46, 47]. Pharyngeal and laryngeal diseases were studied along with other ORL diseases [8, 28-30] and not separately, the reason why these publications can be seen in this section of the chapter.

Data from the 4 abovementioned experimental publications [amelioration of symptoms and clinical condition (and respective scores), modulation of genes involved in tissue repair, innate immune response, antioxidant defence, and inflammation as well as of circulating cytokine and immunoglobulins profiles, reduction of frequency, duration, severity and social impact of upper respiratory tract infections and improvement of nasal mucociliary transport time; Table 1] seem to support pharyngeal and laryngeal diseases as good targets for Spa therapy [8, 28-30]. In line, aetiology of pharyngitis and laryngitis, and drugs used in their treatment [46, 47], sustain that thermal water intervention could be a good non-pharmacological therapeutic option in these conditions. In detail, as already presented, thermal waters appear effective against allergic and nonallergic rhinitis (both conditions can contribute to pharyngitis); thermal waters improve gastroesophageal reflux [48] that associates with laryngitis and pharyngitis; thermal waters are as effective as nasal steroids in the treatment of allergic rhinitis [23] (this class of drugs is also used in chronic laryngitis and allergic rhinitis is linked to pharyngitis).

It is imperative to conduct (much more) studies with different types of thermal waters, along with different types of thermal water administration methods, and short, medium and long treatment periods [short treatment periods (up to 2 weeks) occurred in [8, 29, 30]], accompanied by long follow-up periods [comprising several time points of evaluation within the follow-up; although the follow-up period lasted up to 1 year in 2 studies, very few evaluations were performed within this experimental period [8, 30]], comparing their effects against each other and against other non-pharmacological and pharmacological therapies as well as hypertonic or isotonic saline and placebo, aiming to specifically confirm their applicability and efficacy in pharyngeal and laryngeal diseases treatment and further uncover the biochemical, physiological and molecular mechanisms behind their (putative) beneficial impact. A quite large population per study, extensively characterised, would allow the disclosure of confounding intrinsic and/or extrinsic factors interfering with and/or lessening and/or boosting the thermal water treatment [for example: a) socio-economic profile and lifestyle of the individual determines the decision of experiencing a thermal cure, its duration and the compliance to it, b) distinct disease subgroups (rhinitis, pharyngitis, laryngitis, sinusitis) modulate the thermal cure impact, c) smoking habit interferes with thermal treatment effects, and d) the occurrence of age-related mechanisms/alterations modulates/influences the response to treatment]. The frame of the work by Neri *et al.* fulfils some of these key issues [8].

CONCLUSION

Scientific evidence regarding the use of thermal water therapy upon ORL diseases [mainly, CRS, with or without nasal polyposis, rhinitis (and asthma), after nasal endoscopic surgery, OME and auditory tubal dysfunction (and subsequent rhinogenic deafness)] in children, adults and elderly people is increasing and shows that, when available and possible, it can be indicated as an effective non-pharmacological therapeutic intervention in ORL. Interestingly, standard nasal topical drugs can be scarcely effective if nasal secretions are not sufficiently removed by nasal lavage. Besides their cleansing action, thermal waters can play other roles (see below) that will allow them to be either a co-adjuvant or an alternative to standard pharmacological therapies (or even be helpful in the post-surgery recovery process). This will be particularly relevant if a) the ORL disease occurs in a patient with other diseases/comorbidities and requires additional pharmacological therapies to be added to the drugs already prescribed, b) poor compliance with standard pharmacological ORL therapies occurs, and c) antibiotic resistance and long-term use of corticoids are to be prevented/avoided. Additionally, thermal water treatments in ORL are well-accepted and tolerated, presenting a high safety level [no cases of toxicity or neoplasm occurrence were reported; only very rare, light, self-limited secondary effects were seen (although they can be somehow unpleasant in patients with hyperergic disorders when treated with sulphurous and salso-bromo-iodic thermal waters which are particularly active; a greater sensation of burning and/or irritation of nasal mucosa can occur with the use of undiluted hypertonic thermal waters)], but are still underutilized. There are no specific indications pointing towards the most advantageous form of thermal water application in the different ORL diseases and the same occurs for the most suitable thermal water per clinical condition per age group [4, 5, 7, 8, 10-34].

Thermal waters influence upon inflammatory, immune and redox responses, which can explain the long-term relief observed in the clinical practice in ORL, are now beginning to be unravelled. Still, more studies are needed to ameliorate the design of the clinical interventions, in the rhinology, otology, laryngology and pharyngology fields (as detailed before), that should be viewed as an opportunity to further explore the molecular, enzymatic and cellular mechanisms behind the beneficial effects of thermal water therapy in ORL. For example, it would be interestingly to assess the impact of distinct thermal waters upon arginase 2 as a) modulation of nitric oxide (NO) levels (through modulation of NO production and/or inducible nitric oxide synthase expression as well as the presence of NO scavenging activity) has been recently attributed to different thermal waters in an *in vitro* inflammatory setting (macrophages exposed to lipopolysaccharides) [49], and b) nitric oxide levels seem relevant in CRS and arginase 2 expression is increased in CRS (depending on patient groups and CRS subtypes) [37, 50].

Relevantly for the therapeutic action upon those ORL conditions (considering their anatomical background and aetiology), thermal waters hold several distinct, and interconnected, beneficial effects [according to disease evolution stage and patients age (as well as their comorbidities, habits and life-style)] upon auditory and olfactory senses, and organs lining, flow and resistance as well as secretions ascribed to the a) normalization of the proportion among the different epithelium cellular subsets, regulating epithelial trophism and integrity as well as cellular metabolic activity, b) mechanic clearance of thickened mucus and favourable regulation/modulation of mucus production, mucus consistency/fluidity/viscosity (for example, by the opening of mucoprotein disulphide bonds that lowers mucus viscosity; anticatarrhal action), and mucus biochemical characteristics, c) normalization of mucociliary clearance [depending on the regularisation of epithelium cellularity and integrity along with thermal water antiseptic-type of action (by avoiding organic, inorganic, bacterial, fungal and viral particles from entering the organism, by blocking bacteria adhesins synthesis and by killing bacteria and fungus, e.g., either indirectly by inducing the expression of antimicrobial peptides or directly through thermal water ions and active molecules that have antibacterial and antifungal effects)], d) restoration of the physiological drainage, the micro-environment of the upper airways and the Eustachian tubes (including endotympanic pressure balance) as well as the mucosae of the middle ear and Eustachian wall (the latter as a mechanical consequence of Politzer insufflation), e) decrease of mucosal oedema, improvement of local blood supply and modulation of vessel lumen diameter and capillary permeability (direct vasoactive effect with the reduction of the inflammatory mucosal congestion), and f) favourable timely regulation/modulation of inflammation and (innate and acquired) immune response (beneficially acting upon the release of pro- and anti-inflammatory cytokines and immune-regulatory peptides as well as the production and activation of immune cells along with production of immunoglobulins) as well as of remodelling parameters and antioxidant defence [4, 5, 7, 8, 11, 12, 15-25, 27, 29, 30, 51-53].

Curiously, and in line considering the impact of thermal waters upon the redox regulation, antioxidant effects by mineral water consumption were revealed both in humans and in rats [54-57]. Since nutritional mineral deficiencies contribute to recurrent upper respiratory tract infections in children [29] and nutritional mineral deficiencies can be prevented/ameliorated by mineral waters intake [9, 58], specific hydropinic therapy could also be considered in ORL.

In conclusion, Spa therapy deserves relevant application in the ORL field, in prevention, rehabilitation and treatment. The positive impact found upon inflammation, immune response and redox status could open the way for new possible applications of Spa therapy.

REFERENCES

[1] Porter R. The medical history of waters and spas. Introduction. *Med Hist Suppl.* 1990(10):vii-xii.

[2] Petraccia L, Masciullo SG, Grassi M, Pace A, Lucchetta MC, Valenzi VI, Avino P, Fraioli A. Possibilità crenoterapiche e climatoterapiche nelle malattie ostruttive polmonari croniche. [Spa and climate therapy in chronic obstructive pulmonary diseases]. *Clin Ter.* 2005;156(1-2):23-31.

[3] Nocco PB. Mineralwasser als Heilmittel. [Mineral water as a cure]. *Veroff Schweiz Ges Gesch Pharm.* 2008;29:13-402.

[4] Mirandola P, Gobbi G, Malinverno C, Carubbi C, Ferné FM, Artico M, Vitale M, Vaccarezza M. Impact of sulphurous water politzer inhalation on audiometric parameters in children with otitis media with effusion. *Clin Exp Otorhinolaryngol.* 2013;6(1):7-11.

[5] Passali D, De Corso E, Platzgummer S, Streitberger C, Lo Cunsolo S, Nappi G, Passali GC, Bellussi L. Spa therapy of upper respiratory tract inflammations. *Eur Arch Otorhinolaryngol.* 2013;270(2):565-70.

[6] Mooventhan A, Nivethitha L. Scientific evidence-based effects of hydrotherapy on various systems of the body. *N Am J Med Sci.* 2014;6(5):199-209.

[7] Ciprandi G, Cristofolini M, Mira E. Comano thermal water inhalations in the treatment of allergic rhinitis: preliminary results. *Eur Ann Allergy Clin Immunol.* 2016;48(6):220-223.

[8] Neri M, Sansone L, Pietrasanta L, Kisialiou A, Cabano E, Martini M, Russo MA, Ugolini D, Tafani M, Bonassi S. Gene and protein expression of CXCR4 in adult and elderly patients with chronic rhinitis, pharyngitis or sinusitis undergoing thermal water nasal inhalations. *Immun Ageing.* 2018;15:10.

[9] Costa-Vieira D, Monteiro R, Martins MJ. Metabolic Syndrome features: Is there a modulation role by mineral water consumption? A review. *Nutrients.* 2019;11(5):1141.

[10] Barbieri M, Salami A, Mora F, Casazza A, Sovatzis A, Teglia R, Cordone MP, Mora R. Comportamento delle IGE e IGA sieriche in pazienti con rinite allergica trattata con acque salsobromoiodiche. [Behavior of serum IgE and IgA in patients with allergic rhinitis treated with iodine bromide thermal water]. *Acta Otorhinolaryngol Ital.* 2002;22(4):215-9.

[11] Staffieri A, Abramo A. Sulphurous-arsenical-ferruginous (thermal) water inhalations reduce nasal respiratory resistance and improve mucociliary clearance in patients with chronic sinonasal disease: preliminary outcomes. *Acta Otolaryngol.* 2007;127(6):613-7.

[12] Staffieri A, Marino F, Staffieri C, Giacomelli L, D'Alessandro E, Maria Ferraro S, Fedrazzoni U, Marioni G. The effects of sulfurous-arsenical-ferruginous thermal water nasal irrigation in wound healing after functional endoscopic sinus surgery for chronic rhinosinusitis: a prospective randomised study. *Am J Otolaryngol.* 2008;29(4):223-9.

[13] Passali FM, Crisanti A, Passali GC, Cianfrone F, Bocchi M, Messineo G, Bellussi L, Passali D. Effetti terapeutici dell'acqua termale salsobromoiodica di Salsomaggiore nel trattamento delle flogosi naso-sinusali ricorrenti e croniche. [Efficacy of inhalation therapy with water of Salsomaggiore (Italy) in chronic and recurrent nasosinusal inflammation treatment]. *Clin Ter.* 2008;159(3):175-80.

[14] Passali D, Lauriello M, Passali GC, Passali FM, Cassano M, Cassano P, Bellussi L. Studio clinico per la valutazione dell'efficacia terapeutica dello spray nasale con acqua termale salsobromoiodica isotonica delle Terme di Salsomaggiore nel trattamento delle

patologie rinosinusali. [Clinical evaluation of the efficacy of Salsomaggiore (Italy) thermal water in the treatment of rhinosinusal pathologies]. *Clin Ter.* 2008;159(3):181-8.

[15] Fenu G, Bozzo C, Carai A, Delehaye E, Foddai M, Meloni F, Montella AC. Effects of isotonic salso-bromo-iodine thermal water after sinunasal surgery: a preliminary morphological study. *J Altern Complement Med.* 2010;16(4):341-3.

[16] Salami A, Dellepiane M, Strinati F, Guastini L, Mora R. Sulphurous thermal water inhalations in the treatment of chronic rhinosinusitis. *Rhinology.* 2010;48(1):71-6.

[17] Del Giudice MM, Decimo F, Maiello N, Leonardi S, Parisi G, Golluccio M, Capasso M, Balestrieri U, Rocco A, Perrone L, Ciprandi G. Effectiveness of Ischia thermal water nasal aerosol in children with seasonal allergic rhinitis: A randomised and controlled study. *Int J Immunopathol Pharmacol.* 2011;24(4):1103-1109.

[18] Ottaviano G, Marioni G, Staffieri C, Giacomelli L, Marchese-Ragona R, Bertolin A, Staffieri A. Effects of sulfurous, salty, bromic, iodic thermal water nasal irrigations in nonallergic chronic rhinosinusitis: a prospective, randomised, double-blind, clinical, and cytological study. *Am J Otolaryngol.* 2011;32(3):235-9.

[19] Pagani D, Galliera E, Dogliotti G, De Bernardi di Valserra M, Torretta S, Solimene U, Corsi MM, Pignataro L. Carbon dioxide-enriched water inhalation in patients with allergic rhinitis and its relationship with nasal fluid cytokine/chemokine release. *Arch Med Res.* 2011;42(4):329-33.

[20] Ottaviano G, Marioni G, Giacomelli L, La Torre FB, Staffieri C, Marchese-Ragona R, Staffieri A. Smoking and chronic rhinitis: effects of nasal irrigations with sulfurous-arsenical-ferruginous thermal water: A prospective, randomised, double-blind study. *Am J Otolaryngol.* 2012;33(6):657-62.

[21] Passariello A, Di Costanzo M, Terrin G, Iannotti A, Buono P, Balestrieri U, Balestrieri G, Ascione E, Pedata M, Canani FB, Canani RB. Crenotherapy modulates the expression of proinflammatory cytokines and immunoregulatory peptides in nasal secretions of

children with chronic rhinosinusitis. *Am J Rhinol Allergy.* 2012;26(1):e15-9.

[22] Cantone E, Marino A, Ferranti I, Castagna G, Maione N, Di Rubbo V, Iengo M. Nasal cytological assessment after crenotherapy in the treatment of chronic rhinosinusitis in the elderly. *Int J Immunopathol Pharmacol.* 2014;27(4):683-7.

[23] Passali D, Gabelli G, Passali GC, Magnato R, Platzgummer S, Salerni L, Lo Cunsolo S, Joos A, Bellussi LM. Radioactive Merano SPA treatment for allergic rhinitis therapy. *Int J Otolaryngol.* 2016;2016:2801913.

[24] Costantino M, Lampa E, Nappi G. Effectiveness of sulphur spa therapy with politzer in the treatment of rhinogenic deafness. *Acta Otorhinolaryngol Ital.* 2006;26(1):7-13.

[25] Tozzi A, Blancasio AC, Basagni C, Ricci C, Burzynska J, Battaglia MA. Prevention and cure of rhinogenous deafness at the Thermal Baths "Bagni delle Galleraie." *J Prev Med Hyg.* 2006;47(4):146-50.

[26] Califano L, Salafia F, Mazzone S, D'Ambrosio G, Malafronte L, Vassallo A. A comparative randomised study on the efficacy of a systemic steroid therapy vs. a thermal therapy in otitis media with effusion in children. *Minerva Pediatr.* 2016;68(4):241-9.

[27] La Mantia I, Andaloro C. Effects of salso-bromo-iodine thermal water in children suffering from otitis media with effusion: a randomised controlled pilot study. *Clin Ter.* 2018;169(1):e10-e13.

[28] Costantino M, Rossi F, Lampa E. Cura inalatoria con acqua minerale sulfurea in ambito ORL: studio clinico-sperimentale. [Inhalation therapy with sulphur water in ORL: clinical-experimental study]. *Clin Ter.* 2003;154(6):395-400.

[29] Salami A, Dellepiane M, Crippa B, Mora F, Guastini L, Jankowska B, Mora R. Sulphurous water inhalations in the prophylaxis of recurrent upper respiratory tract infections. *Int J Pediatr Otorhinolaryngol.* 2008;72(11):1717-22.

[30] Magrone T, Galantino M, Di Bitonto N, Borraccino L, Chiaromonte G, Jirillo E. Effects of thermal water inhalation in chronic upper

respiratory tract infections in elderly and young patients. *Immun Ageing.* 2016;13:18.

[31] Olina M, Aluffi Valletti P, Pia F, Toso A, Borello G, Policarpo M, Garavelli PL. Indicazioni idrologiche nella terapia delle faringiti. [Hydrological indications in the therapy of pharyngitis]. *Recenti Prog Med.* 2008;99(6):314-21.

[32] Hermelingmeier KE, Weber RK, Hellmich M, Heubach CP, Mösges R. Nasal irrigation as an adjunctive treatment in allergic rhinitis: a systematic review and meta-analysis. *Am J Rhinol Allergy.* 2012;26(5):e119-25.

[33] Keller S, König V, Mösges R. Thermal water applications in the treatment of upper respiratory tract diseases: A systematic review and meta-analysis. *J Allergy (Cairo).* 2014;2014:943824.

[34] Casale M, Moffa A, Cassano M, Carinci F, Lopez MA, Trecca EMC, Torretta S, Rinaldi V, Pignataro L. Saline nasal irrigations for chronic rhinosinusitis: From everyday practice to evidence-based medicine. An update. *Int J Immunopathol Pharmacol.* 2018;32:2058738418802676.

[35] Eifan AO, Durham SR. Pathogenesis of rhinitis. *Clin Exp Allergy.* 2016;46(9):1139-51.

[36] Sheikh J, Jean T. *Allergic Rhinitis*. 2018. Available at: https://emedicine.medscape.com/article/134825-overview. Accessed on December 16, 2019.

[37] Albu S. Chronic rhinosinusitis - An update on epidemiology, pathogenesis and management. *J Clin Med.* 2020;9(7):2285.

[38] Thomas M. Allergic rhinitis: evidence for impact on asthma. *BMC Pulm Med.* 2006;6 Suppl 1(Suppl 1):S4.

[39] Skoner DP. Allergic rhinitis: definition, epidemiology, pathophysiology, detection, and diagnosis. *J Allergy Clin Immunol.* 2001;108(1 Suppl):S2-8.

[40] Chong LY, Head K, Hopkins C, Philpott C, Glew S, Scadding G, Burton MJ, Schilder AG. Saline irrigation for chronic rhinosinusitis. *Cochrane Database Syst Rev.* 2016;4:Cd011995.

[41] Garavello W, Romagnoli M, Sordo L, Gaini RM, Di Berardino C, Angrisano A. Hypersaline nasal irrigation in children with symptomatic seasonal allergic rhinitis: a randomised study. *Pediatr Allergy Immunol.* 2003;14(2):140-3.

[42] Rosenfeld RM, Culpepper L, Doyle KJ, Grundfast KM, Hoberman A, Kenna MA, Lieberthal AS, Mahoney M, Wahl RA, Woods CR, Jr., Yawn B. Clinical practice guideline: Otitis media with effusion. *Otolaryngol Head Neck Surg.* 2004;130(5 Suppl):S95-118.

[43] Rosenfeld RM, Shin JJ, Schwartz SR, Coggins R, Gagnon L, Hackell JM, Hoelting D, Hunter LL, Kummer AW, Payne SC, Poe DS, Veling M, Vila PM, Walsh SA, Corrigan MD. Clinical practice guideline: Otitis media with effusion (update). *Otolaryngol Head Neck Surg.* 2016;154(1 Suppl):S1-S41.

[44] Higgins TSJ. *Otitis media with effusion.* 2018. Available at: https://emedicine.medscape.com/article/858990-overview#a5. Accessed on April 06, 2020.

[45] World Health of Organization. *Addressing the rising prevalence of hearing loss*. 2018: Geneva.

[46] Grief SN. Upper respiratory infections. *Prim Care.* 2013;40(3):757-70.

[47] Stein DJ, Noordzij JP. Incidence of chronic laryngitis. *Ann Otol Rhinol Laryngol*. 2013;122(12):771-774.

[48] Beer AM, Uebelhack R, Pohl U. Efficacy and tolerability of hydrogen carbonate-rich water for heartburn. *World J Gastrointest Pathophysiol.* 2016;7(1):171-80.

[49] Silva A, Oliveira AS, Vaz CV, Correia S, Ferreira R, Breitenfeld L, Martinez-de-Oliveira J, Palmeira-de-Oliveira R, Pereira CMF, Palmeira-de-Oliveira A, Cruz MT. Anti-inflammatory potential of Portuguese thermal waters. *Sci Rep.* 2020;10(1):22313.

[50] Bommarito L, Guida G, Heffler E, Badiu I, Nebiolo F, Usai A, De Stefani A, Rolla G. Nasal nitric oxide concentration in suspected chronic rhinosinusitis. *Ann Allergy Asthma Immunol.* 2008;101(4):358-62.

[51] Valitutti S, Castellino F, Musiani P. Effect of sulfurous (thermal) water on T lymphocyte proliferative response. *Ann Allergy.* 1990;65(6):463-8.

[52] Braga PC, Sambataro G, Dal Sasso M, Culici M, Alfieri M, Nappi G. Antioxidant effect of sulphurous thermal water on human neutrophil bursts: chemiluminescence evaluation. *Respiration.* 2008;75(2):193-201.

[53] Braga PC, Ceci C, Marabini L, Nappi G. The antioxidant activity of sulphurous thermal water protects against oxidative DNA damage: a comet assay investigation. *Drug Res (Stuttg).* 2013;63(4):198-202.

[54] Benedetti S, Benvenuti F, Nappi G, Fortunati NA, Marino L, Aureli T, De Luca S, Pagliarani S, Canestrari F. Antioxidative effects of sulfurous mineral water: protection against lipid and protein oxidation. *Eur J Clin Nutr.* 2009;63(1):106-12.

[55] Costantino M, Giuberti G, Caraglia M, Lombardi A, Misso G, Abbruzzese A, Ciani F, Lampa E. Possible antioxidant role of SPA therapy with chlorine-sulphur-bicarbonate mineral water. *Amino Acids.* 2009;36(2):161-5.

[56] Pereira CD, Severo M, Araújo JR, Guimarães JT, Pestana D, Santos A, Ferreira R, Ascensão A, Magalhães J, Azevedo I, Monteiro R, Martins MJ. Relevance of a hypersaline sodium-rich naturally sparkling mineral water to the protection against metabolic syndrome induction in fructose-fed Sprague-Dawley rats: A biochemical, metabolic, and redox approach. *Int J Endocrinol.* 2014;2014:384583.

[57] Sokrateva TD, Roussev BH, Nashar MA, Kiselova-Kaneva YD, Mihaylova GM, Todorova MN, Pasheva MG, Tasinov OB, Nazifova-Tasinova NF, Vankova DG, Ivanova DP, Radanova MA, Ts Galunska B, Vlaykova TI, Ivanova DG. Effects of sulphur-containing mineral water intake on oxidative status and markers for inflammation in healthy subjects. *Arch Physiol Biochem.* 2019:1-10.

[58] Neves MO, Marques J, Eggenkamp HGM. Lithium in portuguese bottled natural mineral waters - Potential for health benefits? *Int J Environ Res Public Health.* 2020;17(22):8369.

In: Mineral Water
Editors: Maria João Martins

ISBN: 978-1-68507-458-6

Chapter 4

SPA THERAPIES AND RHEUMATIC DISEASES

Bruno Miguel Fernandes[1,*], MD and Miguel Bernardes[1,2], MD, PhD
[1]Department of Rheumatology,
São João University Hospital Centre, Porto, Portugal
[2]Department of Medicine, Faculty of Medicine,
University of Porto, Porto, Portugal

ABSTRACT

Spa therapies seem to show anti-inflammatory and beneficial redox effects, functional benefits and pain improvement as adjunct therapies for rheumatic diseases, namely Rheumatoid Arthritis, Osteoarthritis and Fibromyalgia. Some data suggest that these therapies may have an effect at a molecular level, acting directly on the local inflammatory mediators involved in rheumatic diseases and, although the exact mechanisms are not fully understood, both physical and chemical aspects may have a role. More *in vitro* and *in vivo* studies, more animal and human studies are

[*] Corresponding Author's E-mail: bfernandesmg@gmail.com.

needed to understand the exact mechanisms of these effects in addition to the long-term results and effectiveness of this kind of therapies.

Keywords: balneotherapy, fibromyalgia, mud therapy, osteoarthritis, rheumatic diseases, rheumatoid arthritis, spa therapy, thermal water bath

INTRODUCTION

Some data suggest the benefits of mineral waters in inflammatory diseases, although the exact mecanisms are still not completely understood [1], given the limitations of *in vitro* studies, namely differences in experimental procedures, high heterogeneity in the research designs, and difficulties in considering all the factors that may be implicated [2].

Both physical properties and chemical components may contribute to the benefits of balneotherapy. Within physical properties, temperature can play a central role, as the ability to change body temperature helps to support healing processes and to relieve pain [3, 4]. Specific chemical components, depending on the composition of the mineral water, may also determine different effects; as an example, low doses of sulphated mineral-medicinal waters seem to have potential cytoprotective, anti-inflammatory and antioxidant effects [5-9]. However, the scarce evidence available shows that the mechanisms behind the beneficial effects in this field are still not fully understood [10].

In several diseases, including osteoarthritis (OA) and fibromyalgia, and also in healthy individuals, some studies have shown a reduction in pro-inflammatory cytokines, like tumour necrosis factor-α [11, 12], interleukin (IL)-1β [12, 13] and IL-6 [14, 15], with balneo and mud therapies. Moreover, an increase in the anti-inflammatory insulin growth factor-1 has been noted [11] with mud therapy. In the same trend, other inflammatory parameters, including C-reactive protein (CRP) [14] and prostaglandin E2 [13], decreased after balneotherapy. These results support a possible anti-inflammatory effect of balneo and mud therapies.

SPA THERAPY AND RHEUMATIC DISEASES

Spa therapy is becoming increasingly popular as an adjunct treatment for rheumatic diseases, with the aim of reducing pain and improving functional mobility [16, 17].

As aforementioned, the mechanisms of action of Spa therapy in rheumatic diseases are not fully clear. Various components have been proposed. Non-specific mechanical effects, particularly mediated by hydrostatic pressure, have shown benefits in muscle tone, joint mobility and pain control [10]. Thermal effects also seem to play a central role: hot stimuli reduce muscle spasm and increase the pain threshold at nerve endings; in addition, heat induces the release of adrenocorticotropic hormone, cortisol, growth hormone and beta-endorphin, which have potential anti-inflammatory and analgesic effects [18, 19]. Moreover, hyperthermia increases the extensibility of tendons and joint capsules, improving mobility and range of motion of the joints [20]. Chemical effects of balneotherapy and mud packs are less studied, and the eternal question remains whether the organic/mineral substances can pass through the skin and act systemically [10]. Also, immunologically, an imunossupressive effect has been proposed [11-15]. Sulphurous thermal water exhibits an inhibitory *in vitro* effect on the mitogen induced proliferation of T lymphocytes in chronic inflammatory diseases [21]. Matrix metalloproteinases (MMPs), produced by chondrocytes and other cells, have a major role in cartilage degradation in joint diseases [22], and a significant reduction in MMP levels has been demonstrated with mud bath therapy in a study enrolling 80 patients with OA [23]. Also, a study including 50 healthy individuals (43 women) suggested that the ingestion of sulphurous mineral water may improve the redox status of the body, given the significantly increased levels of plasmatic total glutathione and total thiols as well as of peripheral blood mononuclear cells γ-glutamyl-cysteinyl ligase gene expression [7]. In line, while a study in 30 rats suggested a possible antioxidant effect of chlorine-sulphur-bicarbonate Spa hydropinic treatments, given the significant reduction of plasmatic reactive oxygen species [8], a study with 40 healthy adults (22 women) revealed a significant decrease of lipid and protein oxidation products and a significant increase of total antioxidant capacity as well as of total thiols, in plasma, after hydropinic therapy with a sulphurous mineral water [9].

In a study in monosodium iodoacetate-induced OA and complete Freund's adjuvant-induced rheumatoid arthritis (RA) murine models, mineral water and mud from the Lake Héviz (Hungary) showed antinociceptive and anti-inflammatory effects [24]. Mud applications, balneotherapy and mineral water consumption have been reported to beneficially impact the lipid profile [10, 25-27]. In line, a significant reduction in plasma homocysteine has been demonstrated with sulphurous thermal baths (temperature not specified) in a group of 20 OA patients (8 women) *versus* 20 OA control patients (9 women) [28]. This is of utmost importance since inflammatory rheumatic diseases have a well-known increased cardiovascular risk [29]. As an example, in a recent study in 60 female RA patients, homocysteine and apolipoprotein (Apo) AI levels, as well as the ApoB/ApoAI ratio, were shown to correlate with the coronary calcium score assessed by computed tomography [30].

Regarding the consumption of mineral waters, there is no evidence in the literature to support a potential impact on the incidence and/or disease activity in inflammatory rheumatic diseases.

SPA THERAPY AND RHEUMATOID ARTHRITIS

RA is an autoimmune disease characterized by synovial inflammation and progressive structural joint damage. Most data on mineral waters in rheumatic inflammatory disease come from RA. Few data are available in fibromyalgia and other inflammatory rheumatic diseases, such as ankylosing spondylitis, non-radiographic axial spondyloarthritis, undifferentiated spondyloarthritis, Sjögren's syndrome, systemic lupus erythematosus, systemic sclerosis, and inflammatory myopathies.

Spa therapy (at 36-37 °C) with salt-rich saline water (1.9 g/L sodium chloride; also contained other minerals/ions, predominantly calcium, magnesium, potassium, bicarbonate and sulphate) seems to have an antioxidant effect in patients with RA, reflected by the increase in nonenzymatic superoxide radical scavenger activity in 15 RA patients (13 women) *versus* 22 RA control (female) patients. It is unknown if this result supports the improved clinical status seen after the Spa therapy [31]. A systematic review from 2016, which included eight studies, showed some improvement in functional capacity, morning stiffness, number of active joints and pain in RA patients with balneotherapy (range of temperatures not mencioned) [32]. However, a Cochrane review concluded that the evidence is insufficient to state that balneotherapy is more effective than no treatment or that one type of bath is more effective than another in RA patients [33] (Table 1). Also of note, a study showed that high concentrations of hydrogen sulphide increased the expression of pro-inflammatory genes in fibroblast-like synoviocytes derived from patients with RA and OA, recommending caution in patients with active RA when undergoing sulphur bath therapy [34].

Table 1. Summary of findings: balneotherapy compared with placebo in Rheumatoid Arthritis

Outcomes	Ilustrative comparative risks		Relative effect (95% confidence interval)	Number of partici-pants (Number of studies)	Quality of the evidence (GRADE)
	Assumed risk	Corres-ponding risk			
	Placebo	Balneotherapy (mud packs)			
Pain intensity (VAS 0-100)	Mean pain intensity was 47	Mean pain intensity was 0.5 higher	-	45 (1)	Very low
Improvement (yes/no based on 5 outcome measures)	522 per 1000	501 per 1000	Relative risk 0.96 (0.54-1.70)	45 (1)	Very low
Tender joints (0-28)	Mean number of tender joints was 12.5	Mean number of tender joints was 4.6 lower	-	45 (1)	Very low
Swollen joints (0-28)	Mean number of swollen joints was 1.9	Mean number of swollen joints was 0.6 higher		45 (1)	Very low

Adapted from [33].

Another important question is whether Spa therapy has a sustained effect on RA patients. One study including 37 patients (35 women) has shown that short- and medium-term beneficial effects of balneotherapy with saline water (at 36-37 °C) with a high concentration of sodium chloride (1.9 g/L; also contained other minerals/ions, predominantly calcium, magnesium, potassium, bicarbonate and sulphate) can be mildly to moderately maintained up to 12 months [35]; however, evidence is scarce and further studies are still needed.

Spa Therapy and Osteoarthritis

OA is the most common rheumatic disease and the main cause of pain, disability and impaired quality of life, affecting mainly elderly individuals [36]. Pathophysiological mechanisms are multifactorial and most of them still remain unknown, but low-grade systemic inflammation seems to play a role in addition to the local release of inflammatory mediators by cartilage, bone and synovium [37].

At the molecular level, one study joining 66 patients (44 women) with chronic back pain secondary to OA disclosed that Spa therapy (local mud packs and bathing in sodium-bicarbonate-alkaline mineral water; at a temperature range of 34-45 °C) increased some circulating proteins [inhibin beta A subunit, activin A receptor type 2B, angiopoietin-1, beta-2-microglobulin, growth differentiation factor 10, C-X-C motif chemokine ligand 5, fibroblast growth factor (FGF) 2, FGF 12, oxidised low-density lipoprotein receptor 1 and MMP13] and decreased others (ApoCIII, IL-23 alpha subunit p19 and syndecan-1), suggesting that Spa therapy may induce changes in proteins involved in gene expression modulation, differentiation, angiogenesis, tissue repair and acute and chronic inflammatory responses [38]. Furthermore, a study including 36 patients (23 women), that looked at the immunological effects of Spa therapy [whole-body mud application (40-42 °C) + mud bath (38-40 °C); bicarbonate and calcium as predominant ions in the mineral-medicinal water of the mud bath] in patients with knee OA, revealed that circulating concentrations of IL-8 and transforming growth factor-β decreased (in correlation with decreased pain and improved knee flexion, respectively), percentage of $CD4^+$ regulatory T cells decreased while $CD8^+$ regulatory T cells and neutrophil functional capacity increased, imputing an anti-inflammatory effect mediated by cytokines, what reflects a bioregulatory effect on the inflammatory and innate responses [39]. Moreover, in recent years, emphasis has been given on the involvement of adipocytokines in inflammation [40], although much remains to be known. In this regard, a study enrolling 46 patients with knee OA showed that cold peloid therapy, combined with physical therapy and balneal factors [general cold mud baths and salt bath in the lake Techirghiol (Romania)], induced circulating adiponectin elevation and improved knee pain, suggesting not only efficacy but also possible correlations with adiponectin levels [41]. On the other hand, other study, that also looked at the impact of Spa therapy (combination of mud packs applied on both knees and bicarbonate-sulphate mineral water baths; at a temperature range of 38-45 ºC) in 30 knee OA patients (16 females), unveiled a slight, but not significant, increase in circulating leptin levels and a significant decrease in circulating adiponectin levels [42]. Not only mineral [43], but also organic elements [44], seem to be responsible for the therapeutic effect of Spa therapy in OA.

Several studies have demonstrated positive clinical effects of Spa therapy on OA. A randomised controlled study showed that balneotherapy (mineral sodium chloride bath, with mineralisation 40-46 g/L) and peloid therapy (temperature range of 36-42 ºC) effectivelly reduced pain and improved the functional status in a study including 92 patients (87% females) with OA of the knee [45]. Another randomised controlled trial in 140 patients with OA of the knee indicated a significant decrease in visual analogue scale (VAS) pain score (pain during movement, at rest, and at night) and in the use of pain medication as well as an improvement in Western Ontario and McMaster Universities Arthritis Index (WOMAC), Lequesne Algofunctional Index (LAFI) and Stanford Health Assessment Questionnaire (HAQ) scores with thermal sulphurous and non-sulphurous waters (at a temperature range of 37-39 ºC), with the sulphurous water baths showing longer-lasting effects than non-sulphurous water baths [46]. Other study, also in knee OA (n=60; 30 females), demonstrated beneficial effects of sulphate-bicarbonate-calcium mineral water baths (at 38 ºC) on painful symptomatology, with a significant improvement on functional capacities and quality of life [47]. Interestingly, one study with 30 women with bilateral OA of the knee compared ultrasound therapy with mineral water (anions and cations in higher amount: chloride, sodium, calcium, magnesium and potassium) versus ultrasound therapy with aqua sonic gel: both groups experienced a significant reduction in pain and significant improvement in WOMAC when compared with preintervention values, with the ultrasound with mineral water group exhibiting a more pronounced impact [48]. Regarding long-term effects, more data are needed, but some studies seem to conclude in favour of a long-term positive effect of Spa therapy (as mud packs and mineral water baths; at a temperature range of 34-45 ºC) in knee OA [49, 50]. Particularly, a systematic review suggests that the improvements with Spa therapy [hot mineral water baths, mud therapy, hot showers, massages and supervised water exercises (information about temperature not provided)] in knee OA remain clinically significant for up to 3 to 6 months, and sometimes 9 months [51].

In hand OA, several randomised controlled studies showed positive effects: sulphurous Spa water (at 37 ºC) was effective for the attenuation of pain [52], thermal mineral water (at a temperature range of 36-38 ºC) combined with magnetotherapy improved pain, function and quality of life [53] and local mud packs + sulphate-calcium-magnesium-fluoride water bath treatments (at a temperature range of 38-43 ºC) provided a positive effect on the painful symptomatology, drugs consumption and functional capacities, that lasted over time [54]. The same results in pain and function were observed with bathing in mineral water extremely rich in sulphide ion (but also with significant amounts of calcium, magnesium, bicarbonate, and sodium chloride; at 36 ºC) for hip OA [55] and with a combination of several Spa treatments for generalised OA (temperature range 35-52 °C; anions and cations in higher amount in the mineral water used in Spa facilities: bicarbonate, sulphate and calcium) [56].

In conclusion, Spa therapy seems to have positive effects in OA with a good safety profile.

SPA THERAPY AND FIBROMYALGIA

Fibromyalgia, characterized by chronic pain and reduced pain threshold, is the second most common rheumatic disease [57]. Pathophysiology of fibromyalgia is not completely understood but is frequently described as a centralized pain state [58]. The best management of this disease remains the combination of pharmacological and non-pharmacological treatments, where Spa therapy may have a role: the last European League Against Rheumatism (EULAR) revised recommendations for the management of fibromyalgia [59] included hydrotherapy/balneotherapy with acupuncture in a group denominated "defined physical therapies" that resulted in a weak strength of recommendation in favour of these strategies.

A randomised clinical trial including 50 patients with fibromyalgia (48 women) that evaluated the impact of baths with mineral-medicinal water (bicarbonate-sodium-alkaline-lithic-fluorinated-silicated water, of medium mineralisation, at 38 °C) from As Burgas (Spain) showed an improvement in the Fibromyalgia Impact Questionnaire (FIQ) [60]. Also, a randomised controlled clinical study including a total of 66 patients with fibromyalgia showed a statistically significant improvement in VAS, tender point count, FIQ and modified fatigue impact scale with thermomineral water baths (at 34.8 °C; anions and cations in higher amount: chloride, bicarbonate, sodium and calcium) from Uğurlu Thermal Plants (Turkey) [61].

Other study, including 120 female fibromyalgia patients, indicated that balneotherapy with oligometallic thermal water (at 42±1 °C; with bicarbonate, chlorine and calcium in higher amount) in combination with exercise therapy had superior and more sustained effects that either therapy alone [62]. Regarding mud therapy, a study with 7 fibromalgia patients suggested that daily mud bathing therapy (at 40 °C) was able to reduce the pain and lowered triglyceride and CRP levels; also, in this study, the analysis of telomere length of peripheral leukocytes revealed a trend of negative correlation between telomere shortening and laboratory data change of haemoglobin and circulating albumin, suggesting a possible anti-aging effect of mud therapy proposed by the extending life-span of circulating leukocytes [63].

Overall, Spa therapy may be one of the suitable non-pharmacological modalities recommended in the management of fibromyalgia patients.

CONCLUSION

Various positive clinical effects of mud packs and mud and mineral water baths have been described. Most of these reported results refer only to short-term effects, which last until the end of the cycle, with little or no information on the possible long-term effects [6]. Also, the great heterogeneity between the most diverse mineral waters makes it difficult to study the individual and/or synergistic effects of its different components. Moreover, the climatic and environmental conditions of the Spas and the fact that they are usually far from the stressful environment of daily life are likely to be potential confounding factors [19].

In conclusion, Spa therapies seem to have positive results as adjunct therapies in inflammatory and non-inflammatory rheumatic diseases. However, more in-depth studies are needed in order to draw solid conclusions.

REFERENCES

[1] Gálvez I, Torres-Piles S, Ortega-Rincón E. Balneotherapy, Immune System, and Stress Response: A Hormetic Strategy? *Int J Mol Sci.* 2018;19(6):1687.

[2] Cheleschi S, Gallo I, Tenti S. A comprehensive analysis to understand the mechanism of action of balneotherapy: why, how, and where they can be used? Evidence from *in vitro* studies performed on human and animal samples. *Int J Biometeorol.* 2020;64(7):1247-61.

[3] Srámek P, Simecková M, Janský L, Savlíková J, Vybíral S. Human physiological responses to immersion into water of different temperatures. *Eur J Appl Physiol.* 2000;81(5):436-42.

[4] Matsumoto T, Nishiyama T, Nishimura N, Kato M, Inukai Y, Sugenoya J, Yamauchi M, Kosaka M. Endocrine responses to heat and cold stress. In: Kosaka M, Sugahara T, Schmidt K L, Simon E, eds. *Thermotherapy for Neoplasia, Inflammation, and Pain*. Tokyo: Springer; 2001:228-41.

[5] Calabrese V, Cornelius C, Dinkova-Kostova AT, Calabrese EJ, Mattson MP. Cellular stress responses, the hormesis paradigm, and vitagenes: novel targets for therapeutic intervention in neurodegenerative disorders. *Antioxid Redox Signal.* 2010;13(11): 1763-811.

[6] Carbajo JM, Maraver F. Sulphurous Mineral Waters: New Applications for Health. *Evid Based Complement Alternat Med.* 2017;2017:8034084.

[7] Sokrateva TD, Roussev BH, Nashar MA, Kiselova-Kaneva YD, Mihaylova GM, Todorova MN, Pasheva MG, Tasinov OB, Nazifova-Tasinova NF, Vankova DG, Ivanova DP, Radanova MA, Ts Galunska B, Vlaykova TI, Ivanova DG. Effects of sulphur-containing mineral water intake on oxidative status and markers for inflammation in healthy subjects. *Arch Physiol Biochem.* 2019:1-10.

[8] Costantino M, Giuberti G, Caraglia M, Lombardi A, Misso G, Abbruzzese A, Ciani F, Lampa E. Possible antioxidant role of SPA therapy with chlorine-sulphur-bicarbonate mineral water. *Amino Acids.* 2009;36(2):161-5.

[9] Benedetti S, Benvenuti F, Nappi G, Fortunati N A, Marino L, Aureli T, De Luca S, Pagliarani S, Canestrari F. Antioxidative effects of sulfurous mineral water: protection against lipid and protein oxidation. *Eur J Clin Nutr*. 2009;63(1):106-12.

[10] Fioravanti A, Cantarini L, Guidelli GM, Galeazzi M. Mechanisms of action of spa therapies in rheumatic diseases: what scientific evidence is there? *Rheumatol Int*. 2011;31(1):1-8.

[11] Bellometti S, Cecchettin M, Galzigna L. Mud pack therapy in osteoarthrosis. Changes in serum levels of chondrocyte markers. *Clin Chim Acta*. 1997;268(1-2):101-6.

[12] Cozzi F, Carrara M, Sfriso P, Todesco S, Cima L. Anti-inflammatory effect of mud-bath applications on adjuvant arthritis in rats. *Clin Exp Rheumatol.* 2004;22(6):763-6.

[13] Ardiç F, Ozgen M, Aybek H, Rota S, Cubukçu D, Gökgöz A. Effects of balneotherapy on serum IL-1, PGE2 and LTB4 levels in fibromyalgia patients. *Rheumatol Int.* 2007;27(5):441-6.

[14] Oyama J, Kudo Y, Maeda T, Node K, Makino N. Hyperthermia by bathing in a hot spring improves cardiovascular functions and reduces the production of inflammatory cytokines in patients with chronic heart failure. *Heart Vessels*. 2013;28(2):173-8.

[15] Basili S, Martini F, Ferroni P, Grassi M, Sili Scavalli A, Streva P, Cusumano G, Musca A, Battista Rini G. Effects of mud-pack treatment on plasma cytokine and soluble adhesion molecule levels in healthy volunteers. *Clin Chim Acta*. 2001;314(1-2):209-14.

[16] Nicholas JJ. Physical modalities in rheumatological rehabilitation. *Arch Phys Med Rehabil.* 1994;75(9):994-1001.

[17] Karagülle M, Kardeş S, Dişçi R, Karagülle MZ. Spa therapy adjunct to pharmacotherapy is beneficial in rheumatoid arthritis: a crossover randomized controlled trial. *Int J Biometeorol*. 2018;62(2):195-205.

[18] Kuczera M, Kokot F. Wp-yw leczenia uzdrowiskowego na uk-ad endokrynny. I: Hormony reakcji stresowej. [Effect of spa therapy on the endocrine system. I. Stress reaction hormones]. *Pol Arch Med Wewn.* 1996;95(1):11-20.

[19] Laatikainen T, Salminen K, Kohvakka A, Pettersson J. Response of plasma endorphins, prolactin and catecholamines in women to intense heat in a sauna. *Eur J Appl Physiol Occup Physiol* 1988;57(1):98-102.

[20] Sukenik S, Flusser D, Abu-Shakra M. The role of spa therapy in various rheumatic diseases. *Rheum Dis Clin North Am*. 1999;25(4): 883-97.

[21] Valitutti S, Castellino F, Musiani P. Effect of sulfurous (thermal) water on T lymphocyte proliferative response. *Ann Allergy*. 1990; 65(6):463-8.

[22] Lohmander LS, Hoerrner L A, Lark MW. Metalloproteinases, tissue inhibitor, and proteoglycan fragments in knee synovial fluid in human osteoarthritis. *Arthritis Rheum*. 1993;36(2):181-9.

[23] Bellometti S, Richelmi P, Tassoni T, Bertè F. Production of matrix metalloproteinases and their inhibitors in osteoarthritic patients undergoing mud bath therapy. *Int J Clin Pharmacol Res*. 2005; 25(2):77-94.

[24] Tékus V, Borbély É, Kiss T, Perkecz A, Kemény Á, Horváth J, Kvarda A, Pintér E. Investigation of Lake Hévíz mineral water balneotherapy and Hévíz mud treatment in murine Osteoarthritis and Rheumatoid Arthritis Models. *Evid Based Complement Alternat Med.* 2018;2018:4816905.

[25] Mizoguchi T. Effects of thermal spring bath on lipids in serum. *Med Balneol Climat.* 1970;33:115-20.

[26] Strauss-Blasche G, Ekmekcioglu C, Leibetseder V, Marktl W. Seasonal variation of lipid-lowering effects of complex spa therapy. *Forsch Komplementarmed Klass Naturheilkd*. 2003;10(2):78-84.

[27] Costa-Vieira D, Monteiro R, Martins MJ. Metabolic Syndrome features: Is there a modulation role by mineral water consumption? A review. *Nutrients*. 2019;11(5):1141.

[28] Leibetseder V, Strauss-Blasche G, Holzer F, Marktl W, Ekmekcioglu C. Improving homocysteine levels through balneotherapy: effects of sulphur baths. *Clin Chim Acta*. 2004;343(1-2):105-11.

[29] Turesson C, Jacobsson L T, Matteson EL. Cardiovascular co-morbidity in rheumatic diseases. *Vasc Health Risk Manag*. 2008; 4(3):605-14.

[30] Bernardes M, Madureira A, Oliveira A, Martins MJ, Lucas R, Costa L, Pereira JG, Ventura F, Ramos I, Martins E. Coronary artery calcium score in female rheumatoid arthritis patients: Associations with apolipoproteins and disease biomarkers. *Int J Rheum Dis*. 2019;22(10):1841-56.

[31] Karagülle M, Kardeş S, Karagülle O, Dişçi R, Avcı A, Durak İ, Karagülle MZ. Effect of spa therapy with saline balneotherapy on oxidant/antioxidant status in patients with rheumatoid arthritis: a single-blind randomized controlled trial. *Int J Biometeorol*. 2017; 61(1):169-180.

[32] Santos I, Cantista P, Vasconcelos C. Balneotherapy in rheumatoid arthritis-a systematic review. *Int J Biometeorol*. 2016;60(8):1287-301.

[33] Verhagen AP, Bierma-Zeinstra SM, Boers M, Cardoso JR, Lambeck J, de Bie R, de Vet HC. Balneotherapy (or spa therapy) for rheumatoid arthritis. *Cochrane Database Syst Rev*. 2015;2015(4): CD000518.

[34] Kloesch B, Liszt M, Krehan D, Broell J, Kiener H, Steiner G. High concentrations of hydrogen sulphide elevate the expression of a series of pro-inflammatory genes in fibroblast-like synoviocytes derived from rheumatoid and osteoarthritis patients. *Immunol Lett*. 2012;141(2):197-203.

[35] Karagülle M, Kardeş S, Karagülle MZ. Long-term efficacy of spa therapy in patients with rheumatoid arthritis. *Rheumatol Int*. 2018;38(3):353-362.

[36] Li Y, Wei X, Zhou J, Wei L. The age-related changes in cartilage and osteoarthritis. *Biomed Res Int*. 2013;2013:916530.

[37] Kapoor M, Martel-Pelletier J, Lajeunesse D, Pelletier J P, Fahmi H. Role of proinflammatory cytokines in the pathophysiology of osteoarthritis. *Nat Rev Rheumatol*. 2011;7(1):33-42.

[38] Angioni MM, Denotti A, Pinna S, Sanna C, Montisci F, Dessole G, Loi A, Cauli A. Spa therapy induces clinical improvement and protein changes in patients with chronic back pain. *Reumatismo*. 2019;71(3):119-31.

[39] Gálvez I, Torres-Piles S, Ortega E. Innate/inflammatory bioregulation and clinical effectiveness of whole-body hyperthermia (balneotherapy) in elderly patients with osteoarthritis. *Int J Hyperthermia.* 2018;35(1):340-7.

[40] Wang K, Xu J, Cai J, Zheng S, Han W, Antony B, Ding C. Serum levels of interleukin-17 and adiponectin are associated with infrapatellar fat pad volume and signal intensity alteration in patients with knee osteoarthritis. *Arthritis Res Ther*. 2016;18(1):193.

[41] Ionescu EV, Tica I, Oprea C, Iliescu DM, Petcu LC, Iliescu MG. Adiponectin correlation with bioclinical benefits of using natural therapeutic factors in knee osteoarthritis. *Acta Endocrinol (Buchar)*. 2017;13(3):308-13.

[42] Fioravanti A, Cantarini L, Bacarelli MR, de Lalla A, Ceccatelli L, Blardi P. Effects of spa therapy on serum leptin and adiponectin levels in patients with knee osteoarthritis. *Rheumatol Int*. 2011; 31(7):879-82.

[43] Morer C, Roques CF, Françon A, Forestier R, Maraver F. The role of mineral elements and other chemical compounds used in balneology: data from double-blind randomized clinical trials. *Int J Biometeorol*. 2017;61(12):2159-73.

[44] Hanzel A, Berényi K, Horváth K, Szendi K, Németh B, Varga C. Evidence for the therapeutic effect of the organic content in Szigetvár thermal water on osteoarthritis: a double-blind, randomized, controlled clinical trial. *Int J Biometeorol.* 2019;63(4):449-458.

[45] Varzaityte L, Kubilius R, Rapoliene L, Bartuseviciute R, Balcius A, Ramanauskas K, Nedzelskiene I. The effect of balneotherapy and peloid therapy on changes in the functional state of patients with knee

joint osteoarthritis: a randomized, controlled, single-blind pilot study. *Int J Biometeorol.* 2020;64(6):955-64.

[46] Branco M, Rêgo NN, Silva PH, Archanjo I E, Ribeiro MC, Trevisani VF. Bath thermal waters in the treatment of knee osteoarthritis: a randomized controlled clinical trial. *Eur J Phys Rehabil Med.* 2016;52(4):422-30.

[47] Fioravanti A, Giannitti C, Bellisai B, Iacoponi F, Galeazzi M. Efficacy of balneotherapy on pain, function and quality of life in patients with osteoarthritis of the knee. *Int J Biometeorol.* 2012;56(4):583-90.

[48] Abdalbary SA. Ultrasound with mineral water or aqua gel to reduce pain and improve the WOMAC of knee osteoarthritis. *Future Sci OA.* 2016;2(1):FSO110.

[49] Fioravanti A, Iacoponi F, Bellisai B, Cantarini L, Galeazzi M. Short- and long-term effects of spa therapy in knee osteoarthritis. *Am J Phys Med Rehabil.* 2010;89(2):125-32.

[50] Harzy T, Ghani N, Akasbi N, Bono W, Nejjari C. Short- and long-term therapeutic effects of thermal mineral waters in knee osteoarthritis: a systematic review of randomized controlled trials. *Clin Rheumatol.* 2009;28(5):501-7.

[51] Forestier R, Erol Forestier F B, Francon A. Spa therapy and knee osteoarthritis: A systematic review. *Ann Phys Rehabil Med.* 2016; 59(3):216-26.

[52] Kovács C, Pecze M, Tihanyi Á, Kovács L, Balogh S, Bender T. The effect of sulphurous water in patients with osteoarthritis of hand. Double-blind, randomized, controlled follow-up study. *Clin Rheumatol.* 2012;31(10):1437-42.

[53] Horváth K, Kulisch Á, Németh A, Bender T. Evaluation of the effect of balneotherapy in patients with osteoarthritis of the hands: a randomized controlled single-blind follow-up study. *Clin Rehabil.* 2012;26(5):431-41.

[54] Fioravanti A, Tenti S, Giannitti C, Fortunati N A, Galeazzi M. Short- and long-term effects of mud-bath treatment on hand osteoarthritis: a randomized clinical trial. *Int J Biometeorol.* 2014;58(1):79-86.

[55] Kovács C, Bozsik Á, Pecze M, Borbély I, Fogarasi A, Kovács L, Tefner IK, Bender T. Effects of sulfur bath on hip osteoarthritis: a randomized, controlled, single-blind, follow-up trial: a pilot study. *Int J Biometeorol.* 2016;60(11):1675-80.

[56] Erol FB, Forestier RJ, Güneri FD, Karagülle MZ, Erdoğan N. Spa therapy for generalized osteoarthritis: an open, observational, preliminary study. *Therapie*. 2015;70(3):273-81.

[57] Clauw DJ. Fibromyalgia: a clinical review. *JAMA*. 2014;311(15): 1547-55.

[58] Woolf CJ. Central sensitization: implications for the diagnosis and treatment of pain. *Pain*. 2011;152(3 Suppl):S2-S15.

[59] Macfarlane GJ, Kronisch C, Dean L E, Atzeni F, Häuser W, Fluß E, Choy E, Kosek E, Amris K, Branco J, Dincer F, Leino-Arjas P, Longley K, McCarthy GM, Makri S, Perrot S, Sarzi-Puttini P, Taylor A, Jones GT. EULAR revised recommendations for the management of fibromyalgia. *Ann Rheum Dis*. 2017;76(2):318-328.

[60] Pérez-Fernández MR, Calvo-Ayuso N, Martínez-Reglero C, Salgado-Barreira Á, Muiño López-Álvarez JL. Efficacy of baths with mineral-medicinal water in patients with fibromyalgia: a randomized clinical trial. *Int J Biometeorol.* 2019;63(9):1161-70.

[61] Koçyiğit BF, Gür A, Altındağ Ö, Akyol A, Gürsoy S. Comparison of education and balneotherapy efficacy in patients with fibromyalgia syndrome: A randomized, controlled clinical study. *Agri*. 2016;28(2):72-8.

[62] Kurt EE, Koçak FA, Erdem HR, Tuncay F, Kelez F. Which Non-Pharmacological Treatment is More Effective on Clinical Parameters in Patients With Fibromyalgia: Balneotherapy or Aerobic Exercise? *Arch Rheumatol*. 2016;31(2):162-9.

[63] Maeda T, Kudo Y, Horiuchi T, Makino N. Clinical and anti-aging effect of mud-bathing therapy for patients with fibromyalgia. *Mol Cell Biochem*. 2018;444(1-2):87-92.

In: Mineral Water
Editors: Maria João Martins
ISBN: 978-1-68507-458-6

Chapter 5

MINERAL WATER CONSUMPTION AND DIET-INDUCED ACID LOAD: PUTATIVE RELEVANCE FOR BONE HEALTH

Cidália D. Pereira*[1,2,*]*, PhD, Cátia Pontes*[1,2]*, PhD, Vânia Ribeiro*[1,2]*, PhD and Maria João Martins*[3,4]*, PhD

[1]School of Health Sciences, Polytechnic of Leiria, Leiria, Portugal
[2]CiTechCare - Centre for Innovative Care and Health Technology, Polytechnic of Leiria, Leiria, Portugal
[3]Department of Biomedicine, Biochemistry Unit, Faculty of Medicine, University of Porto, Porto, Portugal
[4]i3S-Instituto de Investigação e Inovação em Saúde, University of Porto, Porto, Portugal

ABSTRACT

Human diet has been changing towards a pattern with higher ingestion of acidifying nutrients than of alkalising ones, increasing diet-

* Corresponding Author's E-mail: cidalia.pereira@ipleiria.pt.

induced acid load. Although with some controversy, increasing evidence associates the rise of the dietary acid load, which chronically may lead to a low-grade metabolic acidosis, to several (chronic) non-communicable diseases: hypertension, dyslipidaemia, non-alcoholic fatty liver disease, obesity, metabolic syndrome, type 2 diabetes, kidney, cardiovascular and bone diseases, cancer, and asthma in obese children. Mineral water consumption, owing both to its alkali load and minerals and ions content, seems an interesting strategy to counteract diet-induced acid load. Here, we focused on the links with bone metabolism/bone health/bone disease.

Keywords: bicarbonate, bone health, bone metabolism, calcium, chloride, diet-induced acid load, fluoride, magnesium, mineral water, net endogenous acid production, potential renal acid load, sodium

INTRODUCTION

Contemporary diet contains more animal- than plant-based food components associated with high calorie consumption almost from industrialized/processed food, both from animal and plant sources, rich in sodium chloride (NaCl), fats and simple sugars. Additionally, contemporary diet greatly lacks many fresh/natural products, such as roots, tubers, seeds, leafy green vegetables, vegetable fruits, fruits and nuts (which are rich in fibres, vitamins, minerals and phytochemicals), and significantly includes (refined) cereal grains. The switch from more traditional diets, such as the Mediterranean diet, to more westernised dietary patterns has been associated with the observed increasing incidence and development of (chronic) non-communicable diseases, namely obesity, hypertension, dyslipidaemia, metabolic syndrome, type 2 diabetes, kidney and cardiovascular diseases, osteoporosis and cancer [1–4].

Although research has implicated the dietary imbalance between protective ingredients or nutrients and harmful ones on (chronic) non-communicable diseases, as briefly mentioned above, only recently the relationship of these diseases with diet-induced acid load has gained attention [5–14].

In this chapter, we a) summarised evidence regarding the relationship between diet-induced acid load and (chronic) non-communicable diseases incidence and development, and b) aimed to highlight the relevance of mineral water ingestion to counterbalance the dietary acid load, focusing on bone metabolism/bone health.

DIET-INDUCED ACID LOAD AND DISTINCT CLINICAL OUTCOMES

Diet is a major contributor to the body acid load and the dietary acid load reflects endogenous acid-base equilibrium due to the characteristics/composition of the dietary intake [6, 13, 15]. In general, presenting distinct intensity contributions, meat, fish, sea food, cheese, eggs, cereal grains, beans, and nuts contribute to increased acid production while roots, tubers, leafy green vegetables, vegetable fruits, and fruits are alkalising foods. Milk is a less relevant acid precursor food when compared with cheese; fats and sugars have a very small effect on acid-base balance [3, 4, 16–18].

The explanation for these differences relies on the unalike mechanisms of food metabolism. The metabolism of certain amino acids yields hydrogen ions which drop blood pH. So, the quantity of protein-induced acid production will depend on which amino acids are present and their amount: lysine, arginine and histidine are considered acidic, as they generate hydrochloric acid when metabolised, as well as cysteine and methionine, which are converted into sulphuric acid. Protein quality also influences acid production. Animal proteins are richer in sulphur-containing amino acids than plant proteins and have a high amount of phosphorus, both contributing to the acidification of body fluids. An interesting exception is milk whose calcium content counterbalances its phosphorous richness. It is also important to mention that plant proteins have phosphorus in the form of phytate, which is less bioavailable and does not induce the same acidifying metabolic effect. Moreover, when compared with animal proteins, plant proteins are usually richer in glutamate whose metabolism consumes hydrogen ions what produces an alkalising effect [4, 16]. On the other hand, the metabolism of potassium salts, which are mainly found in fruits and vegetables, including citrate and malate as negative ions, also consumes hydrogen ions. As potassium oxalate cannot be metabolised, the consumption of fruits and vegetables containing a high oxalate content is discouraged [4, 16]. Magnesium and calcium are also precursors of bases [17].

In addition, Frasseto *et al.* found that dietary NaCl intake (indexed by urine chloride excretion) and diet net acid load (indexed by renal net acid excretion) independently induced hyperchloremic metabolic acidosis. Dietary chloride intake (a positive index of dietary NaCl intake) was reported to be an (inverse) independent predictor of plasma bicarbonate concentration [19].

Considering the above-mentioned, it is not surprising that the contemporary diet (westernised diet) may promote an acidic environment as the reduced consumption of base-producing products does not compensate the acidic load caused by this type of diet [4, 14, 20].

Two methods are often used for the assessment of the dietary acid load: net endogenous acid production (NEAP) and potential renal acid load (PRAL) [6, 17, 21–24]. Concerning values interpretation, the more negative the NEAP, the more net base-producing the diet [3] and, similarly, the more negative the PRAL, the more alkalising the food [17]. Urinary pH has been considered a simple and cost-effective parameter to assess NEAP. However, although it seems appropriate in large population-based studies, it may not be reliable in populations with age-related renal function decline or chronic kidney disease as well as under renal tubular acidosis [13].

Sebastian *et al.* computationally predicted a NEAP of 48 mEq/day for the current average American diet (as recorded in the third National Health and Nutrition Examination Survey) whereas for retrojected human ancestral preagricultural diets a mean value of about -88 mEq/day was obtained [3]. Although human body has different mechanisms for handling acid-base imbalance, it can be hypothesised that it may not be adapted to this significant diet alteration, yet, what contributes to the incidence and development of (chronic) non-communicable diseases [13, 20]. In this regard, lungs and kidneys, as well as a complex system of intracellular and extracellular buffers, are involved in the maintenance of the acid-base balance, preserving the arterial pH within the optimal range (7.35-7.45). While the lungs eliminate carbon dioxide, the kidneys reabsorb the filtered bicarbonate and maintain the production of bicarbonate with the excretion of non-titrable and titrable acid, through the ammonium system in the urine [18, 25]. However, it is well-known that some diseases may severely compromise those mechanisms and, consequently, the body's ability to manage acid-base equilibrium [16, 25].

Importantly, increasing evidence shows that diet-induced disturbances in the acid-base status may exert a negative impact on health and have been associated with altered bone metabolism/bone health [17, 26–30], impaired insulin signalling/type 2 diabetes [17, 31–38], urolithiasis [17, 39, 40], chronic kidney disease [9, 14, 17, 41–43], hypertension [6, 7, 15, 17, 38, 44, 45], dyslipidaemia [46], non-alcoholic fatty liver disease [8, 17, 47], cardiovascular disease [11, 48, 49], metabolic syndrome [50], cancer [12, 51, 52], obesity [46] and asthma in obese children [53].

Mediterranean and DASH diets have been considered protective for bone health [54] and both diets have a low (negative) PRAL value [13, 55, 56].

In the sections below, we focused on the detrimental relationship, and the associated mechanisms, between diet-induced acid load and bone metabolism/bone health as well as the beneficial putative impact of mineral water consumption through its alkalising effects (and mineral content).

Diet-Induced Acid Load and Bone Metabolism/Bone Health

Although bicarbonate, phosphate, sodium, and potassium on bone surface can be exchanged for acid, calcium is not passively effluxed from bone in response to an acid load; instead this process results from an acid-base balance-induced physiological modulation of bone cells [57].

From both *in vitro* and *in vivo* studies, metabolic acidosis hinders bone mineralisation/growth by physicochemical mineral dissolution, osteoclast survival, bone-resorbing osteoclast activity stimulation (up-regulating key cellular machinery needed for resorption pit formation and, consequently, increasing resorption pit formation and removal of both mineral and organic bone content), osteoblast function inhibition (decreasing specific extracellular matrix proteins gene expression, alkaline phosphatase activity and mineralisation) and hormonal axis modulation [impairment of the growth hormone/insulin-like growth factor I (IGF-1) endocrine axis and increase of glucocorticoids levels]. At about pH 6.8-6.9 osteoclasts are maximally active while osteoblasts are strongly inhibited, while at pH 7.4 the opposite occurs. After being activated by acidosis, osteoclasts can be further stimulated by ATP/ADP, receptor activator for nuclear factor kB ligand, parathyroid hormone (PTH) and 1,25-dihydroxycholecalciferol [17, 21, 57–61].

Even though published data have shown that diets with high NEAP or high PRAL values may lead to the stimulation of bone resorption, the decrease of bone mineral density (BMD) and the loss of bone mass, creating a higher risk of bone fractures [17, 26–29], this link is not unanimously accepted [10, 62, 63] what supports the argument that it is quite unlikely dietary acid load drives the pH of the extracellular fluid below 7.4 [57]. In fact, Buclin *et al.*, in a double cross-over study (comprising four weekly sessions), did not find a change greater than 0.014 units in the pH value of blood from 8 healthy male volunteers (22-31 years) as a consequence of the type of diet. Nevertheless, under this slight pH change, the acid-forming diet significantly increased urinary calcium and C-telopeptide (resorptive marker) excretion by 74% and 19%, respectively, when compared with the diet providing base-forming nutrients (that included sodium bicarbonate-rich mineral water) [64]. In this context, and referring to what was briefly mentioned above, in 24 h cultured osteoclasts a two-times increase in the number of bone resorption pits was observed with 0.05 units interstitial pH reductions (as attainable by diet) [21, 65]. In accordance, in an one-week calvaria culture system, micro-computed tomography values of bone volume density were higher with 24 mM bicarbonate- *versus* 12 mM bicarbonate-treated bone [66]. As so, it seems reasonable that any change in the interstitial pH (with a lesser buffer capacity than plasma) may alter bone microenvironment and, consequently, impact bone metabolism/bone health (the longer the pH change lasts, the stronger the bone effects are) [21].

Dietary acid load-induced hypercalciuria, not compensated by (elevated) intestinal calcium absorption, has been frequently assumed as the most culprit for the loss of bone mineral content. However, a strong negative calcium balance is not the primary cause of the potentially damaging long-term skeletal effects of diet-related acid production in healthy people, there is no clear evidence that the source for the increased calciuria is (exclusively) bone and the adaptive mechanisms that occur in the hormonal regulation of calcium absorption and metabolism allowing adaptation to increased urinary calcium excretion should be taken into consideration [21, 67].

Systemic proton concentrations are linked with total daily acid load. Diet-induced moderately raised systemic proton concentration (but still within the normal range) is often designated low-grade, subclinical or subtle metabolic acidosis [21]. Although it seems possible that some of the aforementioned mechanisms (in the beginning of this chapter section) for metabolic acidosis altering bone metabolism/bone health may also apply as a consequence of (chronic) diet-induced acid load, the evidence of diet-induced acid load upon bone mass and size as well as bone turnover/remodelling/metabolism markers is scarce [21] and obtained only in special populations or populations sub-groups in cross-sectional [10, 28, 29, 68–70] and interventional studies [27, 71, 72]. For example, New *et al.* found, in a cross-sectional study, that a) lower estimates of energy-adjusted NEAP significantly associated with higher hip and spine BMD [in 1056 women (45-54 years); 92% were premenopausal] as well as with higher forearm bone mass [in 62 women (45-54 years)], b) forearm and hip bone mass significantly decreased as quartiles of energy-adjusted NEAP increased, and c) differences remained significant after adjustment for age, menstrual status, height, and weight. Also, lower estimates of energy-adjusted NEAP were significantly linked with lower urinary deoxypyridinoline excretion (in the smaller group) [26]. Gunn *et al.*, in a 3-month randomised interventional comparative study, observed that a) an increased intake of Scarborough Fair dietary mix of vegetables, herbs and fruits significantly associated with a low dietary PRAL and decreased bone formation and resorptive markers, procollagen type I N propeptide and C-terminal telopeptide of type I collagen, respectively, significantly *versus* baseline when considering all postmenopausal women for the former parameter, but significantly in osteopenic postmenopausal women when compared with those with normal BMD for the latter parameter, and b) increased ingestion of fruits, vegetables and herbs, not necessarily the Scarborough Fair dietary mix, significantly decreased urinary calcium excretion and significantly increased urinary pH *versus* control diet (mean age of all women around 60 years; 50 volunteers recruited/group) [27]. Mangano *et al.* found out, in a cross-sectional study based on 2125 individuals (907 women; $\geq$ 60 years) from the National Health and Nutrition Examination Survey 2005-2008, that there was no association between BMD and dietary acid load among adults, when supplemental calcium was taken into consideration. However, in men with low dietary calcium intake an inverse link with PRAL at the proximal femur BMD was found; no interaction was observed in women [69]. However, McLean *et al.*, assessing participants enrolled in the Framingham Osteoporosis Study [(n=1069; mean age 76 years; 62% women; 1988-1989, 1992-1993) + (n=2919; 56% women, mean age 60 years; 1996-2001)], found an inverse association between estimated NEAP, but not PRAL, and femoral neck BMD, independent from total calcium intake, only among older men (neither NEAP nor PRAL were linked with lumbar spine BMD). In addition, increased dietary acid load (estimated NEAP and PRAL) was not associated with lower BMD at any location among middle-aged men and women or older women, regardless of total calcium intake [70].

Although proteins are primary contributors to the acidifying potential of the diet, dietary proteins (primarily from animal sources) may exert an anabolic influence upon bone turnover by increasing IGF-1 levels and suppressing PTH action as well as improving muscle shape and mass (muscularity promotes bone mass and strength). Additionally, by stimulating intestinal calcium absorption, compensation of protein-induced calciuria could occur [17, 21, 57, 73–75]. As an example, Cao *et al.* performed a 15-week randomised cross-over interventional protocol with 16 postmenopausal women [56.9±3.2 years (mean±standard deviation; SD)] to determine the effects of a high- *versus* low-protein (total 118 g/day *versus* total 61 g/day) and high- *versus* low-PRAL (33 mEq/day *versus* -48 mEq/day) diets upon bone metabolism markers along with calcium absorption and retention. Compared with the low-protein and low-PRAL diet, the high-protein and high-PRAL diet significantly increased and significantly decreased participants' circulating IGF-1 and intact PTH concentrations, respectively, and significantly increased fractional intestinal calcium absorption as well as urinary calcium excretion. This dietary protocol did not affect the net difference between the amount of calcium absorbed and excreted in urine nor markers of bone resorption or formation [75].

Considering the evidence hereby described, it seems plausible that chronic diet-induced acid load negatively impacts bone metabolism and, most probably, associates with a greater risk of bone disease development, namely osteoporosis, later in life. But this impact could be masked/impeded by protein consumption. So, both protein intake and dietary acid load should be adequately accounted for in further studies [21]. On the other hand, the measured bone-related outcomes are also vital. While BMD reflects the degree of bone mineralisation, trabecular bone score combines information on connectivity density, trabecular separation, and trabecular number [10], and may be a predictor factor of osteoporotic fractures [76]. Thereby, as suggested by de Jonge *et al.*, dietary acid load could be detrimental to bone health by influencing trabecular integrity without necessarily altering BMD [10].

In addition, there are many other dietary factors not addressed in diets' NEAP or PRAL calculation that are required to and/or modulate bone metabolism/bone health [namely vitamins (A, C, D and K), minerals (zinc, copper, iron and fluoride), fibre, phytochemicals (as phytoestrogens), caffeine, and alcohol] and so hamper the establishment of a definitive relationship between dietary acid load and bone metabolism/bone health [77–80].

Mineral Water Consumption and Diet-Induced Acid Load: An Overview

Considering the aforementioned evidence regarding the link between dietary acid load and (chronic) non-communicable diseases, there is an increasing interest to find strategies, particularly regarding nutrition, that may counterbalance the acid load induced by the actual dietary pattern. In this context, the ingestion of mineral waters and/or alkaline waters has emerged [50, 61, 64, 81–86]. Interestingly, drinking mineral waters or alkaline waters has been used/tested/suggested as a strategy to improve hydration and acid-base balance status, physical exercise performance and exercise-induced metabolic acidosis [61, 82, 83, 87–90].

Heil assessed the influence of the consumption of a mineralised alkaline bottled water upon acid-base balance markers by performing a blind study with 38 healthy participants (18-30 years; 25 women) under free-living conditions. The mineralised alkaline bottled water contained a naturally high-mineral content (potassium, calcium, magnesium, silica and selenium ranging from 0.1 to 23.0 mg/L) along with an unknown amount of Alka-PlexLiquid (a blend of mineral-based alkalising agents) that further increased the water mineral content and was responsible for the water unusual high pH (pH 10) and the enhanced rate of absorption and retention of water in the body. The participants followed a four-week testing phase, all consuming the control water [with a very low mineral content (no significant concentrations of minerals or electrolytes) and pH 7] during weeks 1 and 4 and: a) control water during weeks 2 and 3 (control group) and b) the mineralised alkaline water during weeks 2 and 3 (experimental group). The control and experimental groups self-reported drinking similar amounts of both waters throughout the study (ranging from 2.2 to 2.5 L/day). Heil observed that the consumption of the highly mineralised alkaline water (*versus* control water) was associated with an increase in both urine and blood pH, with daily physical activity and dietary composition remaining stable [83].

Wasserfurth *et al.* studied for the first time the impact of mineral waters with distinct mineral and bicarbonate content and PRAL value upon acid-base status in 129 free-living, healthy adults (18-75 years; 76% women). In a single-centered randomised trial, the participants drank, for 4 weeks, 1.5-2.0 L/day of one of four mineral waters: low-bicarbonate, high-PRAL (LBHP, HCO_3^-: 403.0 mg/L, PRAL: 10.7 mEq/L); medium-high-bicarbonate, medium-PRAL (MBMP, HCO_3^-: 1816.0 mg/L, PRAL: -10.8 mEq/L); high-bicarbonate, low-PRAL (HBLP, HCO_3^-: 2451.0 mg/L, PRAL: -19.3 mEq/L); or medium-high-bicarbonate, low-PRAL (MBLP, HCO_3^-: 1846.0 mg/L, PRAL: -22.1 mEq/L). The consumption of the three mineral waters with medium- or high-bicarbonate content (> 1800.0 mg/L) and with medium- or low-PRAL (< -11 mEq/L) significantly decreased the net acid excretion, assessed in the 24 h urine output: 48% with MBMP, 53% with MBLP and 68% with HBLP. Additionally, an increase in serum bicarbonate values occurred after HBLP (tendency) and MBLP intake (significantly). Furthermore, and in accordance, LBHP intake significantly decreased spot urine pH, while with the consumption of the 3 other waters an increase was observed, but significantly only for MBMP and MBLP. Regular consumption of these mineral waters could be advantageous in avoiding risks linked to a higher dietary acid load. Interestingly, an additional intake of 792 mg for calcium and 362 mg for magnesium was obtained with LBHP and HBLP ingestion, respectively [82]. Considering that the 4 tested mineral waters were classified according to not only their bicarbonate content but also their PRAL value, it seems important to highlight that although the alkaline load of a mineral water can be indirectly assessed by its bicarbonate content (bicarbonate decreases the acid load), mineral waters possess other minerals/ions that contribute to the water alkali or acid load. For example, calcium in mineral waters is most frequently associated with sulphate what increases PRAL. Accordingly, using PRAL, instead of bicarbonate, allows the direct assessment of the acidifying and alkalising components content of mineral waters. As we previously discussed for food, the higher the PRAL, the more acidifying the mineral water [91].

Considering the potential role of mineral waters and/or alkaline waters counterbalancing dietary acid load under free-living conditions in healthy individuals, the question arises regarding its potential role under clinical conditions that may compromise acid-base homeostasis. Thus, which evidence exists regarding mineral water intake and diet-induced acid load upon bone metabolism/bone health?

Mineral Water Consumption, Mineral/Ion Content of Water and Diet-Induced Acid Load: Putative Relevance for Bone Metabolism/Bone Health

There is evidence arguing for the relevance of mineral water consumption in the reduction of decline, maintenance or increase of BMD as well as prevention or reduction of osteoporosis and bone fractures risk [92–97]. Additionally, mineral water intake may a) decrease circulating PTH levels, b) positively modulate urinary and/or circulating bone turnover/remodelling/metabolism parameter values, c) modulate urinary calcium and magnesium excretion, and d) increase, improve or restore bone microstructural properties, circulating minerals/electrolytes levels and urinary acid-base balance markers [94, 97–103]. However, not all the published data relate the favourable bone effects of mineral water consumption to the potential improvement of diet-induced acid load: more relevance has been given to the mineral content of water, as it is highly bioavailable [50, 104–106], than to the mineral water-associated alkali load. In this regard, the calcium content of mineral waters has received great recognition for the bone beneficial effects of mineral water intake [for example in [92, 95, 97, 99, 100, 102]].

Buclin *et al.*, in a dietary intervention already mentioned in this chapter, found that providing base-forming nutrients, where a sodium bicarbonate-rich mineral water was accounted for [2 L of the mineral water providing 4868 mg bicarbonate and a PRAL of -124 mEq/d [91]], had a positive impact on blood and urine pH (while both parameters decreased under an acid-forming diet). None of the dietary regimens tested interfered with calcium absorption from two different calcium supplements. Importantly, both diets not only had similar content of protein, phosphate, calcium and sodium but also provided similar amount of calories. Although these results originate from an acute intervention (each of the 4 sessions lasted 4 days), authors suggested that avoiding high amounts of acid ash-forming food while increasing the intake of alkalising food may be favourable for bone mass maintenance [64].

Roux *et al.* compared the effects of 2 mineral waters (a two-period randomised cross-over study, with 1 L/d of each water consumed during 28 days) containing similarly high-calcium concentration but one was rich in bicarbonate (mg/L: 606 Ca^{2+}, 27 Mg^{2+}, 2179 HCO_3^-, 3.9 SO_4^{2-}) and the other was rich in sulphate and magnesium (mg/L: 559.59 Ca^{2+}, 80 Mg^{2+}, 291.7 HCO_3^-, 1550.5 SO_4^{2-}). All 39 healthy postmenopausal women [younger than 80 years, 64±6 years (mean±SD)] had similar low initial dietary calcium intake (approximately 400 mg/day). Compliance with intervention was high. No significant differences were observed between the 2 mineral water groups except for urine acidosis markers. Compared with baseline, the former mineral water significantly increased circulating ionized calcium and significantly decreased circulating PTH as well as urinary bone resorption markers (excretion ratios of C-terminal telopeptides, total pyridinoline and deoxypyridinoline to creatinine) while the latter mineral water did not significantly modify any of these parameters. But the opposite occurred for circulating bone alkaline phosphatase (being significantly decreased by the high-sulphate and high-magnesium mineral water and not significantly modified by the high-bicarbonate mineral water) [98]. In line with the previous study, Wynn *et al.*, in a randomised dietary intervention, compared the effects of an alkaline mineral water, rich in calcium, magnesium and bicarbonate (per litre: 548 mg Ca^{2+}, 65 mg Mg^{2+}, 2172 mg HCO_3^-, 9 mg SO_4^{2-}, PRAL -11.2 mEq), with that of an acid one, rich in calcium and sulphate (per litre: 520

mg Ca^{2+}, 35 mg Mg^{2+}, 291 mg HCO_3^-, 1160 mg SO_4^{2-}, PRAL +9.2 mEq), upon bone markers in 30 healthy young dieticians or student dieticians [18-45 years, 26.3±7.3 years (mean±SD)] that were sufficient in oestrogen and calcium (and the dietary plan provided 965 mg of calcium). The ingestion of 1.5 L/day (during 28 days) of the former mineral water significantly decreased circulating C-telopeptides and PTH and significantly increased urinary pH and bicarbonate excretion *versus* baseline, while the latter mineral water had no influence. For all these parameters, there were significant differences between the two mineral waters [81]. Importantly, as this study was carried out in women with an excellent compliance with the dietary plan, the alterations observed were mostly certainly due to the differences in water composition [81, 107].

Trying to define the optimal profile of mineral waters for positive bone effects, Wynn *et al.* determined the PRAL values of 150 European mineral waters and examined their calcium content as well as which components were conditioning their acidifying or alkalising power. A great variability in the composition of the different mineral waters was found, being bicarbonate and potassium the components seen in the largest and the smallest quantities, respectively. Seventy per cent of the mineral waters displayed a negative PRAL (presenting an alkalising impact) while the remaining 30% exhibited a positive PRAL (having an acidifying profile). According to the PRAL algorithm, chloride and sulphate were acidifying components while potassium, sodium, calcium and magnesium were alkalising elements. The strongest inverse link found for PRAL was with bicarbonate. A high-calcium content in mineral waters associated with either high-bicarbonate or high-sulphate content [61]. Although with not consistent evidence, sulphate in mineral waters (more acidifying ones) may counterbalance calcium effects because sulphate and acid load are reported to increase urinary calcium excretion [61, 91]. Additionally, as aforementioned, both under calcium insufficiency or sufficiency initial volunteer status, high-calcium, high-sulphate mineral waters had no relevant positive impact on bone metabolism parameters unlike high-calcium and high-bicarbonate mineral waters [81, 98]. Nevertheless, Meunier *et al.*, performing a 6-month randomised double-blind protocol, reported a beneficial bone modulation on 87 healthy postmenopausal women [70.1±4.0 years (mean±SD)] by the ingestion of a high-calcium (596 mg/L) and high-sulphate (1530.0 mg/L) mineral water *versus* a low-calcium (10 mg/L) and low-sulphate (8.1 mg/L) mineral water (1 L/day for both waters; women had a dietary calcium intake below 700 mg/day in both groups). A significant decrease of circulating PTH, osteocalcin and bone alkaline phosphatase as well as circulating and urinary type-1 collagen C-telopeptide was found in the former group *versus* the latter (these parameters remained almost stable or increased with the low-calcium and low-sulphate water) [100]. In all, Wynn *et al.* advise that the best mineral waters for bone metabolism/bone health should be rich in bicarbonate and mineral alkalising cations, including calcium, and low in sulphate (providing positive effects on calcium metabolism besides the impact of low PRAL values). They discovered that 12% of the 150 studied European waters had Ca^{2+} > 200 mg/L and HCO_3^- > 700 mg/L [61].

Besides the calcium, sulphate and bicarbonate content of mineral waters that may contribute directly (by minerals/ions metabolic effects) and/or indirectly (through PRAL/acidifying/alkalising effects), mineral waters also contain relevant concentrations of other minerals/ions (for example magnesium, sodium, chloride or fluoride) that, likewise, may interfere directly and/or indirectly with bone metabolism [61, 101, 107].

In what concerns magnesium-rich waters, Day *et al.* performed a double-blind parallel-group randomised study enrolling 67 postmenopausal women (50-70 years) that drank, over 84 days, 1.5 to 1.8 L/d of a spring water supplemented or not with magnesium bicarbonate. A significant increase of circulating magnesium and urinary pH was observed in the supplemented spring water (650 mg/L HCO_3^-, 120 mg/L Mg^{2+}, pH 8.3-8.5) group *versus* control spring water group [these parameters remained (almost) stable in this group]. Control spring water led towards an increasing trend in circulating PTH while supplemented spring water did not relevantly change it. No significant differences in the change (from day 0 to day 84) between the 2 water groups were seen on bone metabolism biomarkers (urinary n-telopeptides and hydroxyproline as well as circulating osteocalcin and 1,25-dihydroxyvitamin D) [108].

Schoppen *et al.* found that daily consumption of 1 L of a control low-mineralised mineral water *versus* a sodium-rich carbonated mineral water (mg/L: 2094.4 HCO_3^-, 583.0 Cl^-, 49.9 SO_4^{2-}, 7.9 F^-, 43.6 Ca^{2+}, 1116.5 Na^+, 54.7 K^+, 5.7 Mg^{2+}), tested consecutively for 8 weeks, did not affect bone remodelling markers (procollagen I amino-terminal propeptide and β-carboxy-terminal telopeptide of collagen) in 18 healthy postmenopausal women [53±3 years (mean±SD)]. Urinary calcium and phosphorus excretion were significantly lower and higher, respectively, after the intake of the sodium-rich carbonated water *versus* the control mineral water while urinary sodium and chloride excretion did not change. The sodium-rich carbonated mineral water also significantly increased urinary pH [109]. The same research group found that the consumption of 500 mL of the above-mentioned sodium-rich carbonated mineral water with a standard meal (also *versus* the above-mentioned control low-mineralised mineral water) significantly increased urinary sodium excretion without significantly changing the urinary excretion of potassium, calcium, magnesium, chloride and phosphorus in 18 healthy postmenopausal women [110].

In ovariectomised Sprague-Dawley female rats, our group found that a bicarbonate- and sodium-rich mineral water (mg/L: 2013 HCO_3^-, 30.8 Cl^-, 6.4 SO_4^{2-}, 92.5 Ca^{2+}, 591 Na^+, 29.9 K^+, 26.2 Mg^{2+}), ingested *ad libitum* for 10 weeks, induced a significant effect upon microstructural properties of the cancellous (bone volumetric fraction, specific bone surface, bone surface density, trabecular thickness, trabecular spacing, trabecular number, trabecular bone pattern factor and structural model index) and cortical distal femur compartments (medullary volume and cortical endosteal perimeter) as well as upon cancellous distal femur BMD preventing against ovariectomy detrimental effects [94].

While high dietary sodium intake may seem harmful for bone health [111], the ingestion of sodium-rich mineral waters does not seem to have the same effect [94, 109]. In fact, sodium accompanying anions determine/modulate sodium effects. For example, sodium bicarbonate and NaCl distinctly modulate urinary calcium excretion [50, 112], which is in line with the beneficial bone findings by Schoppen *et al.* and Pereira *et al.*

[94, 109]. So, the difference in mineral waters chloride content should be taken into consideration. As previously mentioned, high-chloride waters are associated with a greater PRAL value and, consequently, are more acidic [61]. Interestingly, the sodium-rich mineral water tested by Shoppen *et al.* has a high chloride concentration, 583 mg/L [109, 110], while the sodium-rich mineral water tested by our group has a low chloride content, 30.8 mg/L [94], but both present a (very) high (and similar) bicarbonate level. Questions remain about chloride effects upon bone health [107].

On the other hand, mineral water fluoride content may also seem important as the mineral-rich water tested by Schoppen *et al.* contained higher levels of fluoride than the control water (7.9 mg/L *versus* 0.2 mg/L) [109, 110] and fluoride is known to inhibit NaCl reabsorption in Henle's loop [113] contributing to Schoppen and colleagues findings [10% and 33% increases (non-significant and significant, respectively) of urinary chloride and sodium excretion were found] [110]. Despite this potential fluoride beneficial effect, it is important to mention that the evidence for this element regarding bone health is still controversial owing to differences in studies type/design/duration, fluoride dosage/exposure, and population enrolled along with the range of possible fluoride bone effects. As fluoride accumulates in bone, where it has a biological half-life of several years, and stimulates osteoblast activity, it has been used in osteoporosis treatment. In spite of the fluoride-induced BMD increase at specific locations, fluoride decreases bone tissue strength and elasticity, alters bone tissue crystalline structure and increases skeletal fragility [114–117].

CONCLUSION

Considering all the above information, mineral waters ingestion may be a putative useful strategy to counteract the negative impact of dietary acid load upon bone metabolism/bone health. Importantly, this favourable effect may be more relevant under pathological conditions that compromise body's ability to maintain the acid-base homeostasis. Mineral waters richness in minerals relevant for bone metabolism play a crucial role in bone health that can be potentiated when the mineral water is alkaline or provides a low (negative) PRAL value.

REFERENCES

[1] Cena H, Calder PC. Defining a healthy diet: evidence for the role of contemporary dietary patterns in health and disease. *Nutrients*. 2020;12(2):334.

[2] Hariharan D, Vellanki K, Kramer H. The western diet and chronic kidney disease. *Curr Hypertens Rep*. 2015;17(3):16.

[3] Sebastian A, Frassetto LA, Sellmeyer DE, Merriam RL, Morris RC Jr. Estimation of the net acid load of the diet of ancestral preagricultural *Homo sapiens* and their hominid ancestors. *Am J Clin Nutr*. 2002;76(6):1308–16.

[4] Goraya N, Wesson DE. Kidney response to the spectrum of diet-induced acid stress. *Nutrients*. 2018;10(5):596.

[5] Daneshzad E, Keshavarz SA, Qorbani M, Larijani B, Bellissimo N, Azadbakht L. Association of dietary acid load and plant-based diet index with sleep, stress, anxiety, and depression in diabetic women. *Br J Nutr*. 2020;123(8):901–12.

[6] Chen SW, Ji GY, Jiang Q, Wang P, Huang R, Ma WJ, Chen ZH, Peng JW. Association between dietary acid load and the risk of hypertension among adults from South China: result from nutrition and health survey (2015-2017). *BMC Public Health*. 2019;19(1):1599.

[7] Daneshzad E, Haghighatdoost F, Azadbakht L. Dietary acid load and cardiometabolic risk factors: a systematic review and meta-analysis of observational studies. *Public Health Nutr*. 2019;22(15):2823–34.

[8] Alferink LJM, Kiefte-de Jong JC, Erler NS, de Knegt RJ, Hoorn EJ, Ikram MA, Janssen HLA, Metselaar HJ, Franco OH, Darwish Murad

S. Diet-dependent acid load-the missing link between an animal protein-rich diet and nonalcoholic fatty liver disease? *J Clin Endocrinol Metab*. 2019;104(12):6325–37.

[9] Crews DC, Banerjee T, Wesson DE, Morgenstern H, Saran R, Burrows NR, Williams DE, Powe NR; Centers for Disease Control and Prevention Chronic Kidney Disease Surveillance Team. Race/ethnicity, dietary acid load, and risk of end-stage renal disease among us adults with chronic kidney disease. *Am J Nephrol*. 2018;47(3):174–81.

[10] de Jonge EAL, Koromani F, Hofman A, Uitterlinden AG, Franco OH, Rivadeneira F, Kiefte-de Jong JC. Dietary acid load, trabecular bone integrity, and mineral density in an ageing population: the Rotterdam study. *Osteoporos Int*. 2017;28(8):2357–65.

[11] Han E, Kim G, Hong N, Lee YH, Kim DW, Shin HJ, Lee BW, Kang ES, Lee IK, Cha BS. Association between dietary acid load and the risk of cardiovascular disease: nationwide surveys (KNHANES 2008-2011). *Cardiovasc Diabetol*. 2016;15(1):122.

[12] Park YM, Steck SE, Fung TT, Merchant AT, Elizabeth Hodgson M, Keller JA, Sandler DP. Higher diet-dependent acid load is associated with risk of breast cancer: Findings from the sister study. *Int J Cancer*. 2019;144(8):1834–43.

[13] Scialla JJ, Anderson CAM. Dietary acid load: a novel nutritional target in chronic kidney disease? *Adv Chronic Kidney Dis*. 2013;20(2):141–9.

[14] Banerjee T, Crews DC, Wesson DE, Tilea AM, Saran R, Rios-Burrows N, Williams DE, Powe NR; Centers for Disease Control and Prevention Chronic Kidney Disease Surveillance Team. High dietary acid load predicts esrd among adults with CKD. *J Am Soc Nephrol*. 2015;26(7):1693–700.

[15] Chen SW, Chen ZH, Liang YH, Wang P, Peng JW. Elevated hypertension risk associated with higher dietary acid load: A systematic review and meta-analysis. *Clin Nutr ESPEN*. 2019;33:171–7.

[16] Rodrigues Neto Angéloco L, de Souza GCA, Romão EA, Chiarello PG. Alkaline diet and metabolic acidosis: practical approaches to the nutritional management of chronic kidney disease. *J Ren Nutr.* 2018;28(3):215–20.

[17] Carnauba RA, Baptistella AB, Paschoal V, Hübscher GH. Diet-induced low-grade metabolic acidosis and clinical outcomes: A review. *Nutrients*. 2017;9(6):538.

[18] Osuna-Padilla IA, Leal-Escobar G, Garza-García CA, Rodríguez-Castellanos FE. Dietary acid load: mechanisms and evidence of its health repercussions. *Nefrol* (*English Ed*). 2019;39(4):343–54.

[19] Frassetto LA, Morris RC Jr, Sebastian A. Dietary sodium chloride intake independently predicts the degree of hyperchloremic metabolic acidosis in healthy humans consuming a net acid-producing diet. *Am J Physiol Ren Physiol*. 2007;293(2):F521-5.

[20] Adeva MM, Souto G. Diet-induced metabolic acidosis. *Clin Nutr.* 2011;30(4):416–21.

[21] Remer T, Krupp D, Shi L. Dietary protein's and dietary acid load's influence on bone health. *Crit Rev Food Sci Nutr*. 2014;54(9):1140–50.

[22] Frassetto LA, Todd KM, Morris RC Jr, Sebastian A. Estimation of net endogenous noncarbonic acid production in humans from diet potassium and protein contents. *Am J Clin Nutr*. 1998;68(3):576–83.

[23] Remer T, Manz F. Potential renal acid load of foods and its influence on urine pH. *J Am Diet Assoc*. 1995;95(7):791–7.

[24] Remer T, Manz F. Estimation of the renal net acid excretion by adults consuming diets containing variable amounts of protein. *Am J Clin Nutr*. 1994;59(6):1356–61.

[25] Hamm LL, Nakhoul N, Hering-Smith KS. Acid-base homeostasis. *Clin J Am Soc Nephrol*. 2015;10(12):2232–42.

[26] New SA, MacDonald HM, Campbell MK, Martin JC, Garton MJ, Robins SP, Reid DM. Lower estimates of net endogenous noncarbonic acid production are positively associated with indexes of bone health in premenopausal and perimenopausal women. *Am J Clin Nutr*. 2004;79(1):131–8.

[27] Gunn CA, Weber JL, McGill AT, Kruger MC. Increased intake of selected vegetables, herbs and fruit may reduce bone turnover in post-menopausal women. *Nutrients*. 2015;7(4):2499–517.

[28] Esche J, Johner S, Shi L, Schönau E, Remer T. Urinary citrate, an index of acid-base status, predicts bone strength in youths and fracture risk in adult females. *J Clin Endocrinol Metab*. 2016;101(12):4914–21.

[29] Rahbar A, Larijani B, Nabipour I, Mohamadi MM, Mirzaee K, Amiri Z. Relationship among dietary estimates of net endogenous acid production, bone mineral density and biochemical markers of bone turnover in an Iranian general population. *Bone*. 2009;45(5):876–81.

[30] Wynn E, Lanham-New SA, Krieg MA, Whittamore DR, Burckhardt P. Low estimates of dietary acid load are positively associated with bone ultrasound in women older than 75 years of age with a lifetime fracture. *J Nutr*. 2008;138(7):1349–54.

[31] Abshirini M, Bagheri F, Mahaki B, Siassi F, Koohdani F, Safabakhsh M, Sotoudeh G. The dietary acid load is higher in subjects with prediabetes who are at greater risk of diabetes: a case-control study. *Diabetol Metab Syndr*. 2019;11:52.

[32] Kiefte-de Jong JC, Li Y, Chen M, Curhan GC, Mattei J, Malik VS, Forman JP, Franco OH, Hu FB. Diet-dependent acid load and type 2 diabetes: pooled results from three prospective cohort studies. *Diabetologia*. 2017;60(2):270–9.

[33] Fagherazzi G, Vilier A, Bonnet F, Lajous M, Balkau B, Boutron-Rualt MC, Clavel-Chapelon F. Dietary acid load and risk of type 2 diabetes: the E3N-EPIC cohort study. *Diabetologia*. 2014;57(2):313–20.

[34] Akter S, Kurotani K, Kashino I, Goto A, Mizoue T, Noda M, Sawada N, Tsugane S; Japan Public Health Center–based Prospective Study Group. High dietary acid load score is associated with increased risk of type 2 diabetes in japanese men: the japan public health center-based prospective study. *J Nutr*. 2016;146(5):1076–83.

[35] Akter S, Eguchi M, Kuwahara K, Kochi T, Ito R, Kurotani K, Tsuruoka H, Nanri A, Kabe I, Mizoue T. High dietary acid load is associated with insulin resistance: The Furukawa Nutrition and Health Study. *Clin Nutr*. 2016;35(2):453–9.

[36] Gaede J, Nielsen T, Madsen ML, Toft U, Jorgensen T, Overvad K, Tjonneland A, Hansen T, Allin KH, Pedersen O. Population-based studies of relationships between dietary acidity load, insulin resistance and incident diabetes in Danes. *Nutr J*. 2018;17(1):91.

[37] Mohammadifard N, Karimi G, Khosravi A, Sarrafzadegan N, Jozan M, Zahed P, Haghighatdoost F. High dietary acid load score is not associated with the risk of metabolic syndrome in Iranian adults. *Int J Vitam Nutr Res*. 2021;91(1–2):152–63.

[38] Dehghan P, Abbasalizad Farhangi M. Dietary acid load, blood pressure, fasting blood sugar and biomarkers of insulin resistance among adults: Findings from an updated systematic review and meta-analysis. *Int J Clin Pract*. 2020;74(4):e13471.

[39] Trinchieri A, Maletta A, Lizzano R, Marchesotti F. Potential renal acid load and the risk of renal stone formation in a case-control study. *Eur J Clin Nutr*. 2013;67(10):1077–80.

[40] Trinchieri A, Lizzano R, Marchesotti F, Zanetti G. Effect of potential renal acid load of foods on urinary citrate excretion in calcium renal stone formers. *Urol Res*. 2006;34(1):1–7.

[41] Banerjee T, Crews DC, Wesson DE, Tilea A, Saran R, Rios B Burrows N, Williams DE, Powe NR; Centers for Disease Control and Prevention Chronic Kidney Disease Surveillance Team. Dietary acid load and chronic kidney disease among adults in the United States. *BMC Nephrol*. 2014;15:137.

[42] Ko BJ, Chang Y, Ryu S, Kim EM, Lee MY, Hyun YY, Lee K. Dietary acid load and chronic kidney disease in elderly adults: Protein and potassium intake. *PLoS One*. 2017;12(9):e0185069.

[43] Toba K, Hosojima M, Kabasawa H, Kuwahara S, Murayama T, Yamamoto-Kabasawa K, Kaseda R, Wada E, Watanabe R, Tanabe N, Suzuki Y, Narita I, Saito A. Higher estimated net endogenous acid production with lower intake of fruits and vegetables based on

a dietary survey is associated with the progression of chronic kidney disease. *BMC Nephrol.* 2019;20(1):421.

[44] Akter S, Eguchi M, Kurotani K, Kochi T, Pham NM, Ito R, Kuwahara K, Tsuruoka H, Mizoue T, Kabe I, Nanri A. High dietary acid load is associated with increased prevalence of hypertension: the Furukawa Nutrition and Health Study. *Nutrition.* 2015;31(2):298–303.

[45] Parohan M Sadeghi A, Nasiri M, Maleki V, Khodadost M, Pirouzi A, Sadeghi O. Dietary acid load and risk of hypertension: A systematic review and dose-response meta-analysis of observational studies. *Nutr Metab Cardiovasc Dis.* 2019;29(7):665–75.

[46] Abbasalizad Farhangi M, Nikniaz L, Nikniaz Z. Higher dietary acid load potentially increases serum triglyceride and obesity prevalence in adults: An updated systematic review and meta-analysis. *PLoS One.* 2019;14(5):e0216547.

[47] Krupp D, Johner SA, Kalhoff H, Buyken AE, Remer T. Long-term dietary potential renal acid load during adolescence is prospectively associated with indices of nonalcoholic fatty liver disease in young women. *J Nutr.* 2012;142(2):313–9.

[48] Mazidi M, Mikhailidis DP, Banach M. Higher dietary acid load is associated with higher likelihood of peripheral arterial disease among American adults. *J Diabetes Complications.* 2018;32(6):565–9.

[49] Akter S, Nanri A, Mizoue T, Noda M, Sawada N, Sasazuki S, Tsugane S; Japan Public Health Center–based Prospective Study Group. Dietary acid load and mortality among Japanese men and women: the Japan Public Health Center-based Prospective Study. *Am J Clin Nutr.* 2017;106(1):146–54.

[50] Costa-Vieira D, Monteiro R, Martins MJ. Metabolic Syndrome features: Is there a modulation role by mineral water consumption? A review. *Nutrients.* 2019;11(5):1141.

[51] Shi LW, Wu YL, Hu JJ, Yang PF, Sun WP, Gao J, Wang K, Peng Y, Wu JJ, Zhong GC. Dietary acid load and the risk of pancreatic

cancer: a prospective cohort study. *Cancer Epidemiol Biomarkers Prev*. 2021;30(5):1009–19.

[52] Jafari Nasab S, Rafiee P, Bahrami A, Rezaeimanesh N, Rashidkhani B, Sohrab G, Naja F, Hejazi E, Sadeghi A. Diet-dependent acid load and the risk of colorectal cancer and adenoma: a case-control study. *Public Health Nutr*. 2020;1–8.

[53] Cunha P, Paciência I, Cavaleiro Rufo J, Castro Mendes F, Farraia M, Barros R, Silva D, Delgado L, Padrão P, Moreira A, Moreira P. Dietary acid load: a novel nutritional target in overweight/obese children with asthma? *Nutrients*. 2019;11(9):2255.

[54] Lin PH, Ginty F, Appel LJ, Aickin M, Bohannon A, Garnero P, Barclay D, Svetkey LP. The dash diet and sodium reduction improve markers of bone turnover and calcium metabolism in adults. *J Nutr*. 2003;133(10):3130–6.

[55] Buhlmeier J, Harris C, Koletzko S, Lehmann I, Bauer CP, Schikowski T, von Berg A, Berdel D, Heinrich J, Hebebrand J, Focker M, Standl M, Libuda L. Dietary acid load and mental health outcomes in children and adolescents: results from the GINIplus and LISA birth cohort studies. *Nutrients*. 2018;10(5):582.

[56] Bullo M, Amigo-Correig P, Marquez-Sandoval F, Babio N, Martinez-Gonzalez MA, Estruch R, Basora J, Sola R, Salas-Salvado J. Mediterranean diet and high dietary acid load associated with mixed nuts: effect on bone metabolism in elderly subjects. *J Am Geriatr Soc*. 2009;57(10):1789–98.

[57] Thorpe MP, Evans EM. Dietary protein and bone health: harmonizing conflicting theories. *Nutr Rev*. 2011;69(4):215–30.

[58] Arnett TR. Extracellular pH regulates bone cell function. *J Nutr*. 2008;138(2):415S-8S.

[59] Quade BN, Parker MD, Occhipinti R. The therapeutic importance of acid-base balance. *Biochem Pharmacol*. 2021;183:114278.

[60] Bushinsky DA, Frick KK. The effects of acid on bone. *Curr Opin Nephrol Hypertens*. 2000;9(4):369–79.

[61] Wynn E, Raetz E, Burckhardt P. The composition of mineral waters sourced from Europe and North America in respect to bone health:

composition of mineral water optimal for bone. *Br J Nutr*. 2009;101(8):1195–9.

[62] Fenton TR, Tough SC, Lyon AW, Eliasziw M, Hanley DA. Causal assessment of dietary acid load and bone disease: a systematic review & meta-analysis applying Hill's epidemiologic criteria for causality. *Nutr J*. 2011;10:41.

[63] Jia T, Byberg L, Lindholm B, Larsson TE, Lind L, Michaelsson K, Carrero JJ. Dietary acid load, kidney function, osteoporosis, and risk of fractures in elderly men and women. *Osteoporos Int*. 2015;26(2):563–70.

[64] Buclin T, Cosma M, Appenzeller M, Jacquet AF, Decosterd LA, Biollaz J, Burckhardt P. Diet acids and alkalis influence calcium retention in bone. *Osteoporos Int*. 2001;12(6):493–9.

[65] Arnett T. Regulation of bone cell function by acid-base balance. *Proc Nutr Soc*. 2003;62(2):511–20.

[66] Geng W, Hill K, Zerwekh JE, Kohler T, Müller R, Moe OW. Inhibition of osteoclast formation and function by bicarbonate: Role of soluble adenylyl cyclase. *J Cell Physiol*. 2009;220(2):332–40.

[67] Hanley DA, Whiting SJ. Does a High Dietary Acid Content Cause Bone Loss, and Can Bone Loss Be Prevented With an Alkaline Diet? *J Clin Densitom*. 2013;16(4):420–5.

[68] New SA, MacDonald HM, Campbell MK, Martin JC, Garton MJ, Robins SP, Reid DM. Lower estimates of net endogenous non-carbonic acid production are positively associated with indexes of bone health in premenopausal and perimenopausal women. *Am J Clin Nutr*. 2004;79(1):131–8.

[69] Mangano KM, Walsh SJ, Kenny AM, Insogna KL, Kerstetter JE. Dietary acid load is associated with lower bone mineral density in men with low intake of dietary calcium. *J Bone Miner Res*. 2014;29(2):500–6.

[70] McLean RR, Qiao N, Broe KE, Tucker KL, Casey V, Cupples LA, Kiel DP, Hannan MT. Dietary acid load is not associated with lower bone mineral density except in older men. *J Nutr*. 2011;141(4):588–94.

[71] Bergqvist AGC, Schall JI, Stallings VA, Zemel BS. Progressive bone mineral content loss in children with intractable epilepsy treated with the ketogenic diet. *Am J Clin Nutr*. 2008;88(6):1678–84.

[72] Zwart SR, Rice BL, Dlouhy H, Shackelford LC, Heer M, Koslovsky MD, Smith SM. Dietary acid load and bone turnover during long-duration spaceflight and bed rest. *Am J Clin Nutr*. 2018;107(5):834–44.

[73] Cao JJ. High Dietary Protein Intake and Protein-Related Acid Load on Bone Health. *Curr Osteoporos Rep*. 2017;15(6):571–6.

[74] Rizzoli R, Biver E, Bonjour JP, Coxam V, Goltzman D, Kanis JA, Lappe J, Rejnmark L, Sahni S, Weaver C, Weiler H, Reginster JY. Benefits and safety of dietary protein for bone health-an expert consensus paper endorsed by the European Society for Clinical and Economical Aspects of Osteopororosis, Osteoarthritis, and Musculoskeletal Diseases and by the International Osteoporosis Foundation. *Osteoporos Int*. 2018;29(9):1933–48.

[75] Cao JJ, Johnson LK, Hunt JR. A diet high in meat protein and potential renal acid load increases fractional calcium absorption and urinary calcium excretion without affecting markers of bone resorption or formation in postmenopausal women. *J Nutr*. 2011;141(3):391–7.

[76] Hans D, Goertzen AL, Krieg MA, Leslie WD. Bone microarchitecture assessed by TBS predicts osteoporotic fractures independent of bone density: the Manitoba study. *J Bone Miner Res*. 2011;26(11):2762–9.

[77] Ilich JZ, Kerstetter JE. Nutrition in bone health revisited: a story beyond calcium. *J Am Coll Nutr*. 2000;19(6):715–37.

[78] Ilich JZ, Brownbill RA, Tamborini L, Crncevic-Orlic Z. To drink or not to drink: how are alcohol, caffeine and past smoking related to bone mineral density in elderly women? *J Am Coll Nutr*. 2002;21(6):536–44.

[79] Chang HC, Hsieh CF, Lin YC, Tantoh DM, Ko PC, Kung YY, Wang MC, Hsu SY, Liaw YC, Liaw YP. Does coffee drinking have

beneficial effects on bone health of Taiwanese adults? A longitudinal study. *BMC Public Health*. 2018;18(1):1273.

[80] Whisner CM, Castillo LF. Prebiotics, bone and mineral metabolism. *Calcif Tissue Int*. 2018;102(4):443–79.

[81] Wynn E, Krieg MA, Aeschlimann JM, Burckhardt P. Alkaline mineral water lowers bone resorption even in calcium sufficiency: Alkaline mineral water and bone metabolism. *Bone*. 2009;44(1):120–4.

[82] Wasserfurth P, Schneider I, Strohle A, Nebl J, Bitterlich N, Hahn A. Effects of mineral waters on acid-base status in healthy adults: results of a randomized trial. *Food Nutr Res*. 2019;63:eCollection 2019.

[83] Heil DP. Acid-base balance and hydration status following consumption of mineral-based alkaline bottled water. *J Int Soc Sports Nutr*. 2010;7:29.

[84] Wynn E, Krieg MA, Lanham-New SA, Burckhardt P. Postgraduate Symposium: Positive influence of nutritional alkalinity on bone health. *Proc Nutr Soc*. 2010;69(1):166–73.

[85] Buehlmeier J, Remer T, Frings-Meuthen P, Maser-Gluth C, Heer M. Glucocorticoid activity and metabolism with NaCl-induced low-grade metabolic acidosis and oral alkalization: results of two randomized controlled trials. *Endocrine*. 2016;52(1):139–47.

[86] Mousa HA. Health Effects of Alkaline Diet and Water, Reduction of Digestive-tract Bacterial Load, and Earthing. *Altern Ther Health Med*. 2016;22 (Suppl 1):24–33.

[87] Chycki J, Kurylas A, Maszczyk A, Golas A, Zajac A. Alkaline water improves exercise-induced metabolic acidosis and enhances anaerobic exercise performance in combat sport athletes. *PLoS One*. 2018;13(11):e0205708.

[88] Chycki J, Zając T, Maszczyk A, Kurylas A. The effect of mineral-based alkaline water on hydration status and the metabolic response to short-term anaerobic exercise. *Biol Sport*. 2017;34(3):255–61.

[89] Brancaccio P, Limongelli FM, Paolillo I, D'Aponte A, Donnarumma V, Rastrelli L. Supplementation of Acqua Lete® (Bicarbonate

Calcic Mineral Water) improves hydration status in athletes after short term anaerobic exercise. *J Int Soc Sports Nutr*. 2012;9(1):35.

[90] Presta V, Ambrosini L, Carubbi C, Masselli E, Mirandola P, Arcari ML, Gobbi G, Vitale M. Different Waters for Different Performances: Can We Imagine Sport-Related Natural Mineral Spring Waters? *Water*. 2021;13(2):166.

[91] Burckhardt P. The Effect of the Alkali Load of Mineral Water on Bone Metabolism: Interventional Studies. *J Nutr*. 2008;138(2):435S-7S.

[92] Costi D, Calcaterra PG, Iori N, Vourna S, Nappi G, Passeri M. Importance of bioavailable calcium drinking water for the maintenance of bone mass in post-menopausal women. *J Endocrinol Invest*. 1999;22(11):852–6.

[93] Aptel I, Cance-Rouzaud A, Grandjean H. Association between calcium ingested from drinking water and femoral bone density in elderly women: evidence from the EPIDOS cohort. *J Bone Miner Res*. 1999;14(5):829–33.

[94] Pereira C, Guede D, Durães C, Brandão I, Silva N, Passos E, Bernardes M, Monteiro R, Martins MJ. Differential Modulation of Cancellous and Cortical Distal Femur by Fructose and Natural Mineral-Rich Water Consumption in Ovariectomized Female Sprague Dawley Rats. *Nutrients*. 2019;11(10):2316.

[95] Cepollaro C, Orlandi G, Gonnelli S, Ferrucci G, Arditti JC, Borracelli D, Toti E, Gennari C. Effect of calcium supplementation as a high-calcium mineral water on bone loss in early postmenopausal women. *Calcif Tissue Int*. 1996;59(4):238–9.

[96] Maraver F, Michán A, Corvillo I, Aguilera L. Papel de las aguas minerales ricas en calcio en la osteoporosis. [Role of calcium-rich mineral waters in osteoporosis]. *Med Clin (Barc)*. 2011;137(13):619–20.

[97] Vannucci L, Fossi C, Quattrini S, Guasti L, Pampaloni B, Gronchi G, Giusti F, Romagnoli C, Cianferotti L, Marcucci G, Brandi ML. Calcium Intake in Bone Health: A Focus on Calcium-Rich Mineral Waters. *Nutrients*. 2018;10(12):1930.

[98] Roux S, Baudoin C, Boute D, Brazier M, De La Gueronniere V, De Vernejoul MC. Biological effects of drinking-water mineral composition on calcium balance and bone remodeling markers. *J Nutr Health Aging*. 2004;8(5):380–4.

[99] Guillemant J, Le HT, Accarie C, du Montcel ST, Delabroise AM, Arnaud MJ, Guillemant S. Mineral water as a source of dietary calcium: acute effects on parathyroid function and bone resorption in young men. *Am J Clin Nutr*. 2000;71(4):999–1002.

[100] Meunier PJ, Jenvrin C, Munoz F, de la Gueronnière V, Garnero P, Menz M. Consumption of a high calcium mineral water lowers biochemical indices of bone remodeling in postmenopausal women with low calcium intake. *Osteoporos Int*. 2005;16(10):1203–9.

[101] Burckhardt P. [Mineral waters and bone health]. *Rev Med Suisse Romande*. 2004;124(2):101–3.

[102] Guillemant J, Accarie C, Peres G, Guillemant S. Acute effects of an oral calcium load on markers of bone metabolism during endurance cycling exercise in male athletes. *Calcif Tissue Int*. 2004;74(5):407–14.

[103] Guillemant J, Accarie C, de la Guéronnière V, Guillemant S. Calcium in mineral water can effectively suppress parathyroid function and bone resorption. *Nutr Res*. 2002;22(8):901–10.

[104] Bacciottini L, Tanini A, Falchetti A, Masi L, Franceschelli F, Pampaloni B, Giorgi G, Brandi ML. Calcium bioavailability from a calcium-rich mineral water, with some observations on method. *J Clin Gastroenterol*. 2004;38(9):761–6.

[105] Heaney RP. Absorbability and utility of calcium in mineral waters. *Am J Clin Nutr*. 2006;84(2):371–4.

[106] Heaney RP, Dowell MS. Absorbability of the calcium in a high-calcium mineral water. *Osteoporos Int*. 1994;4(6):323–4.

[107] Quattrini S, Pampaloni B, Brandi ML. Natural mineral waters: chemical characteristics and health effects. *Clin Cases Miner Bone Metab*. 2016;13(3):173–80.

[108] Day RO, Liauw W, Tozer LM, McElduff P, Beckett RJ, Williams KM. A double-blind, placebo-controlled study of the short term

effects of a spring water supplemented with magnesium bicarbonate on acid/base balance, bone metabolism and cardiovascular risk factors in postmenopausal women. *BMC Res Notes*. 2010;3:180.

[109] Schoppen S, Pérez-Granados AM, Carbajal A, de la Piedra C, Pilar VM. Bone remodelling is not affected by consumption of a sodium-rich carbonated mineral water in healthy postmenopausal women. *Br J Nutr*. 2005;93(3):339–44.

[110] Schoppen S, Pérez-Granados AM, Carbajal A, Sarriá B, Navas-Carretero S, Vaquero MP. Sodium-bicarbonated mineral water decreases aldosterone levels without affecting urinary excretion of bone minerals. *Int J Food Sci Nutr*. 2008;59(4):347–55.

[111] Fatahi S, Namazi N, Larijani B, Azadbakht L. The association of dietary and urinary sodium with bone mineral density and risk of osteoporosis: a systematic review and meta-analysis. *J Am Coll Nutr*. 2018;37(6):522–32.

[112] Luft FC, Zemel MB, Sowers JA, Fineberg NS, Weinberger MH. Sodium bicarbonate and sodium chloride: effects on blood pressure and electrolyte homeostasis in normal and hypertensive man. *J Hypertens*. 1990;8(7):663–70.

[113] Rush GF, Willis LR. Renal tubular effects of sodium fluoride. *J Pharmacol Exp Ther*. 1982;223(2):275–9.

[114] Haguenauer D, Welch V, Shea B, Tugwell P, Wells G. Fluoride for treating postmenopausal osteoporosis. *Cochrane Database Syst Rev*. 2000;(4):CD002825.

[115] Riggs BL, Hodgson SF, O'Fallon WM, Chao EY, Wahner HW, Muhs JM, Cedel SL, Melton LJ 3rd. Effect of fluoride treatment on the fracture rate in postmenopausal women with osteoporosis. *N Engl J Med*. 1990;322(12):802–9.

[116] Levy SM, Warren JJ, Phipps K, Letuchy E, Broffitt B, Eichenberger-Gilmore J, Burns TL, Kavand G, Janz KF, Torner JC, Pauley CA. Effects of life-long fluoride intake on bone measures of adolescents: a prospective cohort study. *J Dent Res*. 2014;93(4):353–9.

[117] Thomas D. No association between water fluoridation and bone fractures. *Evid Based Dent*. 2002;3(2):45–6.

In: Mineral Water
Editors: Maria João Martins
ISBN: 978-1-68507-458-6

Chapter 6

Mineral Waters in Dermatology

Carmen Lisboa*[*], *MD, PhD
Department of Pathology, Microbiology Division,
Faculty of Medicine, University of Porto, Porto, Portugal
Department of Dermatology and Venereology,
São João University Hospital Centre, Porto, Portugal

Abstract

Natural mineral water has been recognized for over two centuries to have beneficial effects on skin. There is good understanding of the origin and physico-chemical profile of natural mineral water. Recently, an indigenous microbial population was identified in a specific natural mineral water which has pertinent beneficial dermatological effects. The use of natural mineral waters in Dermatology is mostly based on topical application, in a type of balneotherapy that employs bathing into natural mineral water. The beneficial effects of natural mineral waters are likely to involve (bio)chemical, aseptic, thermal, mechanical, immunological, and cell differentiation aspects. Although there is growing evidence supporting that natural mineral waters, including balneotherapy, are clinically effective in a variety of dermatological disorders, such as

[*] Corresponding Author's E-mail: carlis@med.up.pt.

atopic dermatitis, psoriasis, eczema, seborrheic dermatiotis, ichthyosis, burns sequelae, or sensitive skin, there is still a lack of knowledge on all the diversity of the mechanisms of effectiveness. It is worth noting the growing tendency to use natural mineral waters in Cosmetology, in the form of sprays or vehiculated in dermatological formulations. Nowadays, there has been a worldwide reawakening to the use of natural mineral waters as part of the treatment of chronic inflammatory skin diseases or of the healing process after cosmetic procedures.

Keywords: balneotherapy, cosmetics, dermatology, natural mineral water, skin disease, therapeutic use, thermal water

INTRODUCTION

Natural mineral water refers to water of underground origin emerging from springs or wells. Formed under specific geological conditions, natural mineral water has three fundamental features: it is characterized by its mineral content, trace elements or other constituents, it is bacteriologically pure and has therapeutic potential. The bacteriological purity refers to absence of pathogenic microorganisms that contaminate the water and cause infectious diseases [1] (further detailed in the first chapter of this book, *Natural Mineral Waters: Concept and Classifications*). In fact, recent studies conveyed the importance of some microorganisms present in natural mineral waters that show pertinent beneficial dermatological effects. As an example, *Aquaphilus dolomiae* sounds to be one of the reasons that could explain the benefit in the treatment of inflammatory skin diseases with the unique natural mineral water in which it is found [2-7]. Therefore, in addition to the physico-chemical properties so emphasized previously, each water seems to have a biological identity that contributes to the therapeutic effects on diseases [8]. A fourth characteristic of natural mineral water is the stability of the physicochemical particularities from the source to human exploitation [9]. Nowadays, there is an increasing tendency to study natural mineral waters as a dynamic biological unit [8].

The use of natural mineral waters in Dermatology is mostly based on topical application, in a type of balneotherapy that employs bathing into natural mineral water. Balneophototherapy is a sort of therapy that combines natural mineral water baths with natural or artificial ultraviolet (UV) radiation to provide a synergistic effect [10, 11].

Other treatments utilising natural mineral waters just reemerged, the thermal muds and the pelotherapy, that is application of a peloma (mud with natural mineral water) coupled with heat and humidity. A recent trend is the usage of natural mineral waters in cosmetics in order to obtain "natural" products and effective cosmeceuticals against skin exposome [12].

The use of natural mineral waters, namely thermal waters, by drinking to manage skin conditions will not be addressed in this work. The mechanisms of action are poorly understood, and more studies are needed.

Thalassotherapy, the treatment using sea bathing or exposure to sea air [10], will be occasionally referred to in the text.

Historical Aspects of the Use of Mineral Waters in Dermatology

Although the use of natural springs and public baths was known for centuries, it was in the 1800s that balneotherapy for the management of skin disorders emerged as an important treatment modality, first in Europe and later in the United States of America [13, 14].

Back to the Greek civilization, Hippocrates (460-370 BC) believed that baths could have a strong influence over the humors. Later, Asclepiades (c.124 BC) introduced bathing both as therapeutic and as preventive interventions [13]. Later, the use of water, in baths, springs and thermae as treatment centers, flourished during the Roman Empire. The Roman baths, largely developed all over the Europe, were abandoned with the rise of Christianity until the 16th and 17th centuries. At that time, some physicians directed their attention toward balneotherapy, first in Italy and then England and across other European countries [15, 16]. Well ahead, in the 18th and 19th centuries, the development of resorts and Spas became prevalent both in Europe and in North America. The dermatologists were pioneer in including natural mineral waters in their armamentaria [15].

From the middle of the last century, Europe experienced a decline in the use of natural mineral waters as therapy, including balneotherapy, especially as new and effective pharmacological agents became available. In some European countries, Health Minister halted insurance reimbursement for the treatments, and consequently the use of Spas drastically declined [17].

In the last decades, there has been a resurgence of interest in natural mineral waters, including balneotherapy, as "natural" and complementary therapy to pharmacological agents. Research on the effects of natural mineral waters in skin has been fruitful and numerous scientific papers have been published.

Nowadays, balneotherapy and balneophototherapy have garnered support in the medical community.

Mineral Waters and Balneotherapy in Dermatology

Natural mineral waters, thermal waters, recommended for skin diseases vary in physical and chemical characteristics. Sulphur-rich waters, sulphur being present as a free or combined ion, are particularly used to treat dermatological conditions. Nevertheless, other mineral waters containing other minerals, such as silicate, calcium, selenium, magnesium and/or zinc, are claimed to be efficacious on skin diseases [1].

Table 1 describes mineral characteristics, namely biological effects and therapeutic uses, as well as mineral deficiency and toxicity disorders.

Table 1. Mineral characteristics: biological effects and therapeutic uses. Mineral deficiency and toxicity disorders

Mineral	Biological effects/ Therapeutic uses	Mineral Deficiency	Toxicity disorders
Aluminium	Acute dermatitis		Encephalopathy, Osteomalacia
Arsenic	Psoriasis		Arsenical keratoses
Boron	Cellular renewal; Wound healing		
Calcium	Regulation of epidermal cell growth; Anti-inflammatory action	Dermatitis	Renal calculi
Copper	Antioxidant; Skin barrier recovery		
Iron (chalybeate)	Hypochromic microcytic anaemia	Koilonychia; Nonscarring alopecia; Hypomelanosis of hair	Hemochromatosis
Lithium	Bipolar affective disorders		Psoriasis; Acne
Magnesium	Acute dermatitis; Cellular renewal; Eclampsia		
Manganese	Cellular renewal; Wound healing; Recovery of skin barrier		
Selenium	Seborrheic dermatitis; Tinea versicolor; Antioxidant action; Protection against UVB	Koilonychia; Hypomelanosis of skin and hair	Alopecia; Paronychia; Red discoloration of hair, nail and teeth

Table 1. (Continued)

Mineral	Biological effects/ Therapeutic uses	Mineral Deficiency	Toxicity disorders
Sodium chloride	Hydration of keratin layer in hyperkeratotic disorders		Hypernatremia
Sulphur	Anti-inflammatory action; Anti-infective action in some skin conditions		
Zinc	Antioxidant; Cellular turnover; Immunomodulation		

Adapted from [10, 16].

Inflammatory and Immunological Aspects

The anti-inflammatory and immunomodulatory activities of natural mineral waters have been evaluated both *in vitro* and *in vivo* studies. Natural mineral waters have been successfully used in immune-mediated skin conditions, including psoriasis, atopic dermatitis and contact dermatitis.

Application of sulphur-rich natural mineral waters on the skin has local immunomodulating effects, possibly related to the modification of a) the activity of functional subsets of T lymphocytes and b) the synthesis and/or release of certain cytokines in the skin [18-20].

Avène® thermal water (France), with high concentration of calcium bicarbonate and silicium, reduces cutaneous basophil degranulation in atopic patients [20]. *In vitro*, Avène® thermal water a) inhibits the histamine release induced in mast cells by substance P [21], and b) reduces vasoactive intestinal peptide-induced inflammation in surviving human skin fragments by decreasing tumour necrosis factor-α, percentage and surface of dilated vessels as well as oedema [22].

On the other hand, *in vitro*, La Roche-Posay® thermal water, characterized by a high concentration of selenium along with calcium bicarbonate, silicium, zinc and copper, a) seems to have a suppressive activity on the cytokine production of epidermal Langerhans cells [20], and b) inhibits migration of Langerhans cells [23].

Clinical improvements in subjects with sensitive skin, namely in erythema, itch, scaling and burning, by applying Avène® thermal water have been shown [20]. The ability of the same and other thermal waters to improve skin irritation has been further documented, both in experimental and clinical studies [24-26].

Very recently, *Aquaphilus dolomiae*, a micro-organism present in Avène® thermal water and never described in another medium, was identified. *In vitro*, *Aquaphilus dolomiae* is responsible for significant beneficial pharmacological activities upon inflammation [inhibits/attenuates thymic stromal lymphopoietin, interleukin (IL)-18, IL-4R, monocyte chemoattractant protein-3, macrophage inflammatory protein-3α and macrophage-derived chemokine expression as well as T helper type (Th) 1, Th2, and Th17 cytokine production and protease-activated receptor-2 activation (different results have been found for IL-8)] and innate immunity [activates toll-like receptor (TLR) 2, TLR4 and TLR5 and increases psoriasin, β-defensin-2, cathelicidin and S100 calcium binding protein A7 (antimicrobial peptides and proteins) expression] [3-5, 7].

Free Radical Aspects

Free radicals are implicated in cellular ageing and death as well as cancer development and progression. Some studies have demonstrated that natural mineral waters are effective in reinforcing the defence system against free radicals.

An *in vitro* study showed the antioxidant activity of spring water from La Roche-Posay® in human cutaneous diploid fibroblasts exposed to UVA radiation through the beneficial modulation of lipid peroxidation levels (and lethality) [27]. On the other hand, an *in vivo* study, in the mouse skin, documented the antioxidant and protective effect against lipid peroxidation and skin carcinogenesis induced by UVB radiation afforded by the percutaneous diffusion of La Roche-Posay® thermal water [20]. A human study reported an *in vitro* and *in vivo* increase of corneocyte catalase activity with Vichy® thermal water (very high total mineral content, with high level of carbonates; France) [28]. An *in vitro* protocol with normal human keratinocytes and skin explants disclosed the benefits of the antioxidant properties of Uriage-les-Bains® thermal water (rich in chloride, sulphate and sodium, with other minerals; France), through both *per se* antioxidant activities and increase of catalase activity, by emphasising its DNA protective role against UVB radiation in addition to the tumour suppressor claudin-6 protective role against UVA+UVB radiations [29]. A further human study looked at any influence on the antioxidant system of therapeutic baths using two distinct natural mineral waters (one alkali-chloridic-hydrogen-carbonic and the other slightly iodine-alkali-hydrogen-carbonic; both Hungarian) and it was found that both waters have a beneficial effect on the formation of free radicals as they decrease circulating malondialdehyde levels and catalase, superoxide dismutase and glutathione peroxidase activity values [30].

Effect on Beta-Endorphins Levels

Beta-endorphins are purported to act as immunosuppressive agents. Increased levels of circulating beta-endorphins levels after mud baths and thermal bath therapy have been reported [20].

It has been hypothesized that some stimuli, such as UV radiation or heat, could induce the release of opioid peptides, influencing the pain threshold and cutaneous/plasma neuro-endocrine systems. The endogenous neuropeptides seem to have an immunosuppressive effect by decreasing lymphocytes and natural killer cell proliferation [31, 32]. Some studies aimed to address the placebo effect of balneotherapy. The heat from thermal baths in balneotherapy must be taken into account while assessing their therapeutic effects [33]. Balneotherapy is experienced as pleasant and has a very positive effect removing stress and ameliorating quality of life.

Antibacterial and Antifungal Effects

Sulphur-rich waters have antibacterial and antifungal properties. The antimicrobial activity may be related to pentationic acid ($H_2S_5O_6$), a compound that results from the interaction of sulphur with oxygen radicals in the deeper layers of the epidermis [1, 34]. This activity may explain some degree of effectiveness on infected leg ulcers, tinea versicolor, tinea corporis and tinea capitis. Further studies described an effect of natural mineral waters on *Staphylococcus aureus* colonization [11, 35]. Additionally, senile and chronic forms of pruritus usually induce scratches and patients might benefit from the antiseptic properties of certain waters [1].

Cellular Renewal and Healing of Wounds

According to published data, natural mineral waters rich in some specific elements, such as boron, manganese, copper and zinc, stimulate the migration of keratinocytes and the proliferation of keratinocytes [36-38]. These effects could be implicated in cellular renewal, healing of wounds and recovery of cutaneous barrier. Additionally, modulation of proteins involved in skin barrier function (namely increased involucrin expression and restored filaggrin expression) by *Aquaphilus dolomiae* has been published [4, 7].

Therapeutic Uses

Many skin diseases have been managed using balneology, either solely or as an adjunct to more specific pharmacological treatments. Although the therapeutic properties are not completely understood, it is known that balneotherapy is effective in the treatment of psoriasis and atopic dermatitis. Other dermatological conditions can also be treated by balneotherapy, such as vitiligo, ichthyosis linearis circumflexa, *acne vulgaris*, contact dermatitis, seborrheic dermatitis, chronic wounds, radiation dermatitis, mycosis fungoides and epidermolysis bullosa [11].

Unfortunately, there are no standardized balneotherapy regimens for treating dermatological diseases and each institution uses its own treatment protocol.

Psoriasis

Psoriasis is a chronic immune mediated disorder largely managed using balneology, thalassotherapy and pelotherapy. A study by Pinton *et al.* disclosed a strong reduction of the Psoriasis Area Severity Index (PASI) in patients with moderate *psoriasis vulgaris* after 3 weeks of balneotherapy with La Roche-Posay® thermal water [39]. A few years after this study, two randomised controlled trials with sodium-rich, magnesiac, calcic, sulphate-rich and chloride-rich (France) or arsenical-ferruginous (with high concentration of iron and sulphate, and relevant concentration of arsenic, calcium and magnesium; Italy) natural mineral waters documented a modest or strong effect, respectively, upon psoriasis [40, 41]. Interestingly, in the former randomised intervention, the therapeutic activity was enhanced by combining the natural mineral water with UVB [40]. Balneophototherapy, the balneotherapy combined with phototherapy, further boosts the anti-inflammatory effects of natural mineral waters. Phototherapy may be administered simultaneously or after immersion on natural mineral water [42].

The Dead Sea, in Israel, and Jordan and the Blue Lagoon, in Iceland, are very popular treatment sites for psoriatic patients. The Dead Sea and the Blue Lagoon are peculiar geothermal spots that combined various qualities, namely atmospheric, solar, chemical, thermal, and contain bioactive materials (microorganisms and *algae*) that contribute to the therapeutic effect on psoriasis [43-45].

On the other hand, other studies evaluated the effect of regular saltwater bath in the treatment of psoriasis and reported clinical improvement [46, 47]. The prospective double-blind controlled study by Halevy *et al.* reported no relevant differences between a heated Dead Sea water and regular saltwater bath on psoriasis [46].

It is difficult to extrapolate efficacy of balneotherapy on psoriasis with diverse study designs, various treatment regimens and different hydrogeologic sources of natural mineral waters without randomised placebo-controlled trials.

Nowadays, psoriasis is one of the most frequent skin diseases managed by balneotherapy by its effect on skin inflammation and pruritus [48, 49].

Atopic Dermatitis

Atopic dermatitis management by balneotherapy aims to decrease skin inflammation, reduce colonization of *Staphylococcus aureus* and increase the moisture content of the skin [11, 35]. Children represent an important part of the patients suffering from atopic dermatitis that use balneotherapy as an adjuvant management of skin inflammation, xerosis and pruritus [5].

By the use of a murine model of atopic dermatitis, it has been demonstrated that bathing in natural mineral water had anti-inflammatory activity decreasing Th2 cell differentiation and IL-4 production and had a positive effect on cutaneous barrier homeostasis [50].

In an observational study with atopic dermatitis patients, a significant improvement of Eczema Area and Severity Index scores and Dermatology Life Quality Index was found after balneotherapy [51].

In line, and interestingly, *Aquaphilus dolomiae* has been found beneficial in the management of xerosis and pruritus [52, 53].

Nonetheless, we need randomised placebo-controlled trials with high methodological quality to confirm these results.

Burns

Inflammatory and hypertrophic scars complicating burns are efficiently managed with natural mineral water interventions [54]. Balneotherapy is a treatment option early in the cicatrisation process or later, when scars are already stablished for functional rehabilitation [55, 56]. It could be hypothesized that anti-inflammatory and immunomodulatory aspects would contribute for the beneficial effects on burns sequelae. Balneotherapy is usually used as complementary therapy [54].

Cancer

More recently balneotherapy has a new indication for management of persistent dermatologic adverse events after surgery, chemotherapy and/or radiotherapy to treat breast cancer. Balneotherapy has shown effects on scars, radiodermatitis, xerosis secondary to chemotherapy [57]. Balneotherapy seems to be an effective supportive care for skin adverse events after breast cancer treatment in patients in complete remission after standard treatment [57, 58].

Other Skin Disorders

Different Spa therapies have been used as treatment or adjuvant treatment of a number of other (and unrelated) skin disorders, such as ichthyosis [59], seborrheic dermatitis [60], acne, vitiligo, contact dermatitis, chronic wounds and epidermolysis bullosa [11].

MINERAL WATERS AND COSMETICS

Natural mineral waters play an important role in dermatological approach through its moisturising and cleaning proprieties [19]; their role is increasing as a vehicle in cosmeceuticals [61]. The stability and influence of natural mineral waters, and their oligo-elements in dermo-cosmetic formulations, have been evaluated [62]. Natural mineral waters can be easily used in the form of sprays or vehiculated in dermatological formulations, such as moisturizers and sunscreens [12]. Natural mineral waters, in natura or dispensed in products, have been indicated as adjuvant in treatments of aging skin, rosacea, acne and other dermatoses [34, 62]. For example, sulphur-rich natural mineral waters can be useful to remove excess sebium in oily and mixed skin types and to treat light acne [34]. Additionally, natural mineral waters seem to be useful after cosmetic procedures, such as chemical peels and laser therapy [63, 64].

Reviewing the role of mineralising thermal water combined with hyaluronic acid in a gel texture in improving the skin barrier function against the effects of exposome factors showed that this combined product has a positive effect on skin aging exposome [65]. The skin exposome refers to the numerous external exposures that contribute to cutaneous aging, including solar radiation, air pollution, tobacco smoking, nutrition, stress, sleep deprivation and cosmetic products [66].

CONCLUSION

The benefits of natural mineral waters in Dermatology have been recognized for centuries. In fact, the pioneer dermatologists included natural mineral waters in their armamentaria. Natural mineral waters are dynamic biological units and, in the last decades, we have progressed from empirical usage to scientific studies, experimental and clinical ones, which demonstrate their benefits on a number of skin disorders. There is a trend to use natural mineral waters, namely in balneotherapy, as a complement to conventional pharmacological treatment. Patients' quality of life is improved. The use of natural mineral waters in Cosmetology is a recent tendency with encouraging results.

Yet, there are still a limited number of randomised double-blind controlled studies to demonstrate definitely the role of balneotherapy (therapeutic, preventive, or just as adjuvant to other treatments) in chronic skin diseases. Additionally, the optimal concentrations of minerals and the adequate regimens are still lacking. The cellular and molecular mechanisms underlying the benefits of external application of natural mineral waters on the skin are not completely elucidated. We must emphasize that this treatment modality would receive much more support if its benefits were objectively assessed.

REFERENCES

[1] Matz H, Orion E, Wolf R. Balneotherapy in dermatology. *Dermatol Ther*. 2003;16(2):132-40.

[2] Bourrain M, Villette C, Nguyen T, Lebaron P. *Aquaphilus dolomiae* Gen.Nov., Sp. Nov., isolated from a deeper aquifer. Vie et milieu - *Life and environment*. 2012;62(4):191-5.

[3] Aries MF, Duplan H, Hernandez-Pigeon H, Galliano M, Castex-Rizzi N, Bessou-Touya S, Nguyen T. I-modulia, an Aquaphilus dolomiae extract, stimulates innate immune response through Toll-like receptor activation. *J Am Acad Dermatol.* 2014;70(5 Suppl 1):AB63.

[4] Aries MF, Hernandez-Pigeon H, Vaissière C, Delga H, Caruana A, Lévêque M, Bourrain M, Ravard Helffer K, Chol B, Nguyen T, Bessou-Touya S, Castex-Rizzi N. Anti-inflammatory and

immunomodulatory effects of *Aquaphilus dolomiae* extract on *in vitro* models. *Clin Cosmet Investig Dermatol.* 2016;9:421-34.

[5] Guerrero D, Garrigue E. Eau thermale d'Avène et dermatite atopique. [Avène's thermal water and atopic dermatitis]. *Ann Dermatol Venereol.* 2017;144(Suppl 1):S27-S34.

[6] Zeichner J, Seite S. From Probiotic to Prebiotic Using Thermal Spring Water. *J Drugs Dermatol.* 2018;17(6):657-662.

[7] Galliano MF, Bäsler K, Caruana A, Mias C, Bessou-Touya S, Brandner JM, Duplan H. Protective effect of *Aquaphilus dolomiae* extract-G1, ADE-G1, on tight junction barrier function in a *Staphylococcus aureus*-infected atopic dermatitis model. *J Eur Acad. Dermatol Venereol.* 2020;34(Suppl 5):30-6.

[8] Lebaron P. Les eaux thermales: quand minéralité et signature biologique se combinent pour expliquer leurs propriétés. [Thermal waters: when minerality and biological signature combine to explain their properties]. *Ann Dermatol Venereol.* 2020;147(1s):1s20-1s24.

[9] Faílde RM, Mosqueira LM. *Afecciones dermatológicas y cosmética dermotermal. Técnicas y tecnologías en hidrología médica e hidroterapia.* [*Dermatological conditions and dermothermal cosmetics. Techniques and technologies in medical hydrology and hydrotherapy*]. Madrid: Agencia de evaluación de tecnologías sanitarias. [Madrid: Health Technology Assessment Agency]; 2006.

[10] Routh HB, Bhowmik KR. Basic tenets of mineral water. *Clin Dermatol.* 1996;14:549-50.

[11] Huang A, Seité S, Adar T. The use of balneotherapy in dermatology. *Clin Dermatol.* 2018;36(3):363-8.

[12] Seite S. Thermal waters as cosmeceuticals: La Roche-Posay thermal spring water example. *Clin Cosmet Investig Dermatol.* 2013;6:23-8.

[13] Jackson R. Waters and spas in the classical world. *Med Hist Suppl.* 1990(10):1-13.

[14] Benedetto AV, Millikan LE. Mineral water and spas in the United States. *Clin Dermatol.* 1996;14(6):583-600.

[15] Routh HB, Bhowmik KR, Parish LC, Witkowski JA. Balneology, mineral water, and spas in historical perspective. *Clin Dermatol.* 1996;14(6):551-4.

[16] Nunes S, Tamura SM. A historical review of mineral water. *Surg Cosmet Dermatol.* 2012;4:252-8.

[17] Gambichler T. Balneophototherapy for psoriasis using saltwater baths and UV-B irradiation, revisited. *Arch Dermatol.* 2007;143(5):647-9.

[18] Valitutti S, Castellino F, Musiani P. Effect of sulfurous (thermal) water on T lymphocyte proliferative response. *Ann Allergy.* 1990;65(6):463-8.

[19] Lotti TM, Ghersetich I. Mineral waters: instead of soap or better than soap? *Clin Dermatol.* 1996;14(1):101-4.

[20] Ghersetich I, Freedman D, Lotti T. Balneology today. *J Eur Acad Dermatol Venereol.* 2000;14(5):346-8.

[21] Joly F, Galoppin L, Bordat P, Cousse H, Neuzil E. Calcium and bicarbonate ions mediate the inhibition of mast cell histamine release by Avène spa water. *Fundam Clin Pharmacol.* 2000;14(6):611-3.

[22] Boisnic S, Branchet-Gumila MC, Segard C. Inhibitory effect of Avene spring water on vasoactive intestinal peptide-induced inflammation in surviving human skin. *Int J Tissue React.* 2001; 23(3):89-95.

[23] Staquet MJ, Peguet-Navarro J, Richard A, Schmitt D, Rougier A. *In vitro* effect of a spa water on the migratory and stimulatory capacities of human Langerhans cells. *Eur J Dermatol.* 2002;12(4):LIX-LXI.

[24] Ferreira MO, Costa PC, Bahia MF. Effect of São Pedro do Sul thermal water on skin irritation. *Int J Cosmet Sci.* 2010;32(3):205-10.

[25] Mias C, Maret A, Gontier E, Carrasco C, Satge C, Bessou-Touya S, Coubetergues H, Bennett-Kennett R, Dauskardt RH, Duplan H. Protective properties of Avène Thermal Spring Water on biomechanical, ultrastructural and clinical parameters of human skin. *J Eur Acad Dermatol Venereol.* 2020;34 (Suppl 5):15-20.

[26] Silva A, Oliveira AS, Vaz CV, Correia S, Ferreira R, Breitenfeld L, Martinez-de-Oliveira J, Palmeira-de-Oliveira R, Pereira CMF, Palmeira-de-Oliveira A, Cruz MT. Anti-inflammatory potential of Portuguese thermal waters. *Sci Rep.* 2020;10(1):22313.

[27] Moysan A, Morlière P, Marquis I, Richard A, Dubertret L. Effects of selenium on UVA-induced lipid peroxidation in cultured human skin fibroblasts. *Skin Pharmacol.* 1995;8(3):139-48.

[28] Bruneau F, Bernard D, Ragueneau N, Montastier C. Effect of Vichy water on catalase activity in the stratum corneum. *Int J Cosmet Sci.* 1996;18(6):269-77.

[29] Joly F, Branka J, Lefeuvre L. Thermal Water from Uriage-les-Bains Exerts DNA Protection, Induction of Catalase Activity and Claudin-6 Expression on UV Irradiated Human Skin in Addition to Its Own Antioxidant Properties. *J Cosmet Dermatol Sci Appl.* 2014;4:99-106.

[30] Bender T, Bariska J, Vághy R, Gomez R, Imre K. Effect of balneotherapy on the antioxidant system--a controlled pilot study. *Arch Med Res.* 2007;38(1):86-9.

[31] Nissen J B, Avrach WW, Hansen ES, Stengaard-Pedersen K, Kragballe K. Increased levels of enkephalin following natural sunlight (combined with salt water bathing at the Dead Sea) and ultraviolet A irradiation. *Br J Dermatol.* 1998;139(6):1012-9.

[32] Sacerdote P, Gaspani L, Panerai AE. Role of beta-endorphin in the modulation of immune responses: perspectives in autoimmune diseases. *Adv Exp Med Biol.* 2001;493:137-42.

[33] Ghersetich I, Lotti TM. Immunologic aspects: immunology of mineral water spas. *Clin Dermatol.* 1996;14(6):563-6.

[34] Ghersetich I, Brazzini B, Hercogova J, Lotti TM. Mineral waters: instead of cosmetics or better than cosmetics? *Clin Dermatol.* 2001;19(4):478-82.

[35] Inoue T, Inoue S, Kubota K. Bactericidal activity of manganese and iodide ions against *Staphylococcus aureus*: a possible treatment for acute atopic dermatitis. *Acta Derm Venereol.* 1999;79(5):360-2.

[36] Dreno B. Oligoelements et peau. [Trace elements and skin]. *Dermatol Pratique.* [*Practical Dermatol*]. 1996; 182(1):1-3.

[37] Tenaud I, Leroy S, Chebassier N, Dreno B. Zinc, copper and manganese enhanced keratinocyte migration through a functional modulation of keratinocyte integrins. *Exp Dermatol.* 2000;9(6):407-16.

[38] Chebassier N, Ouijja el H, Viegas I, Dreno B. Stimulatory effect of boron and manganese salts on keratinocyte migration. *Acta Derm Venereol.* 2004;84(3):191-4.

[39] Pinton J, Fridén H, Kettaneh-Wold N, Wold S, Dreno B, Richard A, Bieber T. Clinical and biological effects of balneotherapy with selenium-rich spa water in patients with *psoriasis vulgaris. Br J Dermatol.* 1995;133(2):344-7.

[40] Léauté-Labrèze C, Saillour F, Chêne G, Cazenave C, Luxey-Bellocq ML, Sanciaume C, Toussaint JF, Taïeb A. Saline spa water or combined water and UV-B for psoriasis vs conventional UV-B: lessons from the Salies de Béarn randomized study. *Arch Dermatol.* 2001;137(8):1035-9.

[41] Borroni G, Brazzelli V, Fornara L, Rosso R, Paulli M, Tinelli C, Ciocca O. Clinical, pathological and immunohistochemical effects of arsenical-ferruginous spa waters on mild-to-moderate psoriatic lesions: a randomized placebo-controlled study. *Int J Immunopathol Pharmacol.* 2013;26(2):495-501.

[42] Gambichler T, Küster W, Kreuter A, Altmeyer P, Hoffmann K. Balneophototherapy-combined treatment of *psoriasis vulgaris* and atopic dermatitis with salt water baths and artificial ultraviolet radiation. *J Eur Acad Dermatol Venereol.* 2000;14(5):425-8.

[43] Abels DJ, Rose T, Bearman JE. Treatment of psoriasis at a Dead Sea dermatology clinic. *Int J Dermatol.* 1995;34(2):134-7.

[44] Olafsson JH. The Blue Lagoon in Iceland and psoriasis. *Clin Dermatol.* 1996;14(6):647-51.

[45] Halevy S, Giryes H, Friger M, Grossman N, Karpas Z, Sarov B, Sukenik S. The role of trace elements in psoriatic patients undergoing balneotherapy with Dead Sea bath salt. *Isr Med Assoc J.* 2001;3(11):828-32.

[46] Halevy S, Giryes H, Friger M, Sukenik S. Dead sea bath salt for the treatment of *psoriasis vulgaris*: a double-blind controlled study. *J Eur Acad Dermatol Venereol.* 1997;9(3):237-42.

[47] Gambichler T, Demetriou C, Terras S, Bechara F G, Skrygan M. The impact of salt water soaks on biophysical and molecular parameters in psoriatic epidermis equivalents. *Dermatology.* 2011;223(3):230-8.

[48] Merial-Kieny C, Mengual X, Guerrero D, Sibaud V. Clinical efficacy of Avène hydrotherapy measured in a large cohort of more than 10,000 atopic or psoriatic patients. *J Eur Acad Dermatol Venereol.* 2011;25(Suppl 1):30-4.

[49] Placintescu D. Cure thermale et prise en charge du prurit dans le psoriasis. [Thermal cure and management of pruritus in psoriasis]. *Ann Dermatol Venereol.* 2020;147(1s):1s28-1s32.

[50] Choi YJ, Lee HJ, Lee DH, Woo SY, Lee KH, Yun ST, Kim JM, Kim HJ, Kim JW. Therapeutic effects and immunomodulation of suanbo mineral water therapy in a murine model of atopic dermatitis. *Ann Dermatol.* 2013;25(4):462-70.

[51] Dikova A, Jeliaskoff A, Seite S. An observational study on patients suffering from atopic dermatitis undergoing balneotherapy. *J Am Acad Dermatol.* 2016;76(6 S1):AB41.

[52] Fostini AC, Georgescu V, Decoster CJ, Girolomoni G. A cream based on *Aquaphilus dolomiae* extracts alleviates non-histaminergic pruritus in humans. *Eur J Dermatol.* 2017;27(3):317-318.

[53] Deleuran M, Georgescu V, Jean-Decoster C. An emollient containing *Aquaphilus dolomiae* extract is effective in the management of xerosis and pruritus: An international, real-world study. *Dermatol Ther (Heidelb).* 2020;10(5):1013-1029.

[54] Guerrero D. Cure thermale et séquelles de brûlures. [Thermal cures and sequelae of burns]. *Ann Dermatol Venereol.* 2020;147 (1s):1s33-1s36.

[55] Rochet JM, Zaoui A. [Burn scars: rehabilitation and skin care]. *Rev Prat.* 2002;52(20):2258-63.

[56] Hess CL, Howard MA, Attinger CE. A review of mechanical adjuncts in wound healing: hydrotherapy, ultrasound, negative pressure therapy, hyperbaric oxygen, and electrostimulation. *Ann Plast Surg.* 2003;51(2):210-8.

[57] Dalenc F, Ribet V, Rossi AB, Guyonnaud J, Bernard-Marty C, de Lafontan B, Salas S, Ranc Royo AL, Sarda C, Levasseur N, Massabeau C, Levecq JM, Dulguerova P, Guerrero D, Sibaud V. Efficacy of a global supportive skin care programme with hydrotherapy after non-metastatic breast cancer treatment: A randomised, controlled study. *Eur J Cancer Care (Engl).* 2018;27(1):e12735.

[58] Kwiatkowski F, Mouret-Reynier MA, Duclos M, Leger-Enreille A, Bridon F, Hahn T, Van Praagh-Doreau I, Travade A, Gironde M, Bézy O, Lecadet J, Vasson MP, Jouvency S, Cardinaud S, Roques CF, Bignon YJ. Long term improved quality of life by a 2-week group physical and educational intervention shortly after breast cancer chemotherapy completion. Results of the 'Programme of Accompanying women after breast Cancer treatment completion in Thermal resorts' (PACThe) randomised clinical trial of 251 patients. *Eur J Cancer.* 2013;49(7):1530-8.

[59] Bodemer C, Bourrat E, Mazereeuw-Hautier J, Boralevi F, Barbarot S, Bessis D, Blanchet-Bardon C, Bourdon-Lanoy E, Stalder JF, Ribet V, Guerrero D, Sibaud V. Short- and medium-term efficacy of specific hydrotherapy in inherited ichthyosis. *Br J Dermatol.* 2011;165(5):1087-94.

[60] Comacchi C, Hercogova J. A single mud treatment induces normalization of stratum corneum hydration, transepidermal water loss, skin surface pH and sebum content in patients with seborrhoeic dermatitis. *J Eur Acad Dermatol Venereol.* 2004;18(3):372-4.

[61] Bernstein JE. Dermatologic aspects of mineral water. *Clin Dermatol.* 1996;14(6):567-9.

[62] Segura JH, Camargo Junior FB, Bagatin E, Campos M. Influência da água termal e de seus oligoelementos na estabilidade e eficácia de formulações dermocosméticas. [Influence of thermal water and its

oligoelements in the stability and efficacy of dermocosmetics formulations]. *Surg Cosmet Dermatol.* 2010;2(1):11-7.

[63] Draelos ZD, Ertel KD, Berge CA. Facilitating facial retinization through barrier improvement. *Cutis.* 2006;78(4):275-81.

[64] Tan J, Spada J, Orlandi C, Kerscher M, Anfilova M, Abdulla S, Floriánová A, Preisz K, Altmayer A, Delva C, Kerob D, Goldobina M, Arenbergerová M, Tuz S, Araviiskaia E. Vichy mineralizing water with hyaluronic acid is effective and well tolerated as an adjunct to the management of various dermatoses and after esthetic procedures. *J Cosmet Dermatol.* 2020;19(3):682-8.

[65] Salsberg J, Andriessen A, Abdulla S, Ahluwalia R, Beecker J, Sander M, Schachter J. A review of protection against exposome factors impacting facial skin barrier function with 89% mineralizing thermal water. *J Cosmet Dermatol.* 2019;18(3):815-820.

[66] Wild CP. The exposome: from concept to utility. *Int J Epidemiol.* 2012;41(1):24-32.

In: Mineral Water
Editors: Maria João Martins
ISBN: 978-1-68507-458-6

Chapter 7

WATER - A NEW NON-PHARMACOLOGICAL THERAPEUTIC AGENT AGAINST METABOLIC DYSFUNCTION THROUGH GUT MICROBIOTA MODULATION?

Christophe Espírito Santo[1,2], PhD,
Maria João Martins[3,4], PhD and Inês Brandão[1,2,*], PhD
[1]Centro de Apoio Tecnológico Agro Alimentar (CATAA) de Castelo Branco, Castelo Branco, Portugal
[2]Centre for Functional Ecology, University of Coimbra, Coimbra, Portugal
[3]i3S-Instituto de Investigação e Inovação em Saúde, University of Porto, Porto, Portugal
[4]Department of Biomedicine, Biochemistry Unit, Faculty of Medicine, University of Porto, Porto, Portugal

* Corresponding Author's E-mail: inesbrandao@cataa.pt or inesm.brandao@gmail.com.

Abstract

Dietary patterns have a strong impact upon metabolic health and disease. Nutritional and non-nutritional diet components/features, both from food and beverages, by modulating several biological mechanisms, are implicated in that association. Here, we discuss the relationship between water intake and gut microbiota in metabolic health and disease taking into consideration the following water variables: water mineral/ion and gas composition, water pH, first time of water consumption, water intake volume and water security. This chapter is divided into 3 sections: 1) relevance of water ingestion in metabolic health and disease, 2) role of gut microbiota in metabolic health and disease, and 3) modulation of gut microbiota by water intake.

Keywords: acidic water, alkaline water, diabetes, drinking habits, drinking water, gut microbiota, hydrogen-water, metabolic health, metabolic syndrome, metabolism, mineral water, obesity, water security

Introduction

Water is the source of all life, and this essential liquid continues shaping how organisms evolve and adapt to the environment. Water ingestion is indispensable for human survival and healthy living. Among its many roles, water acts as a building constituent, as a solvent, reaction medium and reactant, as a carrier for nutrients and waste products, as an important constituent in thermoregulation, and as a lubricant and shock absorber [1, 2].

Since ancient times, water has been used for medical purposes. Asclepiades (124 BC), a Greek physician who established in Rome, advocated the use of general hydrotherapy and drinking cures as treatments. Throughout history, drinking cures with medical purposes have been documented, some with impressive recommended volume amounts, up to 10 litres a day [3]. Although water was bottled and transported as early as the first human civilizations, the first commercialized bottled water appeared in 1622 by the Holy Well (United Kingdom) [4]. By the turn of the 18th century, mineral water consumption gained a popularity boost due to the "Hydrologie Medicale" (Medical Hydrology). Scientists were dedicated in studying medical curative properties of many different waters, leading to the development of Spas and the commercialization of many brand waters that we know nowadays [3, 5]. The chemical composition of each spring was studied and empirically related with therapeutic properties. Despite the popularity of water therapeutic use, scientific evidence remains scarce [3].

During the past decades, several studies have focused on exploring the effects of a wide variety of drinking waters, including those related with metabolic health and disease. Also, with the advent of genetic tools in recent years, the knowledge around gut microbiota and its relationship with host health and disease is rapidly expanding. For instance, multiple studies have identified significant changes in the gut microbiota during obesity, diabetes, and other metabolic disorders [6]. Following this, a few studies have commenced to explore associations between particular drinking waters and gut microbiota modulation.

In this chapter we will explore drinking water attributes, such as water mineral/ion and gas composition, water pH, first time of water consumption, water intake volume and water security, and the impact exerted on gut microbiota and subsequent metabolic features.

Water - Implications in Metabolic Health and Disease

The World Health Organization (WHO) has highlighted the public health significance of water composition and pH [7, 8]. In line, the need to promote highly mineralised water consumption has been supported since it could a) make a relevant contribution to mineral/element nutritional needs, b) support/protect mineral/element homeostasis, and c) be helpful in metabolic disease prevention and treatment, by itself or as an adjuvant to pharmacological and/or surgical therapies. Water pH is also crucial to water relevance upon the above-mentioned points [7–16]. The relevance of water alkali load is further discussed in the chapter *Mineral Water Consumption and Diet-Induced Acid Load: Putative Relevance for Bone Health*.

Diabetes is among the 10 most important causes of death, according to WHO [17]. Beneficial modulation of glucose, insulin and leptin homeostasis as well as blood pressure and lipid profile by ingestion of different mineral waters has been published [15, 18–21], emphasising mineral waters direct role upon diabetes-associated metabolic dysfunction. Furthermore, mineral-rich waters intake could be helpful to avoid mineral and electrolyte imbalance or mineral deficiency observed with sodium-glucose cotransporter 2 inhibitor therapy [14] or after bariatric surgery [11], respectively. In this regard, minerals in water are highly bioavailable (reviewed in [15]) and intake of distinct mineral waters has been shown to modulate parathyroid hormone levels [22–26]. Improvement/beneficial modulation of redox and inflammatory status, NF-κB (nuclear factor kappa-light-chain-enhancer of activated B cells) signalling, insulin, leptin, glucocorticoid and aldosterone levels and/or signalling, sirtuin 1 - AMP-activated protein kinase - peroxisome proliferator-activated receptor gamma coactivator 1-α (Sirt1-AMPK-PGC1-α) signalling, endoplasmic reticulum stress and profibrogenic and apoptotic parameters are among the molecular mechanisms described explaining the positive impact of mineral waters consumption upon diabetes and diabetes-associated metabolic dysfunction and its comorbidities [15, 18–21, 27–29].

Similarly, drinking deep sea water (or deep sea water minerals) improves blood pressure, lipid profile and glucose homeostasis by beneficially modulating redox status, inflammatory tumour necrosis factor (TNF)-α signalling, Sirt1-AMPK-PGC1-α signalling, mitochondrial biogenesis and glucose uptake and metabolism as well as by recovering pancreatic islets of Langerhans [30–37], what reinforces the role of minerals in water upon diabetes and diabetes-associated metabolic dysfunction.

Gut Microbiota - Implications in Metabolic Health and Disease

During the last decade, multiple findings unequivocally show the crucial role of the gut microbiota, a community of more than 100 trillion microbial cells in the gastrointestinal tract, in modulating host metabolism and immune responses in health and disease [38]. Because of its major role as an environmental factor affecting host metabolic balance, gut microbiota has been called "a virtual or separate endocrine organ" [38, 39].

An imbalance in the gut microbial composition -termed dysbiosis-, namely shifts in the relative bacterial abundances, could be due to the gain of phatobionts, loss of commensals and/or loss of diversity and is often observed in metabolic disease phenotypes [40, 41]. Among the various driving forces for metabolic disease, overfeeding and westernised diet are environmental factors that have been reportedly associated with dysbiosis of the gut microbiota and detrimental effects in immunometabolism [42, 43]. Indeed, shifts in the intestinal microbiota, and consequently changes in the microbial components [e.g., lipopolysaccharide (LPS)] and produced metabolites [e.g., trimethylamine-N-oxide (TMAO)] crossing the intestinal barrier, appear to interfere with different metabolic organs (e.g., liver and adipose tissue), thus "fueling" a metabolic chronic low-grade inflammation, an important hallmark in the pathophysiology of metabolic diseases [44, 45]. Altered microbial signatures associated with metabolic dysfunction may include an increased ratio of Firmicutes to Bacteroidetes at phylum level, an expansion of Proteobacteria and a decreased *Akkermansia* abundance [46]. In detail, these reported changes in the gut microbiota still lack further corroboration as there are multiple discrepancies and contradictory results in the literature due to methodological differences (e.g., in sample processing) and to insufficent and distinct characterization of recruited subjects, among others [47].

Some studies have provided evidence that metabolic phenotypes are transmissible and modifiable by transplants of faecal microbiota. Transfer of faecal microbiota from healthy human donors to subjects with metabolic syndrome led to the improvement of the insulin resistance phenotype [48]. Transplants of faecal microbiota from lean and obese human twins into germ-free (GF) mice resulted in the transmission of the corresponding donor metabolic phenotypes [49]. Besides, GF mice were shown to be resistant to diet-induced obesity. Depleted microbiota, in either GF or antibiotic-treated mice, resulted in white adipose tissue browning and metabolic improvements, namely enhanced glucose tolerance and insulin sensitivity [50]. Further studies attribute a role for the gut microbiota in the occurrence or prevention of inflammation [41, 51]. For instance, the abundance of *Bifidobacterium*, *Faecalibacterium*, *Ruminococcus* and *Prevotella* was inversely related to several low-grade inflammation markers [e.g, high sensitivity C-reactive protein and interleukin (IL)-6] in humans [51]. In the same line, probiotic supplementation in individuals with overweight and obesity was suggested to be beneficial upon body weight, body adiposity and some cardiovascular risk markers that include inflammation and impaired glucose metabolism [52]. Also, 3-months supplementation with *Akkermansia muciniphila,* one of the most common species in the human gut microbiota and reported as beneficial in reducing gut barrier permeability, led to the amelioration of several metabolic parameters (e.g., insulin resistance, visceral adiposity, circulating lipids, and systemic inflammation markers) in obese and overweight subjects [53, 54]. On the other hand, the introduction of a pro-inflammatory gut microbiota, derived from caspase-1-deficient mice, accelerated systemic inflammation and atherogenesis in low-density lipoprotein-deficient mice. Noteworthy, the pro-inflammatory microbiota was associated with a lower production of microbial-derived anti-inflammatory short-chain fatty acids (SCFAs) [55].

Despite the large amount of evidence, the full extension of underlying mechanisms by which gut microbiota influences energy homeostasis and shapes host metabolism is still unknown [56]. Some of the mechanisms that have been identified include (1) the increase of energy harvesting from diet (e.g., dietary fibre) by the gut microbiota, with a subsequent impact in augmenting host energy availability and fat storage [38, 57, 58], (2) the regulation of multiple metabolic functions and signalling pathways, such as appetite, inflammation, and glucose and lipid metabolism, by microbial metabolites (e.g., SCFAs and succinate) and structural components (e.g., LPS) [59, 60], and (3) the reinforcement and deterioration of the intestinal barrier by the gut microbiota in homeostasis and dysbiosis, respectively. A decrease in the gut barrier function affects metabolic endotoxaemia (i.e., LPS enters the bloodstream through a disturbed intestinal epithelium, increasing plasma LPS levels), hence driving deleterious inflammatory effects [61]. Illustrating some of the aforementioned mechanisms, SCFAs regulate blood sugar levels by modulating the secretion of hormones in different tissues [60]. The activation of free fatty acid receptor 3 by SCFAs was shown to stimulate the secretion of intestinal hormone peptide YY in endocrine cells, improving the uptake of glucose by muscle and adipose tissue and leading to satiety and reduced food intake [62, 63]. *A. muciniphila*-derived extracellular vesicles were reported to reinforce gut barrier function through the regulation of tight junction proteins [64]. Other findings suggest this bacterium could as well stimulate the production of mucus [65]. In contrast, an abnormal proliferation of Proteobacteria was found to induce and sustain unspecific inflammation in the gut without an actual infection, which correlates with various diseases, such as metabolic disease [66–68]. This is probably due to its cell wall structure covered with LPS [68, 69].

Finally, exploring the interactions and signalling pathways between the gut microbiota and the host may provide important clues for improving the gut microbial ecology with a view to prevent or combat a range of diseases, including metabolic disorders like obesity and associated metabolic dysfunction [38, 70]. Table 1 provides several examples of studies reporting associations (direct observations or correlation analyses) between gut microbiota (or its components) and metabolic features.

Table 1. Examples of published associations between gut microbiota and metabolic features

Host/model Ref.	Changes in microbiota	Supplementation/treatment with microbial strain(s) or their components	Associated metabolic features/markers	Type of analysis
Humans: cohort of 53 non-diabetic, insulin-resistant and overweight or obese individuals, recruited in Belgium [71]	↓*Dysosmobacter welbionis* J115T	-	↑BMI* ↑Fasting circulating glucose* ↑HbA1c*	Pearson's correlation matrix, indicated by arrows, between *Dysosmobacter* spp abundance and clinical variables in the cohort
Rodents: C57BL/6J mice [71]	-	↑*Dysosmobacter welbionis* J115T (oral gavage of 1.0×10^9 cultivable, live bacteria/day/ mouse, for at least 6 weeks and up to 13 weeks)	↑Glucose tolerance (OGTT) ↓Fasting circulating insulin, leptin and resistin levels* ↓Insulin resistance index* ↓Weight gain* ↓Adipose tissue expansion (mesenteric, subcutaneous and epididymal fat deposits)* ↓Adipocyte diameter* ↑mRNA Expression of adipose tisssue lipolysis markers (e.g., adipose triglycerides lipase* and hormone sensitive lipase) ↓mRNA Expression of inflammation markers in adipose tissue (e.g., TNF-α*) and macrophages infiltration markers (e.g., Lbp*, Cd68, Cd163* and Cd11b*)	Effects of supplementation in HFD-fed mice

Host/model Ref.	Changes in microbiota	Supplementation/treatment with microbial strain(s) or their components	Associated metabolic features/markers	Type of analysis
Humans: 1914 healthy and obese Chinese subjects (the latter with or without metabolic abnormalities)	↑*Blautia*[1]	-	↑Waistline* ↑Circulating LDL*, HDL* and TC* ↓Diastolic blood pressure*	Spearman correlation analysis, indicated by arrows, between clinical parameters and gut microbiota
	↑*Romboutsia*[1] ↑*Ruminococcus2*[a,c] ↑*Clostridium sensu stricto*[b] ↑*Dorea*[c]	-	↑Waistline* and BMI* ↑Circulating LDL* and TC* [↓Diastolic blood pressure*[a]] [↑Circulating glucose*[b]] [↑Circulating HDL*[c]]	Spearman correlation analysis, indicated by arrows, between clinical parameters and gut microbiota
	↑*Bacteroides*[1]	-	↓Waistline* and BMI* ↓Circulating LDL*	
	↑*Roseburia*[1]	-	↓Waistline* and BMI* ↓Circulating TG*	
[1]Biomarkers discovered for the obese patients with or without metabolic abnormalities [72]	↑*Parabacteroides*[1]	-	↓Waistline* and BMI* ↓Blood pressure* ↓Circulating glucose*, LDL* and TG*	
	↑*Parasutterella*	-	↓Waistline*, BMI* ↓Circulating LDL* and TC*	
	↑*Alistipes*[1] ↑*Clostridium IV*	-	↓Waistline* and BMI* ↓Blood pressure* ↓Circulating glucose* and TG*	
	↑*Butyricicoccus*	-	↓Circulating TG*	

Table 1. (Continued)

Host/model Ref.	**Changes in microbiota**	**Supplementation/treatment with microbial strain(s) or their components**	**Associated metabolic features/markers**	**Type of analysis**
Cell line: 3T3-L1 adipocytes [73]	-	*Acinetobacter baumannii*-derived LPS (100 ng/mL, for 1 or 24 hours)	↓mRNA Expression of leptin* and adiponectin* ↑mRNA Expression of lipocalin-2* and fatty acid binding protein 4* ↑mRNA Expression of macrophage inflammatory protein-2* and monocyte chemotactic protein 1 (chemoattractants) ↑ mRNA Expression of TNF-α* and IL-6*	Observed effects compared with control cells without LPS treatment
Humans: 45 obese Dutch patients undergoing crash diet followed by bariatric surgery [74]	↓*Coriobacteriaceae* ↑Clostridiales	-	↓HbA1c*	Association analysis, indicated by arrows, between clinical parameters and gut microbiota, based on the difference between 6 months after surgery and baseline
Humans: 32 overweight/obese insulin-resistant subjects, recruited in Belgium [53]	-	↑*Akkermansia muciniphila* (10^{10} bacteria pasteurised/day, for 3 months)	↑Insulin sensitivity* ↓Insulinaemia* ↓Circulating TC* ↓Body weight ↓Fat mass ↓Hip circumference	Observed effects, as compared with placebo and/or baseline; randomised single-centre double-blind placebo-controlled pilot study

Host/model Ref.	Changes in microbiota	Supplementation/treatment with microbial strain(s) or their components	Associated metabolic features/markers	Type of analysis
Humans: cohort 67 Mexican women: healthy, obese, and obese with metabolic syndrome	↑Firmicutes*	-	Obese metabolic syndrome *versus* healthy control	Linear discriminant analysis effect size – abundance of bacterial taxa associated with phenotypic categories
	↑*Faecalibacterium** ↓*Bacteroides** ↑*Lachnospiraceae** family (↑*Roseburia**, ↑*Lachnospira* and* ↑*Coprococcus*)* ↓*Erysipelotrichaceae* * family*	-	Obese and obese metabolic syndrome *versus* healthy control	
[2]More abundant in obesity *versus* obesity with metabolic syndrome [75]	↑*Bilophila*[2]	-	↑Body weight*	Association analysis (multivariate association with linear models), indicated by arrows, between clinical parameters and gut microbiota
Humans: 210 healthy Japanese adults with large visceral fat areas [76]	-	↑*Lactobacillus gasseri* SBT2055 (10^6 or 10^7 CFU/g of fermented milk, 200g of fermented milk/day, for 12 weeks)	↓Abdominal visceral fat areas* ↓BMI* ↓Waist and hip circumferences* ↓Body fat mass*	Observed changes from baseline; multi-centre, double-blind, parallel group RCT

*Significant associations/effects; ↓ decrease; ↑ increase; BMI: body mass index; Cd: cluster of differentiation; CFU: colony forming units; HbA1c: glycated haemoglobin; HDL: high-density lipoprotein; HFD: high-fat diet; IL: interleukin; Lbp: lipopolysaccharide binding protein; LDL: low-density lipoprotein; LPS: lipopolysaccharides; OGTT: oral glucose tolerance test; RCT: randomised controlled trial; Ref: reference; TC: total cholesterol; TG: tryglicerides; TNF: tumour necrosis factor.

IMPACT UPON GUT MICROBIOTA OF DIFFERENT WATERS

Recognising the importance of drinking water constituents dates back thousands of years [77]. Despite the empirical evidence regarding the therapeutic actions of multiple waters, like mineral waters, the physiological effects and molecular mechanisms involved are not fully known and unravelled. In recent years, multiple studies contributed to a more rigorous and detailed scientific knowledge on this matter. The biological effects of water consumption have been explored but, to our knowledge, only a few studies have so far addressed the impact of water consumption upon gut microbiota.

Effects of Water Mineral/Ion and Gas Composition on the Gut Microbiota

The effects upon intestinal inflammation and gut microbiota, in both *in vitro* [intestinal epithelial cells stimulated with heat inactivated *Escherichia coli* (*E. coli*) or H_2O_2] and *in vivo* [moderate colitis induced by 1% dextran sulfate sodium (DSS) in male Balbc/J mice] models, of two French mineral waters were recently described [78]. The first water, from Châtel-Guyon (F3 Spring, Puy de Dôme, France), was a calcium and magnesium sulphate, sodium chloride, carbonic and ferruginous water (CGMW), whereas the second one, from Vichy (Antoine and Boussange Springs, Allier, France), was mainly a bicarbonate water, but also rich in chloride, fluoride and sodium; distilled water was used as control water. Both waters, more efficiently CGMW, induced anti-inflammatory effects in cultured intestinal epithelial cells (66-h period of water treatment), namely by limiting IL-8 secretion. In the moderate colitis mouse model (that included 30 animals), both waters, again more efficiently the CGMW, decreased the severity of inflammation induced by DSS and improved the barrier function; CGMW also induced a significant reduction in the number of epithelial lesions. Authors suggested that the mechanism of action behind beneficial anti-inflammatory effects in the intestinal milieu could be the establishment of a more balanced gut microbiota. A 3-week treatment with both waters resulted in a higher proportion of Firmicutes and lower percentages of Proteobacteria and Bacteroidetes, pointing to the establishment of a less colitogenic microbiota composition in the colonic mucosa. Furthermore, CGMW led to significant increases in beneficial bacteria such as segmented filamentous bacteria (SFB) and a bacteria of the *Lactobacillus* family. Intringuingly, *Akkermansia* genus, known to have a favourable impact on metabolic health, was present in greater abundance in untreated mice than in mice receiving CGMW [78]. Overall, although the observed changes in the composition of the microbiota upon CGMW consumption seem to be beneficial to the intestinal environment, it is conceivable that they may exert unfavorable effects on metabolism, in line with several studies already mentioned in Table 1.

The sodium chloride, bicarbonate, calcium, magnesium, sulphate and iron-rich mineral water (L-CMW), from the spring of Lanjarón-Capuchina (Granada, Spain), has been consumed for more than two hundred years to treat digestive disorders. This water consumption was reported to ameliorate intestinal function, with lasting effects for up to 3 months [79, 80]. Although not studying the gut microbiota (but studying a closely associated intestinal structure, namely the intestinal villi and the enterocytes covering their surface), Crespo *et al.* evaluated the effects exerted by L-CMW in 15 male Wistar rats, either after its administration in the diet, for 15 days, or after direct administration into the gastrointestinal tract (intestinal surface) through a catheter; as control, tap water was used during the 15-day treatment period. Changes were found in the intestinal epithelium, specifically in the microscopic pattern of both microvilli absorption from enterocytes and goblet cells secretory ability, which was augmented. Notably, L-CMW also accelerated the epithelial renewal process, stimulating cell extrusion, and importantly, not causing epithelial disruption. The direct administration of L-CMW led to more pronounced effects than the oral route. The reported effects are concominant with the improved intestinal function reported previously [80].

Another study examined the response of BALB/c mice faecal bacterial community to different types of drinking water, including natural water, commercial bottled mineral water (displaying a low mineral content), tap water and purified water [81]. Faeces were cultured with brain heart infusion broth dissolved in the 4 different types of drinking water, under aerobic and anaerobic conditions (each experimental group had 3 biological replicates). The faecal microbiota composition was distinct between each water type and, importantly, as the culture time passed from 1 to 5 days, mineral water, aerobically, led to a progressive microbial α-diversity increase, promoting Bacteroidetes growth. Finally, authors suggested that, given that Bacteroidetes has been previously associated with many diseases (e.g., a lower proportion of Bacteroidetes correlates with metabolic syndrome and liver cirrhosis [82, 83]), mineral water could be used as a strategy in the prevention and cure of these diseases by favouring this phylum [81].

To explore whether gut microbiota could mediate the effects of tap water consumption in human health, solute concentration measurements of domestic tap water samples (from household or place of work, at multiple locations in the United Kingdom) and drinking habits from 85 monozygotic twins [66.8 ± 7.3 years (mean±standard deviation; SD); 84.7% women] were compared with faecal microbiota profiles and health data (from the TwinsUK dataset) [84]. Sodium average daily dose (ADD) significantly associated with microbiota α-diversity (with decreased species richness), whereas dissimilarity between samples significantly associated with chloride, sodium and sulphate ADD. Also, significant associations for chloride, sodium and sulphate (either as water component or as ADD) with abundances of individual microbial taxa were found. Tenericutes was linked with the 3 solutes while sodium ADD associated with Cyanobacteria and Proteobacteria. Finally, the reported results suggest gut microbiota as a potential mediator of health differences linked to water quality [84].

A mineral water of Hita basin (Kyushu island, Japan) has been recognized for its unique composition, extremely high in silicic acid, sodium, potassium, and hydrogen carbonate (1.4 to 6.1-fold of the world average; 2.4 to 4.3-fold of the Japan average) and relatively low in magnesium, calcium, and sulphate (1.6 to 3.0-fold lower than the world average; 2.8-fold lower than the Japan average). Several "antiobesity" properties were observed upon a 6-month intervention in 20 male C57BL6/J mice with this mineral water (*versus* tap water), such as significantly reduced visceral fat accumulation and weight gain despite significantly increased dietary consumption. After an identical 6-month treatment, shifts in the faecal microbiota, with this mineral water (*versus* tap water), were also reported in 8 male ICR mice, namely significant fluctuations of the families *Lactobacillaceae* (increased) and *Clostridiaceae* (decreased) [85].

Again, another study revealed the modulation of the gut microbiota by drinking water. The response of gut bacterial community [faecal and mucosa-adhered (from *jejunum* to *rectum*)] to the ingestion of four different types of drinking water was evaluated in 20 female BALB/c J Unib mice, in a 23-day protocol [86]. The experimental cohort was divided according to the different water sources: autoclaved tap water (control), disinfected water from Rio das Velhas DWTP (Companhia de Saneamento de Minas Gerais/Brazil), tap water and commercial bottled mineral water. The first three waters were submitted to conventional treatment with chlorination. Particularly, a significant increase in *Acinetobacter* and *Staphylococcus* genera, often associated with antibiotic resistance, was reported not only in faecal samples of mice drinking tap water but also in the mucosa-adhered samples of mice from disinfected and tap water groups. Interaction of drinking water and gut microbiota could be a route for dissemination of antibiotic resistance genes, according to authors [86]. Obesity, metabolic syndrome and diabetes may render patients more susceptible to bacterial infections, such as the ones caused by *Staphylococcus*, and are often associated with a poor outcome [87]. Thus, while the spread of antibiotic resistance genes can be a major public health threat, they certainly have a greater impact on people with associated risk factors, such as metabolic disorders.

The molecular level effects on glycaemic control of bicarbonate-rich mineral water consumption (BMW) were investigated in 19 healthy subjects (26-59 years; 12 women) [88]. BMW, obtained from Nagayu hot spring (Taketa, Oita, Japan), contains one of the highest bicarbonate concentrations in Japan, 2485 mg/kg, being also enriched in sulphate, sodium, magnesium, calcium and iron. Tap water (TW; control) was purchased from Nishikawa water treatment plant (Yamagata, Japan). Volunteers drank 500 mL of TW or BMW divided into thrice daily (30-60 min before breakfast, lunch, and dinner). Consumption periods lasted for a week, for each water, and the cycle TW followed by BMW occurred twice. Interestingly, faecal analysis revealed that *Christensenellaceae* family was the most significantly augmented taxon after BMW consumption. The *Dehalobacteriaceae* family was also increased and, curiously, has been previously positively correlated with *Christensenellaceae* [88, 89]. Curiously, and similarly to what was found in this study, *Bifidobacteriaceae* decreased significantly after crash-diet followed by bariatric surgery [74]. These changes in the gut microbiota, together with significant results from the blood metabolome analysis (changes in some glycolysis-related metabolites and amino acids) and the decreased circulating glycoalbumin (one of the indexes of glycaemic control) after BMW consumption, suggest that BMW intake likely has the potential to prevent and/or improve obesity and type 2 diabetes [74, 88, 89].

Finally, as menopause promotes the incidence of metabolic syndrome, a 10-week study in adult Sprague–Dawley ovariectomised (O) female rats, including sham-operated and tap water or mineral water-treated O rats, with or without fructose (30 rats, n=6/group), was conducted concerning faecal microbiota and SCFAs composition/levels [90]. Lower levels of Bacteroidetes and higher levels of Actinobacteria, Proteobacteria and TM7 occurred in tap water-O rats and higher levels of Firmicutes and lower levels of Bacteroidetes were detected in tap water-O-fructose rats *versus* sham-operated rats. Overall, mineral water (bicarbonate- and sodium-rich) reversed changes in tap water-O and tap water-O-fructose groups, with a more pronounced effect in the latter. Tap water-O-fructose presented the highest Firmicutes to Bacteroidetes ratio *versus* the other groups, while mineral water-supplementation, with and without fructose, reduced this ratio. Sham-operated rats revealed the lowest ratio, showing no differences compared with mineral water-O rats. The Principal Coordinates Analysis differentiated mineral water from tap water groups, with sham-operated rats faecal microbiota similar to mineral water groups (mineral water-O and mineral water-O-fructose) faecal microbiota. Moreover, mineral water reduced total SCFA levels observed in the tap water-O-fructose rats. Mineral water groups revealed a tendency for lower body weight gain when compared with tap water groups, more clearly seen with fructose supplementation [90].

Fluoride in drinking distilled water was found to modulate the composition of faecal microbiota as well as its richness and α-diversity in 25 male Wistar rats [91]. A biphasic effect of fluoride in water was found as microbial richness and diversity index firstly augmented with a relative lower fluoride content and then went down with a higher fluoride level. The richness of the 25 mg/L group (group consuming distilled water with 25 mg/L of sodium fluoride *ad libitum*) was the highest and markedly higher than the one from the 100 mg/L fluoride group. The richness of the 150 mg/L group was the lowest and significantly lower than 25 and 50 mg/L groups. Some bacteria seemed to have a protective role against the development of fluorosis whereas others seemed to contribute to disease pathogenesis. Correlation analysis revealed that abundances of *Roseburia* and *Turicibacter*, which negatively correlated with dental fluorosis, were reduced with fluoride exposure concentration. Also, *Clostridium sensu stricto* was negatively correlated with dental fluorosis. *Pelagibacterium*, *Unclassified Ruminococcaceae* and *Unclassified Bdellovibrionales*, which positively associated with the grade of dental fluorosis, presented a similar trend by increasing with fluoride exposure concentration. All these correlations were significant [91]. Interestingly, other studies have reported associations between fluoride exposure and metabolic risk factors [92–97]. For instance, depending on the dose, fluoride has been described to possibly lead to positive or adverse effects upon the circulating lipid profile/lipid homeostasis as well as upon circulating glucose/glucose homeostasis and insulin secretion, action and clearance (reviewed in [15]).

The effects of a 20-day intervention with hydrogen-rich drinking water, *versus* normal drinking water, in chemotherapy-induced neuropathic pain (CINP) were reported in 40 female C57BL/6J mice [98]. Noticeably, the hydrogen-rich drinking water could alleviate hyperalgesia induced by the chemotherapeutic drug oxaliplatin, which can be possibly explained by the observed effects that include gut microbial α-diversity reduction, change in the structure of gut microbiota, reversion of the imbalance of inflammatory cytokines and oxidative stress in dorsal root ganglia, and decreased levels of LPS and toll-like receptor 4 in dorsal root ganglia. For example, at the family level, *Lachnospiraceae*, *Lactobacillaceae* and *Ruminococcaceae* were higher in the faecal samples of mice treated with hydrogen-rich drinking water and the same modulation was found, at the genus level, for *Faecalibacterium*, *Lactobacillus* and *Roseburia*. Based on the reported results [98] and on a previous study indicating hydrogen-rich drinking water could significantly improve the gastrointestinal function and epithelial integrity of mice after total abdominal irradiation [99], authors finally suggested hydrogen-rich drinking water may be considered to protect gastrointestinal function and epithelial integrity by modulating the gut microbiota, thus improving CINP [98].

The changes reported in the gut microbiota [98] could possibly explain the beneficial effects in the gastrointestinal barrier as, among Firmicutes, the *Lachnospiraceae*, *Lactobacillaceae*, and *Ruminococcaceae* species are butyrate and other SCFAs producers by hydrolysing starch and other sugars [100]. In detail, butyrate has a central role in the protection and maintenance of the intestinal barrier function, being a hallmark in the promotion of metabolic health [101, 102]. In line, during a randomised double-blinded placebo-controlled trial enrolling 60 subjects [43.2 ± 10.0 years (mean±SD); 50% women] with metabolic syndrome, supplementation with high concentration hydrogen-rich water (750 mL/day), for 24 weeks, lowered circulating cholesterol and glucose, attenuated circulating glycated haemoglobin (HbA1c), and ameliorated inflammation biomarkers and redox homeostasis as compared with placebo (all these changes being statistically significant). Furthermore, hydrogen-rich water showed a tendency to mildly reduce body mass index (BMI) and waist-to-hip ratio [103]. Altogether, these studies reveal potential roles for hydrogen-rich water and its capacity to modulate gut microbiota, to diminish inflammation, protect the gut barrier integrity, improve cellular function and ameliorate metabolic clinical features [98, 99, 103].

Water pH Effects on the Gut Microbiota

Water pH is a very important parameter due to the direct impact on water content. For example, heavy metals, such as iron, aluminium, lead, copper and cadmium, have increased solubility at low pH [104, 105]. Although small concentrations might not represent a danger for consumption or exert any toxic effect to multicellular organisms, this is totally different for unicellular organisms such as bacteria (the oligodynamic effect) [106–108].

Similar to food products with pH < 4.2 (fruit juices, sodas, energy drinks, among others), acidified water is widely used in animal facilities to prevent pathogenic bacteria development [109]. Here, an overview of studies conducted in animals and Humans using waters at different pH and their effect on gut microbiota are presented.

The effects of HCl- or H_2SO_4-acidified drinking water [tap water (pH 8.4) acidified with HCl to pH 2.5–2.9 (average was 2.8) or with H_2SO_4 to pH 2.8] received from weaning (postnatal day 21) up to 6 months upon gut microbiota of male 129S6/SvEv mice were compared against mice kept on non-acidified tap water [110]. Interestingly, H_2SO_4- and HCl-acidified water led to different results. For instance, H_2SO_4-acidified drinking water markedly reduced faecal α-diversity when compared with both non-acidified drinking water and HCl-acidified drinking water. Also, while HCl-acidified drinking water did not induce changes in the phylum composition, H_2SO_4-acidified drinking water significantly diminished the relative abundance of Bacteroidetes when compared with the other two conditions [110]. These results were most likely due to the prominent role of sulphur in bacterial metabolism. Indeed, hydrogen sulphide released by sulphate-reducing bacteria can be toxic to several bacteria, which could explain a shift in the gut microbiota composition [110–112].

Acidified drinking water [tap water (pH 8.4) acidified with HCl to pH 2.5-2.9 (average pH 2.8)] was tested in a Batten disease (neuronal ceroid lipofuscinoses) mouse model to explore the exerted effects upon gut microbiota and disease state from postnatal day 21 (weaning) up to 6 months [109]. Johnson *et al.* suggested the disease state beneficial effects observed with this water intervention could be mediated through changes in gut microbiota. α-Diversity was very similar, independently of age, comparing male wild-type and *Cln3*$^{-/-}$ mice with and without HCl-acidified drinking water. Faecal samples overall composition of *Cln3*$^{-/-}$ and wild-type mice was noticeably dissimilar and intake of HCl-acidified drinking water differentially modified them. For instance, by 3 months of age, marked differences at the genus level were found between *Cln3*$^{-/-}$ and wild-type mice in the relative abundance of *Alistipes*, *Barnesiella*, *Bacteroides*, *Tannerella*, *Parabacteroides*, *Eubacterium* and *Lactococcus* on both non-acidified and HCl-acidified drinking water, in the relative abundance of *Lachnoclostridium*, *Anaeroplasma* and *Lactobacillus* on non-acidified drinking water only, and in the relative abundance of *Clostridium*, *Turicibacter* and *Akkermansia* on HCl-acidified drinking water only. By 6 months, also at the genus level, a new difference was detected in *Akkermansia* between the mutant mouse strain and its wild-type on non-acidified drinking water. Some of the differences seen at 3 months of age also vanished (*Lactococcus*, after non-acidified drinking water; *Alistipes*, *Parabacteroides*, *Tannerella*, *Clostridium*, *Lactococcus* and *Turicibacter*, after HCl-acidified drinking water). HCl-acidified drinking water in wild-type mice significantly changed the proportion of *Lactobacillus* and *Lactococcus* by 3 months of age, and of *Alistipes*, *Bacteroides*, *Barnesiella*, *Lactobacillus* and *Turicibacter* by 6 months of age. HCl-acidified drinking water in *Cln3*$^{-/-}$ mice only changed the relative abundance of *Turicibacter* and of *Lactococcus* and *Turicibacter* at 3 and 6 months, respectively. Authors proposed that the significant increase in the *Lactococcus* genus abundance in 3-month-old wild-type mice drinking HCl-acidified water could be linked to the superior rotarod performance observed in these mice. Also, the significantly decreased relative abundance of *Lactobacillus* genus in the gut microbiota of $Cln3^{-/-}$ mice drinking non-acidified water could contribute to the neuropathological changes and neurological deficits observed in this disease model [109]. Adding to the putative metabolic relevance of these results, *Tannerella* and *Barnesiella* species (along with *Bifidobacterium*) increased with a prodiabetogenic diet whereas *Akkermansia* species increased with an anti-diabetogenic diet in faeces from non-obese diabetic mice [113].

Another study on acidified drinking water used it as a substitute for antibiotic feed additives for broiler growth promotion. This study was able to show that acidified drinking water treated groups showed significantly improved weight gain, average daily gain and feed conversion ratio (the study included 540 one-day-old male broilers randomly assigned to 5 treatment groups: negative and posivitive controls and 3 acidified drinking water groups; pH reduction of drinking water from 7.8 to 4.2 with a commercial liquid acidifier). This study only used culture-dependent methods, thus, a precise *cecum* microbiota community was not identified, only that aerobic bacterial counts (significantly) and pathogenic bacteria (*E. coli*) (tendency) were reduced in the acidified water fed groups [114].

Sofi and co-authors showed acidity of drinking water is a crucial feature, able to influence gut microbiota and type 1 diabetes (T1D) incidence and progression in mice [115]. HCl-acidified drinking water (pH 3.0-3.2) led to a more rapid disease progression, including insulitis and hyperglycaemia, in female non-obese diabetic (NOD)/ShiLtJ mice compared with neutral pH (pH 7.0-7.2) drinking water (n=10/group; both waters were autoclaved). Switching from acidic to neutral water, for 30 days, at an early age of 3-4 weeks, led to a significantly slower disease progression and lower T1D incidence, and to significant changes both in gut microbiota diversity and abundance of existing bacterial communities. With this drinking water switch, in faecal samples, *Lactobacilli* abundance remained almost unchanged but significantly reduced loads of *Bacteroides* and some of the *Prevotella* genus members were observed. Additionally, acquisition of *Parabacteroides* as well as of additional members of the *Prevotella* genus was described. In distal *ileum* samples, the abovementioned water switch led to a decrease in *Lactobacilli* (from 98% to 79%, approximately). The newly acquired microbiota upon neutral water consumption comprised ~60% of *Eubacterium bioforme* (11.4% of total) and the remaining commensals (~10% of total) belonged to all major phyla (Firmicutes, Bacteroidetes, Tenericutes, and Actinobacteria). On the other hand, switching B6 mice from neutral to acidified drinking water for 2 months resulted in the enrichment of *Lactobacilli* (to 85% of the gut microbiota). The effect of gut colonisation by SFB on T1D, under acidic and neutral pH drinking water conditions, was also investigated in (NOD)/ShiLtJ mice (as described above). Interestingly, SFB colonisation significantly delayed hyperglycaemia in mice that were on acidified but not on neutral drinking water. Also, SFB colonised mice (on acidified or neutral drinking water) showed, in distal *ileum* samples, a nearly similar level of *Lactobacilli* as found in the neutral drinking water group without SFB colonisation. However, the two water groups showed different microbial profiles upon SFB colonisation: while the main non-*Lactobacilli* flora was *Prevotella loescheii* in the HCl-acidified drinking water group (~40%; 8.6% of total), it was primarily *Clostridium* (~50%; 12.1% of total) species in the neutral drinking water group. Authors suggested that HCl-acidified drinking water consumption results in rapid T1D progression via reduction of gut microbiota diversity and by an increment in the proportion of *Lactobacillus* members [115].

Also on NOD/ShiLtJt mice [female (mostly) and male], another study measured the impact of water pH upon gut microbiota and T1D onset from 9–10 weeks up to 30 weeks of age [116]. In this study a complete opposite effect was noticed, as neutral (pH ~ 7) tap water *versus* HCl-acidified (pH ~ 3.2) tap water (both waters were chlorinated and autoclaved) significantly increased T1D incidence while modifying the faecal microbiota by significantly reducing *Lactobacillus sp.* and *Clostridia sp.* (both Firmicutes) at multiple ages. There was no consistent change in the populations of *Bacteroides sp.*, but prior to disease onset a significant increase was found. No differences were observed in weight gain on acidic *versus* neutral drinking water groups [116].

Bidot and co-workers addressed, in 96 female outbred Crl:CD1 (ICR) mice, the usage of different drinking waters normally consumed in animal facilities: tap water, reverse osmosis-treated water and HCl- or H_2SO_4-acidified water (pH range: 2.3-2.7) [117]. All waters were autoclaved prior to usage in the 28-day protocol and had distinct mineral composition (not analysed in the study). Distinct results were obtained for faecal and caecal samples. Significant changes were primarily observed in caecal samples and include an increase of the genus *Akkermansia* with autoclaved water and a low relative abundance of *Lactobacillus sp.* with reverse osmosis-treated water. Authors were able to show that the different drinking waters differently modulated faecal and caecal microbiota probably due to distinct composition and pH. For instance, during the reverse osmosis procedure water passes through a membrane able to filter various compounds, including minerals, ions, disinfectant byproducts, pharmaceutical residues, endocrine-disrupting compounds, and pesticides that could possibly influence gut microbiota composition and physiology in the studied rodents [117].

Finally, the impact of tap water consumption (2 L/day), of alkaline (pH ~ 9) and neutral (pH ~ 7) pH, on human intestinal microbiota and host glucose metabolism was evaluated [118]. This human clinical trial was a randomised non-blind cross-over study (two 2-week intervention periods, separated by a 3-week wash-out period) in 29 healthy, non-smoking Danish men (18-35 years), with a BMI between 20.0 to 27.0 kg/m^2. Water pH was obtained by ion exchange and electrolysis using a validated commercial device. Regarding α-diversity, richness and community structure, abundance or genera in faecal samples as well as incremental area under the curve of the oral glucose tolerance test, this study did not find any significant differences between the 2 water groups. Thus, a change between alkaline and neutral pH drinking water had no significant impact on gut microbiota or glucose regulation in young male adults. Nevertheless, analyses of within intervention changes suggest a potential effect of quantitative or qualitative changes in habitual drinking habits by showing a significant increase in the relative abundance of 9 operational taxonomic units (OTUs) belonging to order Clostridiales, family *Ruminococcaceae*, genus *Bacteroides*, and species *Prevotella copri* [118].

Effects of Other Water Consumption Properties on the Gut Microbiota: First Contact with Drinking Water, Water Intake Volume and Water Security

Further, examining the effects of offering drinking water since birth on the composition of gut microbiota in dairy calves revealed an increment in the species richness and in the abundance of *Faecalibacterium prausnitzii* and *Bifidobacterium breve*, when compared to calves receiving drinking water for the first time at day 17. This modulatory effect on the gut microbiota composition could be linked to growth and development of animals as the increased bacteria are known to improve growth and performance in preweaned calves (as well as antagonistic effects against pathogenic bacteria) [119].

Next, daily water intake was investigated in a 12-week two-arm randomised controlled trial. Fifty-five healthy Japanese subjects (31 women) were enrolled in a dietary intervention comprising 1 bottle (550 mL) of mineral water from the Southern Japanese Alps being consumed after waking up and before bedtime (2 bottles of water on top of habitual fluid intake that increased mean fluid intake from 1.3 L/day to 2.0 L/day). Overall, water supplementation conducted to health benefits such as the significant decrease in systolic blood pressure (SBP), blood urea nitrogen concentration, HbA1c and glycoalbumin as well as the significant rise in body temperature. Additionally, waste materials dilution was favoured and kidney function decline was suppressed. Importantly, changes in faecal microbiota were detected. A slight correlation was seen in the intervention group between the SBP decrease and the *Pseudoflavonifractor capillosus* bacterial count increase (hypothetically, these bacteria may be involved in the mechanism of blood pressure reduction). Other slight correlations were described linking the rise in body temperature from water intake and practically unchanged *Kineothrix sp.*, and reduction in both *Faecalibacterium prausnitzii* and *Ruminococcaceae* OTUs (hypothetically these bacteria could be involved in the mechanism of temperature regulation) [120].

Regarding water security, the characterisation of the gut microbiota of 41 Nicaraguan children (1 month to 5.9 years, male and female) and its relationship with household water security was done by collecting and analysing drinking water samples as well as faecal samples. Household drinking water quality was poor, presenting high levels of coliform contamination in the majority of cases (85%). *Campylobacter* and *Salmonella* were present in high concentrations in water and faecal samples. Faecal microbiota of children from high coliform homes *versus* low coliform homes had a different composition and a reduced diversity. Children exposed to augmented coliform levels in tap water had significantly increased abundances of the order Bdellovibrionales, and the genera *Treponema*, *Vibrio* and *Clostridium* when compared with children living in low coliform homes. Conversely, the order Aeromonadales was increased in children living in low coliform households [121].

CONCLUSION

Herein, several studies were identified suggesting the modulation of the gut microbiota by the ingestion of water with different characteristics, ranging from origin/source, mineral/ion and gaseous composition, pH value, pathogen presence and drinking habits, namely the first contact with drinking water and volume of water intake.

Although some of these studies already begin to unravel the impact of water intake on the gut microbiota, with subsequent expected or even proven changes in the metabolic health and disease, at this point, further scientific efforts are still needed to clarify the exact effects (pinpointing the involved molecular pathways) exerted by a defined and well-characterised water source. Some discrepancies can be found when comparing currently published research, since study design, protocol conditions, water characteristics, among other variables, may differ largely between studies. The issues raised when comparing data regarding gut microbiota profiles in metabolic health and disease also apply.

REFERENCES

[1] Vieira ADN, Kleinermanns K, Martin WF, Preiner M. The ambivalent role of water at the origins of life. *FEBS Lett.* 2020;594(17):2717–33.

[2] Jéquier E, Constant F. Water as an essential nutrient: the physiological basis of hydration. *Eur J Clin Nutr*. 2010;64(2):115–23.

[3] Tubergen A van, Linden S van der. A brief history of spa therapy. *Ann Rheum Dis*. 2002;61(3):273.

[4] Crystal Beverage Company. *History of bottled water*. Available at: https://myownwater.com/blog/history-of-bottled-water. Accessed on October 7, 2021.

[5] Maison des Eaux Minérales Naturelles. *Histoire de l'eau minérale naturelle*. [*History of natural mineral water*]. Available at: https://eaumineralenaturelle.fr/sante-bienfaits/histoire-de-leau-minerale. Accessed on October 7, 2021.

[6] Cani PD. Human gut microbiome: hopes, threats and promises. *Gut*. 2018;67(9):1716–25.

[7] World Health Organization. *Calcium and Magnesium in Drinking-water: Public health significance*. WHO Press Geneva: 2009. Available at: http://apps.who.int/iris/bitstream/10665/43836/1/9789241563550_eng.pdf. Accessed on October 7, 2021.

[8] World Health Organization. *Hardness in Drinking-water. Background document for development of WHO Guidelines for*

Drinking-water Quality. WHO Press Geneva: 2011. Available at: https://www.who.int/water_sanitation_health/dwq/chemicals/hardness.pdf. Accessed on October 7, 2021.

[9] Stene LC, Hongve D, Magnus P, Ronningen KS, Joner G. Acidic drinking water and risk of childhood-onset type 1 diabetes. *Diabetes Care*. 2002;25(9):1534–8.

[10] Rylander R. Drinking water constituents and disease. *J Nutr*. 2008;138(2):423S-5S.

[11] Bal BS, Finelli FC, Shope TR, Koch TR. Nutritional deficiencies after bariatric surgery. *Nat Rev Endocrinol*. 2012;8(9):544–56.

[12] Rasic-Milutinovic Z, Perunicic-Pekovic G, Jovanovic D, Gluvic Z, Cankovic-Kadijevic M. Association of blood pressure and metabolic syndrome components with magnesium levels in drinking water in some Serbian municipalities. *J Water Health*. 2012;10(1):161–9.

[13] Naumann J, Biehler D, Lüty T, Sadaghiani C. Prevention and therapy of type 2 diabetes—what is the potential of daily water intake and its mineral nutrients? *Nutrients*. 2017;9(8):914.

[14] Cianciolo G, De Pascalis A, Capelli I, Gasperoni L, Di Lullo L, Bellasi A, La Manna G. Mineral and electrolyte disorders with SGLT2i therapy. *JBMR Plus*. 2019;3(11):e10242.

[15] Costa-Vieira D, Monteiro R, Martins MJ. Metabolic Syndrome features: Is there a modulation role by mineral water consumption? A review. *Nutrients*. 2019;11(5):1141.

[16] Dore MP, Pes GM, Realdi G. Health properties of the Italian San Martino® mineral-rich water: A self-controlled pilot study. *Biomed Pharmacother*. 2021;138:111509.

[17] World Health Organization. *Noncommunicable diseases*. Available at: https://www.who.int/data/gho/data/themes/noncommunicable-diseases. Accessed on August 25, 2021.

[18] Sadik NAH, El-Seweidy MM, Shaker OG. The antiapoptotic effects of sulphurous mineral water and sodium hydrosulphide on diabetic rat testes. *Cell Physiol Biochem*. 2011;28(5):887–98.

[19] Costantino M, Giampaolo C, Filippelli A. Effetti della crenoterapia idropinica sullo stress ossidativo. [Effects of drinking spa therapy on oxidative stress]. *Clin Ter*. 2012;163(1):e13-7.

[20] Pereira CD, Severo M, Araújo JR, Guimarães JT, Pestana D, Santos A, Ferreira R, Ascensão A, Magalhães J, Azevedo I, Monteiro R, Martins MJ. Relevance of a hypersaline sodium-rich naturally sparkling mineral water to the protection against metabolic syndrome induction in fructose-fed Sprague-Dawley rats: A biochemical, metabolic, and redox approach. *Int J Endocrinol*. 2014;2014:384583.

[21] Lalovic D, Jakovljevic V, Radoman K, Bradic J, Jeremic N, Vranic A, Milosavljevic I, Jeremic J, Srejovic I, Turnic TN, Zivkovic V, Stanojevic D, Bolevich S, Djuric DM. The impact of low mineral content water on cardiac function in diabetic rats: Focus on oxidative stress. *Mol Cell Biochem*. 2020;472(1–2):135–44.

[22] Guillemant J, Le H-T, Accarie C, du Montcel ST, Delabroise AM, Arnaud MJ, Guillemant S. Mineral water as a source of dietary calcium: Acute effects on parathyroid function and bone resorption in young men. *Am J Clin Nutr*. 2000;71(4):999–1002.

[23] Guillemant J, Accarie C, De La Guéronnière V, Guillemant S. Calcium in mineral water can effectively suppress parathyroid function and bone resorption. *Nutr Res* 2002;22(8):901–10.

[24] Guillemant J, Accarie C, Peres G, Guillemant S. Acute effects of an oral calcium load on markers of bone metabolism during endurance cycling exercise in male athletes. *Calcif Tissue Int*. 2004;74(5):407–14.

[25] Meunier PJ, Jenvrin C, Munoz F, de la Gueronnière V, Garnero P, Menz M. Consumption of a high calcium mineral water lowers biochemical indices of bone remodeling in postmenopausal women with low calcium intake. *Osteoporos Int*. 2005;16(10):1203–9.

[26] Wynn E, Krieg M-A, Aeschlimann J-M, Burckhardt P. Alkaline mineral water lowers bone resorption even in calcium sufficiency:

Alkaline mineral water and bone metabolism. *Bone*. 2009;44(1):120–4.

[27] Das JK, Severo M, Pereira CD, Patrício E, Magalhães J, Monteiro R, Neves D, Martins MJ. Natural mineral-rich water ingestion by ovariectomized fructose-fed Sprague-Dawley rats: Effects on sirtuin 1 and glucocorticoid signaling pathways. *Menopause*. 2017;24(5):563–73.

[28] Pereira CD, Severo M, Neves D, Ascensão A, Magalhães J, Guimarães JT, Monteiro R, Martins MJ. Natural mineral-rich water ingestion improves hepatic and fat glucocorticoid-signaling and increases sirtuin 1 in an animal model of metabolic syndrome. *Horm Mol Biol Clin Investig*. 2015;21(2):149–57.

[29] Pereira CD, Passos E, Severo M, Vitó I, Wen X, Carneiro F, Gomes P, Monteiro R, Martins MJ. Ingestion of a natural mineral-rich water in an animal model of metabolic syndrome: Effects in insulin signalling and endoplasmic reticulum stress. *Horm Mol Biol Clin Investig*. 2016;26(2):135-50.

[30] Sheu M-J, Chou P-Y, Lin W-H, Pan CH, Chien YC, Chung YL, Liu FC, Wu CH. Deep sea water modulates blood pressure and exhibits hypolipidemic effects via the AMPK-ACC pathway: An in vivo study. *Mar Drugs*. 2013;11(6):2183–202.

[31] Fu Z-Y, Yang F Lo, Hsu H-W, Lu Y-F. Drinking deep seawater decreases serum total and low-density lipoprotein–cholesterol in hypercholesterolemic subjects. *J Med Food*. 2012;15(6):535–41.

[32] Lu C, Ou H, Day C, Chen HI, Pai PY, Lee CY, Chen RJ, Chang RL, PadmaViswanadha V, Hsieh DJ, Huang CY. Deep sea minerals ameliorate diabetic-induced inflammation via inhibition of TNFα signaling pathways. *Environ Toxicol*. 2020;35(4):468–77.

[33] Ha B, Shin E, Park J-E, Shon Y. Anti-diabetic effect of balanced deep-sea water and its mode of action in high-fat diet induced diabetic mice. *Mar Drugs*. 2013;11(11):4193–212.

[34] Ha BG, Park J-E, Shin EJ, Shon YH. Modulation of glucose metabolism by balanced deep-sea water ameliorates

hyperglycemia and pancreatic function in streptozotocin-induced diabetic mice. *PLoS One*. 2014;9(7):e102095.

[35] Ha BG, Park J-E, Cho H-J, Shon YH. Stimulatory effects of balanced deep sea water on mitochondrial biogenesis and function. *PLoS One*. 2015;10(6):e0129972.

[36] Ha BG, Moon D-S, Kim HJ, Shon YH. Magnesium and calcium-enriched deep-sea water promotes mitochondrial biogenesis by AMPK-activated signals pathway in 3T3-L1 preadipocytes. *Biomed Pharmacother*. 2016;83:477–84.

[37] Ha B, Jung S, Jang Y, Jeon B, Shon Y. Mineral-enriched deep-sea water modulates lactate metabolism via PGC-1α-mediated metabolic reprogramming. *Mar Drugs*. 2019;17(11):611.

[38] Boulangé CL, Neves AL, Chilloux J, Nicholson JK, Dumas M-E. Impact of the gut microbiota on inflammation, obesity, and metabolic disease. *Genome Med*. 2016;8(1):42.

[39] Clarke G, Stilling RM, Kennedy PJ, Stanton C, Cryan JF, Dinan TG. Minireview: Gut microbiota: The neglected endocrine organ. *Mol Endocrinol*. 2014;28(8):1221–38.

[40] Levy M, Kolodziejczyk AA, Thaiss CA, Elinav E. Dysbiosis and the immune system. *Nat Rev Immunol*. 2017;17(4):219–32.

[41] Scheithauer TPM, Rampanelli E, Nieuwdorp M, Vallance BA, Verchere CB, van Raalte DH, Herrema H. Gut microbiota as a trigger for metabolic inflammation in obesity and type 2 diabetes. *Front Immunol*. 2020;11:571731.

[42] Martinez KB, Leone V, Chang EB. Western diets, gut dysbiosis, and metabolic diseases: Are they linked? *Gut Microbes*. 2017;8(2):130–42.

[43] Moszak M, Szulińska M, Bogdański P. You are what you eat - The relationship between diet, microbiota, and metabolic disorders - A review. *Nutrients*. 2020;12(4):1096.

[44] Tilg H, Zmora N, Adolph TE, Elinav E. The intestinal microbiota fuelling metabolic inflammation. *Nat Rev Immunol*. 2020;20(1):40–54.

[45] Mohammad S, Thiemermann C. Role of metabolic endotoxemia in systemic inflammation and potential interventions. *Front Immunol*. 2021;11:594150.

[46] Li X, Watanabe K, Kimura I. Gut microbiota dysbiosis drives and implies novel therapeutic strategies for diabetes mellitus and related metabolic diseases. *Front Immunol*. 2017;8:1882.

[47] Magne F, Gotteland M, Gauthier L, Zazueta A, Pesoa S, Navarrete P, Balamurugan R. The Firmicutes/Bacteroidetes ratio: A relevant marker of gut dysbiosis in obese patients? *Nutrients*. 2020;12(5):1474.

[48] Vrieze A, Van Nood E, Holleman F, Salojärvi J, Kootte RS, Bartelsman JF, Dallinga-Thie GM, Ackermans MT, Serlie MJ, Oozeer R, Derrien M, Druesne A, Van Hylckama Vlieg JE, Bloks VW, Groen AK, Heilig HG, Zoetendal EG, Stroes ES, de Vos WM, Hoekstra JB, Nieuwdorp M. Transfer of intestinal microbiota from lean donors increases insulin sensitivity in individuals with metabolic syndrome. *Gastroenterology*. 2012;143(4):913-6.e7.

[49] Ridaura VK, Faith JJ, Rey FE, Cheng J, Duncan AE, Kau AL, Griffin NW, Lombard V, Henrissat B, Bain JR, Muehlbauer MJ, Ilkayeva O, Semenkovich CF, Funai K, Hayashi DK, Lyle BJ, Martini MC, Ursell LK, Clemente JC, Van Treuren W, Walters WA, Knight R, Newgard CB, Heath AC, Gordon JI. Gut microbiota from twins discordant for obesity modulate metabolism in mice. *Science*. 2013;341(6150):1241214.

[50] Suárez-Zamorano N, Fabbiano S, Chevalier C, Stojanović O, Colin DJ, Stevanović A, Veyrat-Durebex C, Tarallo V, Rigo D, Germain S, Ilievska M, Montet X, Seimbille Y, Hapfelmeier S, Trajkovski M. Microbiota depletion promotes browning of white adipose tissue and reduces obesity. *Nat Med*. 2015;21(12):1497–501.

[51] van den Munckhof ICL, Kurilshikov A, ter Horst R, Riksen NP, Joosten LAB, Zhernakova A, Fu J, Keating ST, Netea MG, de Graaf J, Rutten JHW. Role of gut microbiota in chronic low-grade

inflammation as potential driver for atherosclerotic cardiovascular disease: A systematic review of human studies. *Obes Rev*. 2018;19(12):1719–34.

[52] Pontes KSDS, Guedes MR, Cunha MRD, Mattos SS, Barreto Silva MI, Neves MF, Marques BCAA, Klein MRST. Effects of probiotics on body adiposity and cardiovascular risk markers in individuals with overweight and obesity: A systematic review and meta-analysis of randomized controlled trials. *Clin Nutr*. 2021;40(8):4915–31.

[53] Depommier C, Everard A, Druart C, Plovier H, Van Hul M, Vieira-Silva S, Falony G, Raes J, Maiter D, Delzenne NM, de Barsy M, Loumaye A, Hermans MP, Thissen JP, de Vos WM, Cani PD. Supplementation with *Akkermansia muciniphila* in overweight and obese human volunteers: A proof-of-concept exploratory study. *Nat Med*. 2019;25(7):1096–103.

[54] Brandão I, Martins MJ, Monteiro R. Metabolically healthy obesity - Heterogeneity in definitions and unconventional factors. *Metabolites*. 2020;10(2):48.

[55] Brandsma E, Kloosterhuis NJ, Koster M, Dekker DC, Gijbels MJJ, van der Velden S, Ríos-Morales M, van Faassen MJR, Loreti MG, de Bruin A, Fu J, Kuipers F, Bakker BM, Westerterp M, de Winther MPJ, Hofker MH, van de Sluis B, Koonen DPY. A proinflammatory gut microbiota increases systemic inflammation and accelerates atherosclerosis. *Circ Res*. 2019;124(1):94–100.

[56] Cuevas-Sierra A, Ramos-Lopez O, Riezu-Boj JI, Milagro FI, Martinez JA. Diet, gut microbiota, and obesity: Links with host genetics and epigenetics and potential applications. *Adv Nutr*. 2019;10(suppl_1):S17–30.

[57] Turnbaugh PJ, Ley RE, Mahowald MA, Magrini V, Mardis ER, Gordon JI. An obesity-associated gut microbiome with increased capacity for energy harvest. *Nature*. 2006;444(7122):1027–131.

[58] Samuel BS, Shaito A, Motoike T, Rey FE, Backhed F, Manchester JK, Hammer RE, Williams SC, Crowley J, Yanagisawa M, Gordon JI. Effects of the gut microbiota on host adiposity are

modulated by the short-chain fatty-acid binding G protein-coupled receptor, Gpr41. *Proc Natl Acad Sci.* 2008;105(43):16767–72.

[59] Canfora EE, Meex RCR, Venema K, Blaak EE. Gut microbial metabolites in obesity, NAFLD and T2DM. *Nat Rev Endocrinol.* 2019;15(5):261–73.

[60] He J, Zhang P, Shen L, Niu L, Tan Y, Chen L, Zhao Y, Bai L, Hao X, Li X, Zhang S, Zhu L. Short-chain fatty acids and their association with signalling pathways in inflammation, glucose and lipid metabolism. *Int J Mol Sci.* 2020;21(17):6356.

[61] Bischoff SC, Barbara G, Buurman W, Ockhuizen T, Schulzke JD, Serino M, Tilg H, Watson A, Wells JM. Intestinal permeability – a new target for disease prevention and therapy. *BMC Gastroenterol.* 2014;14(1):189.

[62] Batterham RL, Cowley MA, Small CJ, Herzog H, Cohen MA, Dakin CL, Wren AM, Brynes AE, Low MJ, Ghatei MA, Cone RD, Bloom SR. Gut hormone PYY(3-36) physiologically inhibits food intake. *Nature.* 2002;418(6898):650–4.

[63] van den Hoek AM, Heijboer AC, Corssmit EPM, Voshol PJ, Romijn JA, Havekes LM, Pijl H. PYY3-36 reinforces insulin action on glucose disposal in mice fed a high-fat diet. *Diabetes.* 2004;53(8):1949–52.

[64] Chelakkot C, Ghim J, Ryu SH. Mechanisms regulating intestinal barrier integrity and its pathological implications. *Exp Mol Med.* 2018;50(8):1–9.

[65] Paone P, Cani PD. Mucus barrier, mucins and gut microbiota: The expected slimy partners? *Gut.* 2020;69(12):2232–43.

[66] Hotamisligil GS. Inflammation and metabolic disorders. *Nature.* 2006;444(7121):860–7.

[67] Lupp C, Robertson ML, Wickham ME, Sekirov I, Champion OL, Gaynor EC, Finlay BB. Host-mediated inflammation disrupts the intestinal microbiota and promotes the overgrowth of Enterobacteriaceae. *Cell Host Microbe.* 2007;2(2):119–29.

[68] Hiippala K, Jouhten H, Ronkainen A, Hartikainen A, Kainulainen V, Jalanka J, Satokari R. The potential of gut commensals in

reinforcing intestinal barrier function and alleviating inflammation. *Nutrients*. 2018;10(8):988.

[69] Rizzatti G, Lopetuso LR, Gibiino G, Binda C, Gasbarrini A. Proteobacteria: A common factor in human diseases. *Biomed Res Int*. 2017;2017:1–7.

[70] Brown JM, Hazen SL. The gut microbial endocrine organ: Bacterially derived signals driving cardiometabolic diseases. *Annu Rev Med.* 2015;66:343–59.

[71] Le Roy T, Moens de Hase E, Van Hul M, Paquot A, Pelicaen R, Régnier M, Depommier C, Druart C, Everard A, Maiter D, Delzenne NM, Bindels LB, de Barsy M, Loumaye A, Hermans MP, Thissen JP, Vieira-Silva S, Falony G, Raes J, Muccioli GG, Cani PD. *Dysosmobacter welbionis* is a newly isolated human commensal bacterium preventing diet-induced obesity and metabolic disorders in mice. *Gut*. 2021 [Online ahead of print].

[72] Zeng Q, Li D, He Y, Li Y, Yang Z, Zhao X, Liu Y, Wang Y, Sun J, Feng X, Wang F, Chen J, Zheng Y, Yang Y, Sun X, Xu X, Wang D, Kenney T, Jiang Y, Gu H, Li Y, Zhou K, Li S, Dai W. Discrepant gut microbiota markers for the classification of obesity-related metabolic abnormalities. *Sci Reports*. 2019;9(1):13424.

[73] Unno Y, Sato Y, Nishida S, Nakano A, Nakano R, Ubagai T, Ono Y. *Acinetobacter baumannii* lipopolysaccharide influences adipokine expression in 3T3-L1 adipocytes. *Mediators Inflamm*. 2017;2017:9039302.

[74] Paganelli FL, Luyer M, Hazelbag CM, Uh HW, Rogers MRC, Adriaans D, Berbers RM, Hendrickx APA, Viveen MC, Groot JA, Bonten MJM, Fluit AC, Willems RJL, Leavis HL. Roux-Y gastric bypass and sleeve gastrectomy directly change gut microbiota composition independent of surgery type. *Sci Reports*. 2019;9(1):10979.

[75] Chávez-Carbajal A, Nirmalkar K, Pérez-Lizaur A, Hernández-Quiroz F, Ramírez-Del-Alto S, García-Mena J, Hernández-Guerrero C. Gut microbiota and predicted metabolic pathways in

a sample of mexican women affected by obesity and obesity plus metabolic syndrome. *Int J Mol Sci.* 2019;20(2):438.

[76] Kadooka Y, Sato M, Ogawa A, Miyoshi M, Uenishi H, Ogawa H, Ikuyama K, Kagoshima M, Tsuchida T. Effect of *Lactobacillus gasseri* SBT2055 in fermented milk on abdominal adiposity in adults in a randomised controlled trial. *Br J Nutr.* 2013;110(9):1696–703.

[77] World Health Organization. *Health risks from drinking demineralised water*. WHO Press Geneva: 2004. Available at: https://www.who.int/water_sanitation_health/dwq/nutrientschap12.pdf. Accessed on August 21, 2021.

[78] Barnich N, Rodrigues M, Sauvanet P, Chevarin C, Denis S, Le Goff O, Faure-Imbert D, Hanh T, Roques CF, Chassaing B, Alric M. Beneficial effects of natural mineral waters on intestinal inflammation and the mucosa-associated microbiota. *Int J Mol Sci.* 2021;22(9):4336.

[79] Maraver F. Lanjarón (Balneario y Aguas). [Spa and waters]. *Bol Soc Española Hidrol Medica.* [*Bulletin of the Spanish Society of Medical Hydrology*]. 1987;2(3):137–40.

[80] Crespo P-V, Campos F, Leal M, Maraver F. Effects of sodium chloride-rich mineral water on intestinal epithelium. experimental study. *Int J Environ Res Public Health.* 2021;18(6):3261.

[81] Zhou K, Liu W, Chen Z, Yang D, Qiu Z, Feng H, Li C, Jin M, Li J, Xu Q, Shen Z. The effect of different drinking water in culture medium on feces microbiota diversity. *J Water Health.* 2021;19(2):267–77.

[82] Chen Y, Yang F, Lu H, Wang B, Chen Y, Lei D, Wang Y, Zhu B, Li L. Characterization of fecal microbial communities in patients with liver cirrhosis. *Hepatology.* 2011;54(2):562–72.

[83] Zong-Jie L, Zhen C. Effects of metabolic syndrome on intestinal flora, inflammatory factors, and infants of pregnant patients. *Clin Lab*. 2020;66(10).

[84] Bowyer RCE, Schillereff DN, Jackson MA, Le Roy C, Wells PM, Spector TD, Steves CJ. Associations between UK tap water and

gut microbiota composition suggest the gut microbiome as a potential mediator of health differences linked to water quality. *Sci Total Environ*. 2020;739:139697.

[85] Yahiro T, Hara T, Matsumoto T, Ikebe E, Fife-Koshinomi N, Xu Z, Hiratsuka T, Iha H, Inomata M. Long-Term Potable Effects of Alkalescent Mineral Water on Intestinal Microbiota Shift and Physical Conditioning. *Evid Based Complement Altern Med*. 2019;2019:2710587.

[86] Dias MF, Reis MP, Acurcio LB, Carmo AO, Diamantino CF, Motta AM, Kalapothakis E, Nicoli JR, Nascimento AMA. Changes in mouse gut bacterial community in response to different types of drinking water. *Water Res*. 2018;132:79–89.

[87] Scully IL, McNeil LK, Pathirana S, Singer CL, Liu Y, Mullen S, Girgenti D, Gurtman A, Pride MW, Jansen KU, Huang PL, Anderson AS. Neutrophil killing of *Staphylococcus aureus* in diabetes, obesity and metabolic syndrome: A prospective cellular surveillance study. *Diabetol Metab Syndr*. 2017;9(1):76.

[88] Murakami S, Goto Y, Ito K, Hayasaka S, Kurihara S, Soga T, Tomita M, Fukuda S. The consumption of bicarbonate-rich mineral water improves glycemic control. *Evid Based Complement Altern Med*. 2015;2015:824395.

[89] Goodrich JK, Waters JL, Poole AC, Sutter JL, Koren O, Blekhman R, Beaumont M, Van Treuren W, Knight R, Bell JT, Spector TD, Clark AG, Ley RE. Human genetics shape the gut microbiome. *Cell*. 2014;159(4):789.

[90] Pereira CD, Collado MC, Passos E, Azevedo I, Monteiro R, Martins MJ. Comment to: Luo et al. (2013) *Int J Cardiol*. 168(4):4454–6. *Int J Cardiol*. 2014;172(2):512–4.

[91] Zhong N, Ma Y, Meng X, Sowanou A, Wu L, Huang W, Gao Y, Pei J. Effect of fluoride in drinking water on fecal microbial community in rats. *Biol Trace Elem Res*. 2022 Jan;200(1):238-246.

[92] Amini H, Taghavi Shahri SM, Amini M, Ramezani Mehrian M, Mokhayeri Y, Yunesian M. Drinking water fluoride and blood

pressure? An environmental study. *Biol Trace Elem Res.* 2011;144(1-3):157–63.

[93] Afolabi OK, Oyewo EB, Adekunle AS, Adedosu OT, Adedeji AL. Oxidative indices correlate with dyslipidemia and pro-inflammatory cytokine levels in fluoride-exposed rats. *Arh Hig Rada Toksikol.* 2013;64(4):521–9.

[94] Yousefi M, Yaseri M, Nabizadeh R, Hooshmand E, Jalilzadeh M, Mahvi AH, Mohammadi AA. Association of hypertension, body mass index, and waist circumference with fluoride intake; water drinking in residents of fluoride endemic areas, Iran. *Biol Trace Elem Res.* 2018;185(2):282–8.

[95] Sun L, Gao Y, Zhang W, Liu H, Sun D. Effect of high fluoride and high fat on serum lipid levels and oxidative stress in rabbits. *Environ Toxicol Pharmacol.* 2014;38(3):1000–6.

[96] Pereira AG, Chiba FY, de Lima Coutinho Mattera MS, Pereira RF, de Cássia Alves Nunes R, Tsosura TVS, Okamoto R, Sumida DH. Effects of fluoride on insulin signaling and bone metabolism in ovariectomized rats. *J Trace Elem Med Biol.* 2017;39:140–6.

[97] Liu Y, Téllez-Rojo M, Sánchez BN, Ettinger AS, Osorio-Yáñez C, Solano M, Hu H, Peterson KE. Association between fluoride exposure and cardiometabolic risk in peripubertal Mexican children. *Environ Int.* 2020;134:105302.

[98] Lian N, Shen M, Zhang K, Pan J, Jiang Y, Yu Y, Yu Y. Drinking hydrogen-rich water alleviates chemotherapy-induced neuropathic pain through the regulation of gut microbiota. *J Pain Res.* 2021;14:681-91.

[99] Xiao H, Li Y, Luo D, Dong JL, Zhou LX, Zhao SY, Zheng QS, Wang HC, Cui M, Fan SJ. Hydrogen-water ameliorates radiation-induced gastrointestinal toxicity via MyD88's effects on the gut microbiota. *Exp Mol Med.* 2018;50(1):e433.

[100] Vacca M, Celano G, Calabrese FM, Portincasa P, Gobbetti M, De Angelis M. The controversial role of human gut Lachnospiraceae. *Microorganisms.* 2020;8(4):573.

[101] Coppola S, Avagliano C, Calignano A, Canani RB. The protective role of butyrate against obesity and obesity-related diseases. *Molecules*. 2021;26(3) :682.

[102] Brahe LK, Astrup A, Larsen LH. Is butyrate the link between diet, intestinal microbiota and obesity-related metabolic diseases? *Obes Rev*. 2013;14(12):950–9.

[103] LeBaron TW, Singh RB, Fatima G, Kartikey K, Sharma JP, Ostojic SM, Gvozdjakova A, Kura B, Noda M, Mojto V, Niaz MA, Slezak J. The effects of 24-week, high-concentration hydrogen-rich water on body composition, blood lipid profiles and inflammation biomarkers in men and women with Metabolic Syndrome: A randomized controlled trial. *Diabetes, Metab Syndr Obes Targets Ther*. 2020;13:889–96.

[104] Król A, Mizerna K, Bożym M. An assessment of pH-dependent release and mobility of heavy metals from metallurgical slag. *J Hazard Mater.* 2020;384:121502.

[105] Riba I, Delvalls TÁ, Forja JM, Gómez-Parra A. The influence of pH and salinity on the toxicity of heavy metals in sediment to the estuarine clam *Ruditapes philippinarum. Environ Toxicol Chem*. 2004;23(5):1100–7.

[106] Nägeli KW. Über oligodynamische Erscheinungen in lebenden Zellen. [About oligodynamic phenomena in living cells]. In: *Neue Denkschriften der Allg Schweizerischen Gesellschaft für die Gesamte Naturwiss*. [*New memoranda of the Allg Swiss Society for the whole of natural science*]. Zurich: Zürcher & Furrer; 1893-1895:1–51.

[107] Kraemer H. The Oligodynamic Action of Copper Foil on Certain Intestinal Organisms. In: *Proceedings of the American Philosophical Society American Philosophical Society.* Philadelphia: American Philosophical Society; 1905:51–65.

[108] Dupont CL, Grass G, Rensing C. Copper toxicity and the origin of bacterial resistance - New insights and applications. *Metallomics.* 2011;3(11):1109–18.

[109] Johnson TB, Langin LM, Zhao J, Weimer JM, Pearce DA, Kovács AD. Changes in motor behavior, neuropathology, and gut microbiota of a Batten disease mouse model following administration of acidified drinking water. *Sci Rep.* 2019;9(1):14962.

[110] Whipple B, Agar J, Zhao J, Pearce DA, Kovács AD. The acidified drinking water-induced changes in the behavior and gut microbiota of wild-type mice depend on the acidification mode. *Sci Rep*. 2021;11(1):2877.

[111] Carbonero F, Benefiel AC, Alizadeh-Ghamsari AH, Gaskins HR. Microbial pathways in colonic sulfur metabolism and links with health and disease. *Front Physiol*. 2012;3:448.

[112] Deplancke B, Hristova KR, Oakley HA, McCracken VJ, Aminov R, Mackie RI, Gaskins HR. Molecular ecological analysis of the succession and diversity of sulfate-reducing bacteria in the mouse gastrointestinal tract. *Appl Environ Microbiol*. 2000;66(5):2166–74.

[113] Marietta EV, Gomez AM, Yeoman C, Tilahun AY, Clark CR, Luckey DH, Murray JA, White BA, Kudva YC, Rajagopalan G. Low incidence of spontaneous type 1 diabetes in non-obese diabetic mice raised on gluten-free diets is associated with changes in the intestinal microbiome. *PLoS One*. 2013; 8(11):e78687.

[114] Hamid H, Shi HQ, Ma GY, Fan Y, Li WX, Zhao LH, Zhang JY, Ji C, Ma QG. Influence of acidified drinking water on growth performance and gastrointestinal function of broilers. *Poult Sci*. 2018;97(10):3601–9.

[115] Sofi MH, Gudi R, Karumuthil-Melethil S, Perez N, Johnson BM, Vasu C. pH of drinking water influences the composition of gut microbiome and type 1 diabetes incidence. *Diabetes*. 2014;63(2):632-44.

[116] Wolf KJ, Daft JG, Tanner SM, Hartmann R, Khafipour E, Lorenz RG. Consumption of acidic water alters the gut microbiome and decreases the risk of diabetes in nod mice. *J Histochem Cytochem*. 2014;62(4):237-50.

[117] Bidot WA, Ericsson AC, Franklin CL. Effects of water decontamination methods and bedding material on the gut microbiota. *PLoS One*. 2018;13(10):e0198305.

[118] Hansen TH, Thomassen MT, Madsen ML, Kern T, Bak EG, Kashani A, Allin KH, Hansen T, Pedersen O. The effect of drinking water pH on the human gut microbiota and glucose regulation: Results of a randomized controlled cross-over intervention. *Sci Reports*. 2018;8(1):16626.

[119] Wickramasinghe HKJP, Anast JM, Schmitz-Esser S, Serão NVL, Appuhamy JADRN. Beginning to offer drinking water at birth increases the species richness and the abundance of *Faecalibacterium* and *Bifidobacterium* in the gut of preweaned dairy calves. *J Dairy Sci*. 2020;103(5):4262–74.

[120] Nakamura Y, Watanabe H, Tanaka A, Yasui M, Nishihira J, Murayama N. Effect of Increased Daily Water Intake and Hydration on Health in Japanese Adults. *Nutrients*. 2020;12(4):1191.

[121] Piperata BA, Lee S, Mayta Apaza AC, Cary A, Vilchez S, Oruganti P, Garabed R, Wilson W, Lee J. Characterization of the gut microbiota of Nicaraguan children in a water insecure context. *Am J Hum Biol*. 2020;32(1):e23371.

In: Mineral Water
Editors: Maria João Martins
ISBN: 978-1-68507-458-6

Chapter 8

INFLUENCE OF MINERAL WATERS UPON MEMBRANE TRANSPORTERS

***Fátima Martel*[*], PhD**
Department of Biomedicine, Biochemistry Unit,
Faculty of Medicine, University of Porto, Porto, Portugal
i3S-Instituto de Investigação e Inovação em Saúde,
University of Porto, Porto, Portugal

ABSTRACT

Membrane transporters present in our body are involved in the transport of most substances across cell and intracellular membranes. They are therefore determinants of the biological activity, biodistribution, absorption and excretion of both endogenous and exogenous compounds, of both natural and synthetic origin, in our body. The activity of these membrane proteins is therefore of fundamental importance for cell, tissue, organ and body homeostasis and changes in the activity of these proteins often lead to disease. Over the last several years, considerable progress has been made regarding the molecular identification and functional characterization of membrane transporters.

[*] Corresponding Author's E-mail: fmartel@med.up.pt.

However, very little is known concerning the effect of mineral waters on specific membrane transport mechanisms. In this chapter, we summarise knowledge concerning the interaction of mineral waters with specific membrane transporters. It is concluded that mineral waters are able to interact with some membrane transporters and can therefore affect the biological activity of these proteins. These effects can be of relevance for the biological effects of the mineral waters.

Keywords: inorganic element, membrane transporter, mineral water, organic compound

INTRODUCTION

The majority of solutes, including endogenous compounds, nutrients, xenobiotics, toxins and drugs, use membrane transporters in order to cross biological membranes. So, membrane transporters, by mediating the passage of most solutes across biological membranes, are an essential component of cell, tissue, organ and body homeostasis. Accordingly, under some physiological and pathophysiological conditions, the expression and transport activity of specific membrane transporters are changed, affecting the transport of specific substances across membranes.

The minerals present in mineral waters may interact with membrane transport mechanisms in several distinct ways. First, the minerals can be themselves transported across cell membranes by using specific ion channels or membrane transport proteins. So, membrane transport activity influences absorption, distribution, biological effects, metabolism and excretion of minerals present in mineral waters. Second, the minerals present in mineral waters can influence the expression and/or activity of specific membrane transporters. Namely: (1) the activity of many membrane transporters depends on the presence of specific ions, e.g., Na^+, Cl^- or HCO_3^-. For instance, sodium/glucose cotransporter 1 (SGLT1)-mediated transport of glucose depends on a Na^+ gradient and Na^+ is transported together with glucose across the cell membrane; (2) the activity of many membrane transporters is dependent on the pH, which can be modulated by the minerals present in mineral waters; (3) carrier-transported minerals present in mineral waters will affect the ability of the carrier to transport these minerals from other food sources, and (4) some inorganic ions are specific allosteric modulators of membrane transporters. For instance, the glutamate transport mediated by excitatory amino acid transporters is inhibited by Zn^{2+} [1].

Over the last several years, considerable progress has been made regarding the molecular identification and functional characterization of membrane transporters. However, very little is known concerning the effect of mineral waters on specific membrane transport mechanisms. Mineral waters are claimed to possess preventive and therapeutic effects in a number of pathologies including gastrointestinal [2, 3], renal [4], cardiovascular, cerebrovascular [5, 6], neurologic [7], obstetric-gynecologic, hematological, rheumatic, dermatological, respiratory [8], metabolic [9] and osteoporotic [10] (see other chapters). It is very plausible that the effect of mineral waters on membrane transporters may contribute to their health effects. In this review, we will summarise current knowledge concerning the effect of mineral waters on membrane transporters.

EFFECT ON MEMBRANE TRANSPORT OF ORGANIC COMPOUNDS

Effect on Butyrate Transport

The short-chain fatty acid butyrate is a main end-product of anaerobic bacterial fermentation of dietary fibre within the human colon. Butyrate plays a key role in colonic epithelium homeostasis, possessing multiple important roles at that level. Namely, butyrate (1) is the main energy source for the intestinal epithelial cells; (2) promotes growth and proliferation of normal intestinal epithelial cells; (3) inhibits inflammation; (4) inhibits oxidative stress; (5) improves the colonic defence barrier function; (6)

stimulates mucus secretion; (7) stimulates fluid and electrolyte absorption and (8) inhibits colon carcinogenesis [11, 12].

The acute (20 min), sub-acute (2 h) and chronic (48 h) effects of three distinct commercial mineral waters (Pedras Salgadas®, Vidago® and Melgaço®) on the *in vitro* uptake of butyrate by a human intestinal epithelial cell line (Caco-2 cells) was studied [13]. Pedras Salgadas® and Vidago® are mineral-rich waters, while Melgaço® is a medium-mineral content water and, according to the predominant chemical element, Pedras Salgadas® and Vidago® waters are classified as sodium-bicarbonate-fluorate-carbonic waters, whereas Melgaço® is a bicarbonate-fluorate-carbonic water (Figure 1) [8, 13].

	Pedras Salgadas®	**Vidago®**	**Melgaço®**
Total dissolved solids (mg/L)	1973	1870	711
Electrical conductivity (µS/cm)	2260	2370	909
pH	6.16	6.16	5.72
Free CO_2 (g/L)	3.9	3.4	5.1
Na^+ (mg/L)	641	627	82.2
K^+ (mg/L)	31.2	46.8	3.4
Ca^{2+} (mg/L)	106	82	137
Mg^{2+} (mg/L)	26.1	15.2	30.3
Li^+ (mg/L)	2.1	2.9	0.61
Mn^{2+} (mg/L)	0.215	0.224	0.245
Sr^{2+} (mg/L)	0.54	0.49	2.3
NH_4^+ (mg/L)	< 0.05	0.35	< 0.05
F^- (mg/L)	1.5	1.1	1.1
Cl^- (mg/L)	31.2	34.8	12.1
HCO_3^- (mg/L)	2135	2013	763
SO_4^{2-} (mg/L)	5.3	6.3	6.1
SiO_2 (mg/L)	60.4	46.4	53.8
NO_3^- (mg/L)	0.18	0.25	< 0.12

Figure 1. Chemical composition of the mineral waters Pedras Salgadas®, Vidago®, and Melgaço® used by [13].

Table 1. Effect of mineral waters on the transport of organic compounds

Mineral water	Solute/Transporter	Cell/animal/model	Effect	Ref.
Melgaço®, Vidago®, Pedras Salgadas®	Butyrate cellular uptake	Human intestinal epithelial cell line *in vitro* (Caco-2 cells)	↓: Melgaço® and Pedras Salgadas® (20 min) ↑: Vidago® (20 min) and Vidago® and Melgaço® (48 h)	[13]
Melgaço®, Vidago®, Pedras Salgadas®	O-Methyl-glucose cellular uptake	Human intestinal epithelial cell line *in vitro* (Caco-2 cells)	↓: Melgaço® (20 min and 48 h) ↑: Pedras Salgadas® (48 h)	[13]
Avène®	Renal elimination of lactulose and mannitol	Humans (atopic dermatitis patients)	↓	[28]
Two bicarbonated waters	ppTG	Healthy postmenopausal women	↓	[30]
Bicarbonated water	ppTG	Moderately hypercholesterolae-mic young male and female adults	↓	[31]
Volcic®, Evian®, Vittel®, Contrex®	Oleic acid cellular uptake	Hamster isolated enterocytes *in vitro*	↓	[35]

Table 1. (Continued)

Mineral water	Solute/Transporter	Cell/animal/model	Effect	Ref.
Avène®	ABCA12 expression	Normal human keratinocytes *in vitro*	↑	[40]
Balneotherapy with alcalinic salso-sulphidric ozonised water	SERT activity	Humans (healthy)	↑ Affinity of SERT for 5-HT	[45, 46]
Contrex®	Alendronate intestinal absorption (24 h)	Rats	↓	[47]
Evian®, Contrex®	Risedronate intestinal absorption (24 h)	Rats	↓	[48]

↓ decrease; ↑ increase; 5-HT: serotonin; ABCA12: ATP-binding cassete sub-family A member 12; Ref: reference; SERT: serotonin transporter (SLC6A4 gene); ppTG: postprandial triglyceride levels.

Vidago® water caused an increase in the uptake of butyrate, both acutely and chronically, Melgaço® water acutely decreased and chronically increased butyrate uptake, and Pedras Salgadas® decreased butyrate uptake, when acutely tested (Table 1). Moreover, uptake of butyrate was decreased after acute exposure to $MgCl_2$, $MgSO_4$ and $CaCl_2$. So, it was concluded that these minerals might be involved in the negative effect of these waters in relation to butyrate uptake [13].

Uptake of butyrate by Caco-2 cells is mainly mediated by the monocarboxylate transporter 1 (MCT1) [14, 15]. Given the beneficial effect of butyrate on human intestinal health, MCT1-mediated transport of butyrate into colonocytes is fundamental for the regulation of colon homeostasis. One of the important effects of butyrate at the colonic level is the prevention and inhibition of colon carcinogenesis. In this context,

MCT1 is considered a tumour suppressor [16, 17]. From the results of Gonçalves *et al.* [13], it can thus be concluded that modulation of butyrate uptake by mineral waters may interfere with the protective effect of fibre consumption/butyrate in relation to colorectal cancer.

Effect on Glucose Transport

Glucose is the main fuel that provides energy for normal activity in humans, its major source being the carbohydrates in food. Glucose derived from food and absorbed at the intestinal level plays an important role in the regulation of plasma glucose levels. Glucose homeostasis is essential to human health and a dysregulation in this process can increase the risk of obesity, type 2 diabetes, and cardiovascular events as well as lead to a higher mortality [18, 19]. So, knowledge on the factors affecting the intestinal absorption of glucose is of major importance. In this context, the acute (20 min), sub-acute (2h) and chronic (48h) effects of 3 distinct mineral waters (Pedras Salgadas®, Vidago® and Melgaço®) on the *in vitro* uptake of the glucose analogue 3-O-methyl-glucose (OMG) by Caco-2 cells was evaluated [13].

Both acutely and chronically, Melgaço® mineral water decreased OMG uptake, while chronic exposure to Pedras Salgadas® increased it (Table 1). The inhibitory effect of the Melgaço® mineral water upon OMG glucose suggests that ingestion of this water may reduce the intestinal absorption of glucose, thus having beneficial effects on pathologies such as type 2 diabetes and obesity. This observation is most interesting because there is an increase in the intestinal absorption of glucose in diabetes and obesity, through increased expression of SGLT1 and GLUT2 [20, 21].

Moreover, by testing the effects of some mineral salts upon OMG uptake, it was concluded that both SO_4^{2-} and F^- appear to have an inhibitory effect upon this parameter, and that Mg^{2+} appears to have no effect [13]. In this context, a previous work found F^- to reduce glucose uptake by isolated epithelial cells of rat intestine [22]. As to Na^+, a stimulatory effect of this ion on glucose intestinal absorption is very well documented [20,

23]. So, given the fact that Melgaço® mineral water has a much lower concentration of Na^+, comparatively with Pedras Salgadas®, it is possible that Na^+ is responsible for the stimulatory effect of Pedras Salgadas® mineral water on OMG uptake.

Fluoride, chloride, sodium, bicarbonate, sulphate/H_2S/H_2S donors, magnesium and calcium are present in relevant amounts in mineral waters linked to positive effects upon parameters associated with glucose homeostasis [9]. Accordingly, bicarbonate-sulphur mineral waters are indicated in diabetes, because they decrease glycaemia, polydipsia, and polyuria, and reduce insulin requirements [8]. So, it was hypothesized that a reduction on glucose intestinal absorption might contribute to the anti-diabetic effect of sulphur waters [13].

Effect on Lactulose and Mannitol Transport

A number of tests based on the passive absorption of sugars or sugar-derived compounds are used to assess intestinal permeability which is changed in disorders such as inflammatory bowel disease, acute pancreatitis or liver cirrhosis [24, 25]. The urinary lactulose/mannitol ratio is the most frequently used test of intestinal permeability used in clinical practice [26]. These probe compounds are passively absorbed from the intestine (by paracellular and transcellular routes, respectively), and are not extensively metabolised, being excreted unchanged in urine in proportion to the quantities absorbed [27].

Interestingly, a fraction of atopic dermatitis patients present an increase in the intestinal permeability to lactulose. During 18 days, these patients followed a medical Spa treatment course, including topical application and oral ingestion of Avène® spring water, a low mineral water (Figure 2). At the end of the treatment period, the lactulose concentration in urine diminished dramatically and urine mannitol was also found to be reduced over the cure period, although to a lesser extent (Table 1). It was thus concluded that low mineral water normalises the intestinal permeability of patients with atopic dermatitis [28].

Cations (mg/L)		Anions (mg/L)	
Mg^{2+}	22.5	HCO_3^-	234.8
Na^+	4.9	Cl^-	5.2
K^+	0.7	SO_4^{2-}	14.8
Ca^{2+}	44.3	NO_3^-	2.0
Mn^{2+}	20.0		

Figure 2. Chemical composition of Avène® spring water used in the study [28].

Effect on Lipid Transport

Food Lipids

The use of postprandial triglyceride (ppTG) levels as a cardiovascular disease risk indicator has gained recent popularity. ppTG refers to the rise in circulating blood triglycerides (TG) after the consumption of a meal. ppTG is the result of an increase in both intestine-derived chylomicrons and liver-derived VLDL [29]. A ppTG-lowering effect was noted for several bicarbonated mineral waters (Figures 3a and 3b) in randomised, cross-over studies involving healthy postmenopausal women [30] and moderately hypercholesterolaemic young adults [31] (Table 1). Because *chylomicra* TG derive mainly from dietary absorbed fatty acids which, in turn, result from digestion of food TG, this observation suggests that sodium-bicarbonated mineral water may decrease TG digestion and/or fatty acid intestinal absorption and/or chylomicron exocytosis [9, 32].

Oleic Acid

Several epidemiological studies indicate that the incidence of colon cancer is positively correlated with the dietary fat intake and negatively correlated with the intake of calcium [33, 34]. In this context, Goré *et al.* decided to investigate the effect of 4 distinct commercial mineral waters, with very different Ca^{2+} contents (Figure 3c), upon fatty acid absorption, by using *in vitro* isolated hamster enterocytes. Interestingly, they verified that the cellular uptake of oleic acid (1 min) was markedly reduced when Hanks medium was substituted by mineral waters, and that the ionic composition of these waters (Figure 3c) was correlated with the decrease of initial rates of oleic acid uptake (Table 1) [35].

a)

Component	Bicarbounated mineral water 1 mg/L (mmol/L)	Bicarbounated mineral water 2 mg/L (mmol/L)
DM	2872	2865
HCO_3^-	2094.4 (34.34)	2013 (32.99)
Cl^-	583.0 (16.44)	592 (16.7)
SO_4^{2-}	49.9 (0.52)	42.9 (0.45)
F^-	7.9 (1.0)	1.4 (0.07)
Ca^{2+}	43.6 (1.09)	52.1 (1.30)
Mg^{2+}	5.7 (0.24)	9.7 (0.40)
Na^+	1116.5 (48.57)	948 (41.3)
K^+	54.7 (1.4)	47.7 (1.22)

b)

	Bicarbounated water[a] mg/L (mmol/L)
HCO_3^-	2,120 (34.75)
Cl^-	597 (16.84)
SO_4^{2-}	45.3 (0.47)
F^-	0.9 (0.05)
Ca^{2+}	32.0 (0.80)
Mg^{2+}	9.4 (0.39)
Na^+	1,102 (47.91)
K^+	49.5 (1.27)

[a]Contains 3.9 g/L of CO_2.

c)

Ions (mg/L)	Water 1 (Volvic)	Water 2 (Evian)	Water 3 (Vittel)	Water 4 (Contrex)	Hank's medium
Ca^{2+}	9.9	78	202	467	50
Mg^{2+}	6.1	24	36	84	19.7
Na^+	9.4	5.0	-	7.0	3164
K^+	5.7	1.0	-	3.0	227
Cl^-	8.4	4.5	306	7.0	5139
SO_4^{2-}	6.9	10	402	1192	79
HCO_3^-	65.3	357	750	377	0
Total ion	109	309	750	1850	9790
pH	7.0	7.2	7.4	7.2	7.3
Osmolarity (mOsm/kg H_2O)	1	6	11	24	276

Figure 3. Chemical composition of the waters used in the studies to evaluate the effects on lipid transport. (a) Mineral components of the two bicarbonated waters tested by [30]; (b) Chemical composition of the bicarbonated water used by [31]; (c) Chemical composition of the mineral waters and Hanks' medium used by [35].

Further experiments to investigate the mechanism involved in the inhibitory effect of the mineral waters on oleic acid cellular uptake led the authors to conclude that the ion-induced inhibition of oleic acid uptake is not due to the formation of insoluble soaps but rather to a direct effect on the fatty acid transport in membranes, and that the action of mineral waters on the uptake of oleic acid by intestinal cells can be ascribed to the simultaneous and synergetic presence of several ions (notably Ca^{2+} and Mg^{2+}) and absence of others (notably Na^+ and Cl^-) [35].

Protein-mediated fatty acid uptake systems, i.e., fatty acid transporters, are believed to be the dominant means by which fatty acids are taken up on the apical membrane of enterocytes. A large number of fatty acid transporters have been identified, including fatty acid translocase (FAT/CD36), plasma membrane-associated fatty acid-binding protein (FABPpm), and a family of fatty acid transport proteins 1–6 (FATP1–6) [36]. The stimulatory effect of Na^+ upon fatty acid uptake is most probably related to the fact that intestinal fatty acid uptake is dependent on the presence of extracellular Na^+ [37, 38]. As to the other ions, nothing is known concerning their interaction with fatty acid membrane transporters.

Effect on Epidermoside Transport

The ABCA12 (ATP-binding cassette sub-family A member 12) gene is active in some types of skin cells and in several other tissues, such as testis, placenta, lung, stomach, and fetal brain and liver. This transporter appears to be essential for normal development of the skin, and it is known to transport epidermoside, a glucosylceramide, out of the keratinocytes of the stratum corneum of the epidermis [39].

Interestingly, *in vitro* incubation of normal human keratinocytes with a cell culture medium made with Avène® spring water led to an overexpression of ABCA12 [40] (Table 1).

Effect on SERT-Mediated Serotonin Transport

Serotonin (5-hydroxytryptamine, 5-HT) signaling in the central nervous system modulates several physiological functions, including sleep, mood, anxiety, appetite, affection, impulsivity, cognition as well as memory, and perception [e.g., 41]. Accordingly, dysregulation of 5-HT signaling has been linked to several central nervous system-associated disorders, such as depression, obsessive-compulsive disorder, anxiety disorders, and autism spectrum disorder [42].

The transporter protein that mediates 5-HT reuptake into the presynaptic terminals, once released in the synaptic cleft (SERT), is an important determinant of 5-HT signaling. SERT inhibitors are very effective antidepressants and are also therapeutically approved for the management of conditions such as anxiety disorders, *bulimia nervosa* and neuropathic pain [43]. Since blood platelets and neurons share a similar reuptake system of 5-HT, platelet SERT has become a useful peripheral model of presynaptic serotonergic activity [44].

Interestingly, balneotherapy treatment of healthy subjects in alcalinic salso-sulphidric ozonised water at 36 °C, performed in a single small pool for 20 min, caused an increase in the affinity of SERT for 5-HT (Table 1). This effect was not observed in subjects bathing in normal water. So, it was suggested that SERT modifications may be related to a specific effect of ozonised water and, perhaps, also to the increased sense of well-being [45, 46].

Effect on Bisphosphonates Transport

Bisphosphonates are antiosteoporotic agents prescribed for patients with osteoporosis. Their bioavailability is known to be reduced by high levels of metal cations (Ca^{2+}, Mg^{2+}, etc.). However, standards for these cations in water used for taking bisphosphonates have not been defined yet. In this regard, two studies examined the effect of mineral waters on the intestinal absorption of two different bisphosphonates.

Alendronate

Akagi *et al.* examined the effect of several distinct waters [ultrapure water, tap water, deep ocean water, Evian® and Contrex® mineral waters (Figure 4)] on the bioavailability of the second-generation bisphosphonate, alendronate, following oral administration in rats. Intestinal absorption of alendronate was determined based on 24-h urinary excretion of its unchanged form. Of the waters tested, only Contrex® was found to decrease alendronate absorption when compared with ultrapure water (Table 1). So, authors concluded that the absorption of alendronate is affected by the Ca^{2+} concentration of mineral water, and that, consequently, mineral water containing high levels of Ca^{2+} is not recommended when alendronate is taken [47].

Water	Ca^{2+} (mg/L)	Mg^{2+} (mg/L)	Total hardness (mg/L)
Ultrapure water	0	0	0
Tap water	13	4	48
"Amami no mizu" (Deep-Seawater)	68	215	1067
Evian®	83	20	289
Contrex®	469	77	1493

Figure 4. Chemical composition of the waters used in the works by [47] and [48].

Risedronate

Itoh *et al.* studied the effect of the same waters (Figure 4) on the bioavailability of the third-generation bisphosphonate, risedronate, following oral administration in rats. The 24-h urinary recovery of risedronate, reflecting its intestinal absorption, was significantly reduced by Evian® and Contrex® mineral waters (when compared with both ultrapure and tap water) (Table 1). By examining the effect of $CaCl_2$ and $MgCl_2$ on risedronate absorption, it was concluded that absorption of risedronate declines as the Ca^{2+} concentration of mineral waters increases. So, it was inferred that consumption of mineral waters containing high levels of calcium (80 mg/L or above), such as Evian® and Contrex®, is not recommended when taking risedronate [48].

EFFECT ON THE MEMBRANE TRANSPORT OF INORGANIC ELEMENTS

Effect on Na^+, K^+-ATPase Activity

Mineral water Naftusia® and its components (macrosalt analog and bitumen fraction) caused an *in vitro* inhibition in Na^+, K^+-ATPase activity of the mucous small intestine membrane (Table 2) [49]. The effect of this mineral water was also assessed *in vivo* in rats. Similarly to what was observed *in vitro*, Naftusia® mineral water induced sodium accumulation in the small intestine epithelium that was a result of Na^+, K^+-pump inhibition. However, in contrast, artificial salt Naftusia® analog (ASNA) activated the Na^+, K^+-ATPase (Table 2) [50].

Table 2. Effect of mineral waters on the transport of inorganic elements

Mineral water	Solute/ Transporter	Cell/animal/model	Effect	Ref.
Naftusia®	Na^+, K^+-ATPase activity	Mucous small intestinal membrane *in vitro*	↓	[49]
Naftusia®	Na^+, K^+-ATPase activity	Rats	↓	[50]
Marina®	Na^+, K^+-ATPase activity	Human erythrocytes (chronic active hepatitis or atherosclerosis patients)	↑	[51]
Contrex®	Ca^{2+} urinary excretion	Healthy young women	Ca^{2+} renal excretion ↑ than with milk	[63]
Avène®	TRPV6 Ca^{2+} channel expression and activity	Normal human keratinocyte cell line *in vitro* (NHC cells)	↑	[66]

Mineral water	Solute/ Transporter	Cell/animal/model	Effect	Ref.
Hita tenryosui® **Rokko®** **Evian®**	AQP-mediated water permeability	Oocytes expressing AQP *in vitro*	↑ AQP1- and AQP2-mediated water transport: Hita tenryosui®	[70]
Hita tenryosui®	AQP-mediated water permeability	Humans (healthy)	= AQP1 and AQP9 expression in granular leukocytes	[70]
Vichy®	AQP expression	Human epidermal keratinocytes *in vitro*	↑ AQP3 expression	[71]
Evian® **Volvic®**	Aluminium intestinal absorption	Rats	=	[75]
Spatone®	Iron uptake (ferritin formation)	Human intestinal epithelial cell line *in vitro* (Caco-2 cells)	↑ Ferritin formation	[76]

↓ decrease; ↑ increase; = no effect; AQP: aquaporin; Ref: reference; TRPV6: transient receptor potential vanilloid subfamily member 6.

Finally, the effect of Marina®, an artificially mineralised water containing K^+ and Mg^{2+} ions, on the Na^+, K^+-ATPase activity in erythrocytes of chronic active hepatitis or atherosclerosis patients was investigated by a double-blind method. Treatment lasted 7 days and daily intake of Marina® was 4 x 200 mL before meals [51]. It was verified that the intake of Marina® restored the normal activity of the Na^+, K^+-ATPase (Table 2), that was decreased in chronic active hepatitis and atherosclerosis patients [52, 53]. Moreover, restoration of the Na^+, K^+-ATPase activity brought about the normalisation of vital clinical indices [51].

Effect on Ca^{2+} Transport

Ca^{2+} Urinary Excretion

The increasing incidence of osteoporosis and the consequent bone fractures have encouraged a consideration of food factors in their prevention, notably the dietary intake of Ca^{2+}. Milk and milk products serve as a reference for Ca^{2+} intake [54]. Nevertheless, some mineral waters or Ca^{2+}-enriched beverages are increasingly recommended as sources of Ca^{2+} in the replacement of milk and dairy products. This is because other major foods (meat, fish, cereals, fruits) are poor in Ca^{2+} or contain Ca^{2+} but often with a low bioavailability [54] and because minerals from water are well-absorbed and highly bioavailable [55-58]. Indeed, because of their chemical presentation forms in water, minerals can be more readily and easily absorbed, and so more bioavailable, from water than from food [55, 56, 58].

The intestinal bioavailability of Ca^{2+} from Ca^{2+}-rich mineral waters is equivalent [56, 59, 60, 61] or even higher [57-59, 62] than that of milk Ca^{2+}. However, the effect of associated anions on Ca^{2+} urinary loss was not known and was addressed by comparing, under ordinary conditions of consumption, milk and a Ca^{2+} and SO_4^{2-}-rich mineral water (Contrex®) as the Ca^{2+} provider in a large number of women consuming the same quantity of Ca^{2+} from the two sources, in a cross-over study lasting for an extended period [63]. The urinary excretion of Ca^{2+} was found to be higher (0.5 mmol/day more) with Contrex® water than with milk (Table 2). According to the authors, the acidogenic action of SO_4^{2-} was responsible for this increased calciuria, because a moderate chronic metabolic acidosis, induced by different nutritional factors, leads to a higher urinary excretion of Ca^{2+} and Mg^{2+} [9, 64, 65]. Thus, despite an equal Ca^{2+} intake, and assuming a similar intestinal absorption, these results suggest that Ca^{2+} balance is better with milk consumption than with $CaSO_4$-rich water [63].

TRPV6-Mediated Ca^{2+} Transport

In another study, the effect of Avène® spring water upon Ca^{2+} transport by a human keratinocyte cell line (NHK) was assessed. Treatment of NHK with Avène® spring water led to an enhanced transient receptor potential vanilloid subfamily member 6 (TRPV6) Ca^{2+} channel-mediated constitutive Ca^{2+} entry, which was associated with an increase in TRPV6 expression and abundance at the cell membrane (Table 2). Authors concluded that treatment with Avène® spring water induced an enhanced constitutive Ca^{2+} entry mediated by TRPV6 channel leading to an acceleration of human keratinocytes differentiation [66].

Interestingly, Avène® spring water was found to increase the fluidity of plasma membrane of *in vitro* cultured human skin fibroblasts [67]. This property could be of interest, as membrane fluidity impacts on the expression of receptors, enzyme activities, and cell transport processes [40].

Effect on Aquaporin Activity

Aquaporins (AQPs) are intrinsic membrane proteins functioning as water channels that mediate water entrance and exit to maintain cellular water balance [68]. AQPs are present in plasma membrane, vacuole and endoplasmic reticulum membranes, and 13 AQP isoforms have been described in humans [68]. Besides water molecules, AQPs can also conduct a wide range of nonpolar and polar solutes, such as urea, glycerol, carbon dioxide, nitric oxide, ammonia, hydrogen peroxide, antimonite, arsenite, boron and silicon [69]. The permeability of most AQPs is dynamically regulated at different levels.

Kitagawa *et al.* investigated the *in vitro* effect of 3 distinct mineral waters on water permeability in oocytes expressing distinct AQPs. The mineral waters tested were from Hita city in Japan (Hita tenryosui® water), delicious mineral water from Kobe city in Japan (Rokko® water), and mineral water from Evian-les-Bains in France (Evian® water). Interestingly, in comparison with tap water from Yokohama city in Japan, Hita tenryosui® mineral water induced an increase in AQP1- and AQP2-mediated water permeability, being devoid of effect on water permeability mediated by AQP3, 4, 5 and 7 (Table 2). However, when tested in human healthy volunteers (1000 mL/day, during four weeks), Hita tenryosui® mineral water did not affect the relative expression levels of AQP1 and AQP9 in granular leukocytes [70].

Additionally, the *in vitro* effect of Vichy® thermal spring water on the transcriptome of human epidermal keratinocytes was investigated. Among other genes, an increase in AQP3 gene expression was found (Table 2) [71]. AQP3 is expressed in the basal and spinous epidermal cells, and is the most abundant skin aquaglyceroporin. Of interest, glycerol transport by AQP3 is involved in the metabolism of lipids in skin as well as in the regulation of proliferation and differentiation of keratinocytes [72].

Effect on Aluminium Transport

Aluminium is a ubiquitous existing naturally and widely used metal. Due to good physical and chemical property, aluminium is being tremendously utilized in many fields of our daily life, such as vaccine adjuvant, antacids, food additives, skin care products, cosmetics, and cooking wares, and may be present as an element or contaminant in a lot of foods, including infant formulae, milk products, juice, wine, sea foods, and tea, and in drinking water due to the water treatment process, or naturally coming from weathering rocks and soils, or released from rocks and soils caused by pollution-induced acid rain [73]. Many factors, such as silicon, citrate, iron, etc., can affect absorption of aluminium in humans [73], which occurs through the respiratory and digestive systems and skin. Aluminium affects human health, especially by causing central nervous system (cognitive) impairment. Not surprisingly, Alzheimer's disease and other neurodegenerative disorders have been related with aluminium exposure [73, 74]. An important role of silicon in aluminium bioavailability has been suggested. By virtue of its universal presence in the environment, it represents a major element in the formation of aluminium complexes, namely aluminium silicates. Theoretically, silicon should therefore also bind the aluminium contained in the intestinal lumen and prevent this trace element from being absorbed in excessive amounts.

So, such a protective effect of silicon would be of major importance since it could prevent aluminium intoxication by the oral route [73, 74].

In this context, a study was conducted to examine the effect of silicon present in mineral waters on aluminium intestinal absorption, by using an *in vivo* rat model. Two distinct mineral waters with different silicon content were used [Evian® mineral water (6 mg/L elemental Si) and Volvic® mineral water (14 mg/L elemental Si)] and the effect of an oral gavage with these waters on the 48 h-aluminium intestinal absorption was examined. It was concluded that the provision of large amounts of silicon in the drinking water failed to modify physiological intestinal aluminium absorption under basal conditions or after its stimulation by citrate (Table 2) [75].

Effect on Iron Transport

Iron deficiency anaemia (IDA) is a global public health problem. Treatment with the standard of care ferrous iron salts is commonly poorly tolerated, leading to noncompliance and ineffective correction of IDA. Employing supplements with higher bioavailability might permit lower doses of iron to be used with fewer side effects, thus improving treatment efficacy. In this context, a recent study compared the iron bioavailability from ferrous sulphate tablets and alternative commercial iron products, including a naturally iron-rich mineral water. *In vitro* iron uptake was measured using Caco-2 cells, with ferritin formation as a surrogate marker. Interestingly, iron from a naturally iron-rich mineral water (Spatone®) showed equivalent or better bioavailability compared with iron from ferrous iron sulphate tablets (Table 2). If these results are confirmed *in vivo*, at-risk groups of IDA could be offered a greater choice of more bioavailable and potentially better tolerated iron preparations [76].

CONCLUSION

Membrane transporters involved in the transfer of inorganic and organic solutes are important determinants of cell, tissue, organ and body homeostasis. For instance, they control synaptic transmission, fluid composition and nutrient and drug absorption. Considerable progress has been made in the last decades regarding the molecular identification and functional characterization of transporters, but still very few studies examined the effect of mineral waters on membrane transporters. From the studies already undertaken, it can be concluded that mineral waters are able to interfere with the expression and/or activity of distinct membrane transporters. Additionally, mineral waters possess bacterial communities distinct from tap water [77], and mineral waters can alter the composition of the intestinal microbiota [78-80]. Recent years have seen a surge in publications reporting correlations between the gut microbiota and various medical conditions such as inflammatory bowel disease, colorectal cancer, allergies, autism, kidney stones and metabolic diseases (obesity, type 2 diabetes and dyslipidaemia) [81]. Among the several effects correlating changes in the intestinal microbiota and metabolic disease, an increase in the intestinal absorption of nutrients such as glucose (involving an increase in SGLT1 and GLUT2 activity) and fatty acids (involving an increase in fatty acid translocase (FAT/CD36) activity) has been found, which could result in an increased nutrient absorption by the host [81]. Finally, the effect of mineral waters may not be restricted to membrane transporters, as an extract of *Aquaphilus dolomiae*, a microorganism component of Avène® spring water, was recently found to reinforce the barrier function and to strongly protect tight junction barrier disruption induced by bacterial infection and inflammation in human cultured keratinocytes [82]. So, more investigation in this area should be conducted, because these effects can be of relevance for the biological effects of the mineral waters and for their protective effects regarding human pathologies.

REFERENCES

[1] Mitrovic AD, Plesko F, Vandenberg RJ. Zn(2+) Inhibits the anion conductance of the glutamate transporter EEAT4. *J Biol Chem.* 2001;276(28):26071-6.

[2] Fornai M, Colucci R, Antonioli L, Ghisu N, Tuccori M, Gori G, Blandizzi C, Del Tacca M. Effects of a bicarbonate-alkaline mineral water on digestive motility in experimental models of functional and inflammatory gastrointestinal disorders. *Methods Find Exp Clin Pharmacol.* 2008;30(4):261-9.

[3] Dupont C, Campagne A, Constant F. Efficacy and safety of a magnesium sulfate-rich natural mineral water for patients with functional constipation. *Clin Gastroenterol Hepatol.* 2014;12 (8):1280-7.

[4] Karagülle O, Smorag U, Candir F, Gundermann G, Jonas U, Becker AJ, Gehrke A, Gutenbrunner C. Clinical study on the effect of mineral waters containing bicarbonate on the risk of urinary stone formation in patients with multiple episodes of CaOx-urolithiasis. *World J Urol.* 2007;25(3):315-23.

[5] Vaskonen T. Dietary minerals and modification of cardiovascular risk factors. *J Nutr Biochem.* 2003;14(9):492-506.

[6] Tubek S. Role of trace elements in primary arterial hypertension: is mineral water style or prophylaxis? *Biol Trace Elem Res.* 2006; 114(1-3):1-5.

[7] Gillette-Guyonnet S, Andrieu S, Nourhashemi F, de La Guéronnière V, Grandjean H, Vellas B. Cognitive impairment and composition of drinking water in women: findings of the EPIDOS study. *Am J Clin Nutr*. 2005;81(4):897-902.

[8] Petraccia L, Liberati G, Masciullo SG, Grassi M, Fraioli A. Water, mineral waters and health. *Clinical Nutr.* 2006;25:377-85.

[9] Costa-Vieira D, Monteiro R, Martins MJ. Metabolic Syndrome features: Is there a modulation role by mineral water consumption? A review. *Nutrients.* 2019;11(5):1141.

[10] Pereira C, Guede D, Durães C, Brandão I, Silva N, Passos E, Bernardes M, Monteiro R, Martins MJ. Differential modulation of cancellous and cortical distal femur by fructose and natural mineral-rich water consumption in ovariectomized female Sprague Dawley rats. *Nutrients.* 2019;11(10):2316.

[11] Hamer HM, Jonkers D, Venema K, Vanhoutvin S, Troost FJ, Brummer RJ. Review article: the role of butyrate on colonic function. *Aliment Pharmacol Ther.* 2008;27(2):104-19.

[12] Gonçalves P, Martel F. Butyrate and colorectal cancer: the role of butyrate transport. *Curr Drug Metab.* 2013;14(9):994-1008.

[13] Gonçalves P, Araújo J R, Martel F. Effect of some natural mineral waters in nutrient uptake by Caco-2 cells. *Int J Vitam Nutr Res.* 2010;80(2):131-43.

[14] Gonçalves P, Araújo JR, Pinho MJ, Martel F. Modulation of butyrate transport in Caco-2 cells. *Naunyn Schmiedebergs Arch Pharmacol.* 2009;379(4):325-36.

[15] Hadjiagapiou C, Schmidt L, Dudeja PK, Layden TJ, Ramaswamy K. Mechanism(s) of butyrate transport in Caco-2 cells: role of monocarboxylate transporter 1. *Am J Physiol Gastrointest Liver Physiol.* 2000;279(4):G775-80.

[16] Lambert DW, Wood IS, Ellis A, Shirazi-Beechey SP. Molecular changes in the expression of human colonic nutrient transporters during the transition from normality to malignancy. *Br J Cancer.* 2002;86(8):1262-69.

[17] Cuff M, Dyer J, Jones M, Shirazi-Beechey S. The human colonic monocarboxylate transporter isoform 1: its potential importance to colonic tissue homeostasis. *Gastroenterology.* 2005;128(3):676-86.

[18] Bano G. Glucose homeostasis, obesity and diabetes. *Best Pract Res Clin Obstet Gynaecol.* 2013;27(5):715-26.

[19] Merino B, Fernández-Díaz CM, Cózar-Castellano I, Perdomo G. Intestinal fructose and glucose metabolism in health and disease. *Nutrients.* 2019;12(1): E94.

[20] Wright EM, Hirayama BA, Loo DF. Active sugar transport in health and disease. *J Intern Med.* 2007;261(1):32-43.

[21] Kellett GL, Brot-Laroche E, Mace OJ, Leturque A. Sugar absorption in the intestine: the role of GLUT2. *Annu Rev Nutr.* 2008;28:35-54.

[22] Shayiq RM, Kidwai AM. Effect of fluoride on uptake of D-glucose by isolated epithelial cells of rat intestine. *Environ Res.* 1986;41(2):388-99.

[23] Drozdowski LA, Thompson ABR. Intestinal sugar transport. *World J Gastroenterol.* 2006;12(11):1657-70.

[24] Penalva JC, Martínez A, Esteban A. Intestinal permeability alteration in acute pancreatitis. *Pancreatology.* 2002;2:167-187.

[25] Welcker K, Martin A, Kölle P, Siebeck M, Gross M. Increased intestinal permeability in patients with inflammatory bowel disease. *Eur J Res.* 2004;9(10):456-60.

[26] Dastych M, Novotná H, Cíhalová J. Lactulose/mannitol test and specificity, sensitivity, and area under curve of intestinal permeability parameters in patients with liver cirrhosis and crohn's disease. *Dig Dis Sci.* 2008; 53(10):2789-92.

[27] Bjarnason I, Macpherson A, Hollander D. Intestinal permeability: an overview. *Gastroenterology*. 1995;108(5):1566-81.

[28] Dupuy P, Cassé M, André F, Dhivert-Donnadieu H, Pinton J, Hernandez-Pion C. Low-salt water reduces intestinal permeability in atopic patients. *Dermatology.* 1999;198(2):153-5.

[29] Dias CB, Moughan PJ, Wood LG, Singh H, Garg ML. Postprandial lipemia: factoring in lipemic response for ranking foods for their healthiness. *Lipids Health Dis.* 2017;16(1):178-89.

[30] Schoppen S, Pérez-Granados AM, Carbajal A, Sarriá B, Sánchez-Muniz FJ, Gómez-Gerique JA, Pilar Vaquero M. Sodium bicarbonated mineral water decreases postprandial lipaemia in postmenopausal women compared to a low mineral water. *Br J Nutr.* 2005;94(4):582-7.

[31] Toxqui L, Pérez-Granados AM, Blanco-Rojo R, Vaquero MP. A sodium-bicarbonated mineral water reduces gallbladder emptying and postprandial lipaemia: a randomised four-way crossover study. *Eur J Nutr.* 2012;51(5):607-14.

[32] Lee DPS, Low JHM, Chen JR, Zimmermann D, Actis-Goretta L, Kim JE. The influence of different foods and food ingredients on acute postprandial triglyceride response: a systematic literature review and meta-analysis of randomized controlled trials. *Adv Nutr* 2020;11(6):1529-43.

[33] Appleton GVN, Davies PW, Bristol JB, Williamson RCN. Inhibition of intestinal carcinogenesis by dietary supplementation with calcium. *Br J Surg*. 1987;74(6):523-35.

[34] Song M, Garrett WS, Chan AT. Nutrients, foods, and colorectal cancer prevention. *Gastroenterology*. 2015;148:1244-60.e16.

[35] Goré J, Hoinard C, Antoine JM, Couet C. Effect of calcium and mineral waters on oleic-acid uptake by isolated hamster enterocytes. *Reprod Nutr Develop*. 1994;34(5):439-48.

[36] Wang TY, Liu M, Portincasa P, Wang DQ-H. New insights into the molecular mechanism of intestinal fatty acid absorption. *Eur J Clin Invest.* 2013;43(11):1203-1223.

[37] Stremmel W. Uptake of fatty acids by jejunal mucosal cells is mediated by a fatty-acid binding membrane protein. *J Clin Invest.* 1988;82(6):2001-10.

[38] Goré J, Hoinard C. Linolenic acid transport in hamster intestinal cells is carrier-mediated. *J Nutr*. 1993;123(1):66-73.

[39] Ishibashi Y, Kohyama-Koganeya A, Hirabayashi Y. New insights on glucosylated lipids: metabolism and functions. *Biochim Biophys Acta*. 2013;1831(9):1475-85.

[40] Merial-Kieny C, Castex-Rizzi N, Selas B, Mery S, Guerrero D. Avène thermal spring water: an active component with specific properties. *J Eur Acad Dermatol Venereol.* 2011;25(Suppl. 1):2-5.

[41] Olivier B. Serotonin: a never-ending story. *Eur J Pharmacol*. 2015; 753:2-18.

[42] Murphy DL, Lesch KP. Targeting the murine serotonin transporter: insights into human neurobiology. *Nature Rev Neurosci.* 2008;9(2):85-96.

[43] Barakat A, Hamdy MM, Elbadr MM. Uses of fluoxetine in nociceptive pain management: a literature overview. *Eur J Pharmacol.* 2018;829:12-25.

[44] Yubero-Lahoz S, Robledo P, Farré M, de la Torre R. Platelet SERT as a peripheral biomarker of serotonergic neurotransmission in the central nervous system. *Curr Med Chem.* 2013;20(11):1382-96.

[45] Marazziti D, Baroni S, Giannaccini G, Catena Dell'Osso M, Consoli G, Picchetti M, Carlini M, Massimetti G, Provenzano S, Galassi A. Thermal balneotherapy induces changes of the platelet serotonin transporter in healthy subjects. *Prog Neuropsychopharmacol Biol Psychiatry.* 2007;31(7):1436-9.

[46] Baroni S, Marazziti D, Consoli G, Picchetti M, Catena-Dell'Osso M, Galassi A. Modulation of the platelet serotonin transporter by thermal balneotherapy: a study in healthy subjects. *Eur Rev Med Pharmacol Sci.* 2012;16(5):589-93.

[47] Akagi Y, Sakaue T, Yoneyama E, Aoyama T. Influence of mineral water on absorption of oral alendronate in rats. *Yakugaku Zasshi.* 2011;131(5):801-7.

[48] Itoh A, Akagi Y, Shimomura H, Aoyama T. Interaction between bisphosphonates and mineral water: study of oral risedronate absorption in rats. *Biol Pharm Bull.* 2016;39(3):323-8.

[49] Vavilova GL, Kastrikina TF. Digestive and transport enzymes of the small intestine under the action of low-mineralized water "Naftusya" and its components. *Fiziol Zh.* 1989;35(1):13-7.

[50] Prokopenko ON, Kharlamova ON, Iaremenko MS. Direct and indirect effects of mineral water Naftusia and its components on the sodium-potassium pump of the small-intestinal epithelium in rats. *Fiziol Zh.* 1990;36(2):56-63.

[51] Ponomarenko E, Pokrotnieks J, Jirgensons J, Seleznevs J, Danilans A, Shubnikova N, Kalvins I. Modulation of Na, K-ATPase activity by immunoglobulins-III. Influence of an ATPase activity regulating agent "Marina" on Na, K-ATPase activity in patients with various chronic disturbances. *Zhonghua Yi Xue Za Zhi* (Taipei). 2001;64(11):617-20.

[52] Koter M, Franiak I, Strychalska K, Broncel M, Chojnowska-Jezierska J. Damage to the structure of erythrocyte plasma membranes in patients with type-2 hypercholesterolemia. *Int J Biochem Cell Biol.* 2004;36(2):205-15.
[53] Kuralay F, Tanyalçin T, Kutay F, Yuce G, Ersoz G, Batur Y. Erythrocyte membrane Na^+,K^+ ATPase activity can be a marker of liver histopathology. *Biochem Mol Biol Int.* 1996;40(4):769-77.
[54] Guéguen L, Pointillar, A. The bioavailability of dietary calcium. *J Am Coll Nutr.* 2000;19(2 Suppl):119S-136S.
[55] Kiss SA, Forster T, Dongo A. Absorption and effect of the magnesium content of a mineral water in the human body. *J Am Coll Nutr*. 2004;23(6):758s-62s.
[56] World Health Organization. *Calcium and magnesium in drinking-water. Public health significance.* Geneva: WHO Press; 2009.
[57] Heaney RP. Absorbability and utility of calcium in mineral waters. *Am J Clin Nutr.* 2006;84(2):371-4.
[58] Quattrini S, Pampaloni B, Brandi ML. Natural mineral waters: chemical characteristics and health effects. *Clin Cases Miner Bone Metab.* 2016;13(3):173-80.
[59] Halpern GM, Van de Water J, Delabroise AM, Keen CL, Gershwin ME. Comparative uptake of calcium from milk and a calcium-rich mineral water in lactose intolerant adults: implications for treatment of osteoporosis. *Am J Prevent Med.* 1991;7:379-83.
[60] Guillemant J, Le HT, Accarie C, du Montcel ST, Delabroise AM, Arnaud MJ, Guillemant S. Mineral water as a source of dietary calcium: acute effects on parathyroid function and bone resorption in young men. *Am J Clin Nutr.* 2000;71(4):999-1002.
[61] Bacciottini L, Tanini A, Falchetti A, Masi L, Franceschelli F, Pampaloni B, Giorgi G, Brandi ML. Calcium bioavailability from a calcium-rich mineral water, with some observations on method. *J Clin Gastroenterol.* 2004;38(9):761-6.
[62] Greupner T, Schneider I, Hahn A. Calcium bioavailability from mineral waters with different mineralization in comparison to milk and a supplement. *J Am Coll Nutr.* 2017;36(5):386-90.

[63] Brandolini M, Guéguen L, Boirie Y, Rousset P. Higher calcium urinary loss induced by a calcium sulphate-rich mineral water intake than by milk in young women. *Br J Nutr.* 2005;93(2):225-31.

[64] Lemann J Jr, Gray RW, Maierhofer WJ, Cheung HS. The importance of renal net acid excretion as a determinant of fasting urinary calcium excretion. *Kidney Int.* 1986;29(3):743-6.

[65] Remer T, Dimitriou T, Manz F. Dietary potential renal acid load and renal net acid excretion in healthy, free-living children and adolescents. *Am J Clin Nutr.* 2003;77(5):1255-60.

[66] Lehen'kyi V, Vandenberghe M, Belaubre F, Julié S, Castex-Rizzi N, Skryma R, Prevarskaya N. Acceleration of keratinocyte differentiation by transient receptor potential vanilloid (TRPV6) channel activation. *J Eur Acad Dermatol Venereol.* 2011;25(Suppl 1):12-8.

[67] Cézanne L, Gaboriau F, Charveron M, Morlière P, Tocanne JF, Dubertret L. Effects of the Avène spring water on the dynamics of lipids in the membranes of cultured fibroblasts. *Skin Pharmacol.* 1993;6(3):231-40.

[68] Verkman AS. Mammalian aquaporins: diverse physiological roles and potential clinical significance. *Mol Med.* 2008;10:e13.

[69] Hachez C, Chaumont F. Aquaporins: a family of highly regulated multifunctional channels. *Adv Exp Med Biol.* 2010;679:1-17.

[70] Kitagawa Y, Liu C, Ding X. The influence of natural mineral water on aquaporin water permeability and human natural killer cell activity. *Biochem Biophys Res Commun.* 2011;409(1):40-5.

[71] Tacheau C, Weisgerber F, Fagot D, Bastien P, Verdier MP, Liboutet M, Sore G, Bernard BA. Vichy thermal spring water (VTSW), a cosmetic ingredient of potential interest in the frame of skin ageing exposome: an *in vitro* study. *Int J Cosmetic Sci.* 2018;40(4):377-387.

[72] Hara-Chikuma M, Verkman AS. Roles of aquaporin-3 in the epidermis. *J Invest Dermatol.* 2008;128(9):2145-51.

[73] Klotz K, Weistenhöfer W, Neff F, Hartwig A, van Thriel C, Drexler H. The health effects of aluminum exposure. *Dtsch Arztebl Int.* 2017;114(39):653-9.

[74] Niu Q. Overview of the relationship between aluminum exposure and health of human being. *Adv Exp Med Biol.* 2018;1091:1-31.

[75] Drüeke TB, Jouhanneau P, Banide H, Lacour B, Yiou F, Raisbeck G. Effects of silicon, citrate and the fasting state on the intestinal absorption of aluminium in rats. *Clin Sci (Lond).* 1997;92(1):63-7.

[76] Christides T, Wray D, McBride R, Fairweather R, Sharp P. Iron bioavailability from commercially available iron supplements. *Eur J Nutr*. 2015 Dec;54(8):1345-52.

[77] Sala-Comorera L, Caudet-Segarra L, Galofré B, Lucena F, Blanch AR, García-Aljaro C. Unravelling the composition of tap and mineral water microbiota: divergences between next-generation sequencing techniques and culture-based methods. *Int J Food Microbiol*. 2020;334:108850.

[78] Pereira CD, Collado MC, Passos E, Azevedo I, Monteiro R, Martins MJ. Comment to: Luo *et al*. (2013) *Int. J. Cardiol.* 168(4):4454-6. *Int J Cardiol*. 2014;172(2):512-4.

[79] Dias MF, Reis MP, Acurcio LB, Carmo AO, Diamantino CF, Motta AM, Kalapothakis E, Nicoli JR, Nascimento AMA. Changes in mouse gut bacterial community in response to different types of drinking water. *Water Res.* 2018;132:79-89.

[80] Yahiro T, Hara T, Matsumoto T, Ikebe E, Fife-Koshinomi N, Xu Z, Hiratsuka T, Iha H, Inomata M. Long-term potable effects of alkalescent mineral water on intestinal microbiota shift and physical conditioning. *Evid Based Complement Alternat Med.* 2019; 2710587.

[81] Woting A, Blaut M. The intestinal microbiota in metabolic disease. *Nutrients.* 2016;8(4):202.

[82] Galliano MF, Bäsler K, Caruana A, Mias C, Bessou-Touya S, Brandner JM, Duplan H. Protective effect of *Aquaphilus dolomiae* extract-G1, ADE-G1, on tight junction barrier function in a *Staphylococcus aureus*-infected atopic dermatitis model. *J Eur Acad Dermatol Venereol.* 2020;34(Suppl 5):30-36.

ABOUT THE EDITOR

Maria João Martins is an Assistant Professor at the Department of Biomedicine, Biochemistry Unit, from the Faculty of Medicine, and Senior Researcher at the Instituto de Inovação e Investigação em Saúde (i3S). Both institutions integrate the University of Porto (Porto, Portugal).

Her research interests lie in the broad areas of Biochemistry, Metabolism and Nutrition. In particular, her most recent research interests include the study of metabolic dysfunction amelioration by mineral waters consumption.

Her scientific and pedagogical activity originated 65 publications in national and international journals, including full papers, reviews, letters to the editor and editorials [60 of them indexed (WOS, PubMed and/or SCOPUS)], and 18 chapters in national and international books (3 of them indexed). She co-edited 1 international book and performed as the Lead Guest Editor in 2 special issues of 2 international indexed journals. She (co-)supervised several national and international PhD, MSc, BSc and undergraduate students.

LIST OF CONTRIBUTORS

António Miguéis	Otorhinolaryngology University Clinic, Faculty of Medicine, University of Coimbra, Coimbra, Portugal
Bruno Miguel Fernandes	Department of Rheumatology, São João University Hospital Centre, Porto, Portugal
Carmen Lisboa	Department of Pathology, Microbiology Division, Faculty of Medicine, University of Porto, Porto, Portugal; Department of Dermatology and Venereology, São João University Hospital Centre, Porto, Portugal
Cátia Pontes	School of Health Sciences, Polytechnic of Leiria, Leiria, Portugal; CiTechCare - Centre for Innovative Care and Health Technology, Polytechnic of Leiria, Leiria, Portugal
Cidália D. Pereira	School of Health Sciences, Polytechnic of Leiria, Leiria, Portugal; CiTechCare - Centre for Innovative Care and Health Technology, Polytechnic of Leiria, Leiria, Portugal
Christophe Espírito Santo	Centro de Apoio Tecnológico Agro Alimentar (CATAA) de Castelo Branco, Castelo Branco, Portugal; Centre for Functional Ecology, University of Coimbra, Coimbra, Portugal

Fátima Martel	Department of Biomedicine, Biochemistry Unit, Faculty of Medicine, University of Porto, Porto, Portugal; i3S-Instituto de Investigação e Inovação em Saúde, University of Porto, Porto, Portugal
Francisco Armijo	Professional School of Medical Hydrology, Complutense University, Madrid, Spain
Francisco Maraver	Professional School of Medical Hydrology, Complutense University, Madrid, Spain
Helena Castro	Termas de São Jorge, Santa Maria da Feira, Portugal
Inês Brandão	Centro de Apoio Tecnológico Agro Alimentar (CATAA) de Castelo Branco, Castelo Branco, Portugal; Centre for Functional Ecology, University of Coimbra, Coimbra, Portugal
João Filipe Simões	Otorhinolaryngology Department, Centre Hospitalier de Mouscron, Réseau Santé Louvain, Mouscron, Belgium
Luís Taborda-Barata	NuESP-Planetary Health Study Group, Faculty of Health Sciences, University of Beira Interior, Covilhã, Portugal; CICS-Health Sciences Research Centre, University of Beira Interior, Covilhã, Portugal; Department of Allergy and Clinical Immunology, Cova da Beira University Hospital Centre, Covilhã, Portugal
Maria Augusta Vieira Coelho	Department of Biomedicine, Pharmacology and Therapeutics Unit, Faculty of Medicine, University of Porto, Porto, Portugal
Marco Contoli	Department of Morphology, Surgery and Experimental Medicine, University of Ferrara, Italy
Maria João Martins	Department of Biomedicine, Biochemistry Unit, Faculty of Medicine, University of Porto, Porto, Portugal; i3S-Instituto de Investigação e Inovação em Saúde, University of Porto, Porto, Portugal

Miguel Bernardes	Department of Rheumatology, São João University Hospital Centre, Porto, Portugal; Department of Medicine, Faculty of Medicine, University of Porto, Porto, Portugal
Vânia Ribeiro	School of Health Sciences, Polytechnic of Leiria, Leiria, Portugal; CiTechCare - Centre for Innovative Care and Health Technology, Polytechnic of Leiria, Leiria, Portugal

INDEX

#

1,25-dihydroxycholecalciferol, 138
1,25-dihydroxyvitamin D, 147
5-hydroxytryptamine (5-HT), 232, 237, 238

A

A. muciniphila, 193
abdominal visceral fat, 197
abundance, 2, 3, 191, 192, 199, 206, 207, 209, 210, 226, 243
academic performance, 79
accounting, 17, 93
acid, 14, 20, 38, 40, 42, 96, 134, 135, 136, 137, 138, 139, 141, 142, 143, 144, 145, 146, 149, 150, 151, 152, 153, 154, 155, 156, 157, 158, 159, 162, 173, 177, 185, 193, 196, 201, 219, 229, 231, 235, 236, 237, 244, 246, 250, 253
acid load, 134, 138, 139, 141, 142, 143, 146, 151, 153, 156, 158
acid-base balance, 135, 137, 138, 142, 144, 156, 157, 159
acid-base equilibrium, 135, 137
acid-base homeostasis, 144, 150, 152
acid-base imbalance, 136
acid-base status, 137, 143, 153, 159
acid rich in calcium and sulphate, 145
acidic, 135, 136, 149, 188, 207, 209, 213, 225
acidic water, 188, 225
acidified drinking water, 205, 206, 207, 208, 225
acidified water, 205, 207
acidifying, 133, 135, 140, 143, 146, 147
acidity, 42, 61, 154, 207
acidosis, 136, 138, 139, 142, 145, 152, 159, 242
acidulous, 7, 16, 19
Acinetobacter, 201, 220
Acinetobacter baumannii, 220
acne, 169, 174, 177
acne vulgaris, 174
acoustic impedance, 97

Actinobacteria, 202, 208
active joints, 119
activity, ix, 21, 32, 33, 48, 63, 68, 100, 105, 106, 113, 118, 119, 138, 143, 149, 159, 170, 171, 172, 173, 174, 175, 181, 227, 228, 232, 233, 238, 240, 241, 243, 246, 251, 252, 253, 255
acupuncture, 123
acute, 90, 93, 120, 145, 161, 169, 181, 214, 230, 232, 233, 234, 249, 250, 252
adaptation, 139
adaptive, 36, 139
additives, 98
adenoma, 156
adhesion, 126
adipocytokines, 121
adiponectin, 121, 129, 196
adipose tissue, 191, 192, 193, 194, 217
adiposity, 192, 218, 221
adjustment, 139
adolescents, 156, 163, 253
ADP, 138
adrenocorticotropic hormone, 117
adult, 62, 80, 84, 91, 93, 98, 99, 101, 104, 108, 117, 140, 143, 150, 151, 152, 153, 154, 155, 156, 159, 197, 202, 209, 221, 226, 231, 235, 252
adults, 80, 93, 98, 99, 104, 117, 140, 143, 150, 151, 152, 154, 155, 156, 159, 197, 209, 221, 226, 231, 235, 252
adverse effects, 49, 81, 82, 83, 84, 90, 94, 95, 96, 97, 204
adverse events, 82, 89, 176
adverse side effects, 88, 89
aerobic, 131, 200, 207
aerobic bacteria, 207
Aeromonadales, 211
aerosol, 34, 45, 47, 48, 70, 75, 82, 85, 86, 87, 90, 93, 94, 99, 101, 102, 109
aerosols, 75
aetiology, 93, 98, 103, 105
affective disorder, 169
age, 35, 46, 51, 75, 80, 81, 82, 83, 86, 88, 89, 90, 92, 93, 95, 96, 98, 99, 101, 102, 104, 105, 128, 136, 139, 153, 206, 207, 208
ageing population, 151
aggressive reactions, 86
agonist, 32
airflow limitation, 30, 31, 35
airflow obstruction, 32
airway epithelial cells, 40
airway inflammation, 36, 39, 48, 54, 56, 70, 71, 85
airway wall, 36, 56
airway wall and parenchyma, 36
airways, 31, 33, 34, 35, 36, 37, 42, 44, 46, 56, 57, 60, 68, 75, 78, 90, 94, 97, 106
Akkermansia, 191, 192, 196, 199, 206, 207, 209, 218
Akkermansia muciniphila, 192, 196, 218
albumin, 124
alcalinic salso-sulphidric ozonised, 232, 238
alcohol, 102, 142, 158
alcohol abuse, 102
aldosterone, 162, 190
alendronate, 232, 238, 251
algae, 175
algorithm, 55, 146
Alistipes, 206
alkali load, 134, 144, 160, 190
alkali-chloridic-hydrogen-carbonic, 172
alkaline, 14, 95, 138, 142, 143, 144, 145, 147, 150, 152, 157, 159, 188, 209, 214

alkaline mineral water, 120, 145, 159, 214, 215, 247
alkaline phosphatase, 138, 145, 147
alkaline rich in calcium, magnesium and bicarbonate, 145
alkaline water, 142, 144, 159, 188
alkalinity, 159
alkalising, 133, 135, 136, 137, 142, 143, 145, 146, 147
allergen, 80
allergens, 80
allergic rhinitis, 44, 69, 77, 78, 79, 80, 81, 84, 88, 89, 90, 91, 103, 107, 108, 109, 110, 111, 112
allergy, 29, 54, 55, 61, 68, 70, 81, 99, 102, 107, 110, 111, 112, 113, 127, 180, 258
alopecia, 169
alters, 149, 225
aluminium, 169, 205, 241, 244, 245, 254
aluminium transport, 244
alveolar, 31, 35, 58, 70
alveolar macrophages, 58, 70
amino, 113, 126, 135, 148, 202, 229
amino acid, 113, 126, 135, 202, 229
amino acids, 113, 126, 135, 202
ammonia, 243
ammonium, 137
AMP-activated protein kinase, 190
anabolic, 140
anaerobic, 159, 160, 200, 229
anaerobic bacteria, 229
Anaeroplasma, 206
analgesic, 117
ancestors, 150
anaemia, 169, 245
angiogenesis, 120
animal proteins, 135, 151
anion, 9, 10, 11, 12, 13, 39, 122, 123, 148, 242, 247
anion and cation contents, 9
anions, 10, 122, 123, 148, 242
ankylosing spondylitis, 118
antacids, 244
antibacterial, 37, 83, 99, 106, 173
antibacterials, 83
antibiotic, 78, 81, 83, 84, 88, 94, 97, 105, 192, 201, 207
antibiotic consumption, 97
antibiotic ointment, 88
antibiotic resistance, 105, 201
antibiotics, 78, 81, 83, 84, 94
antidepressants, 238
anti-diabetogenic diet, 207
antifungal, 106, 173
antihistamines, 83, 94, 99
anti-infective, 170
anti-inflammatory, 43, 44, 47, 48, 49, 81, 87, 106, 112, 115, 116, 117, 118, 121, 126, 169, 170, 174, 175, 176, 178, 181, 192, 198
antimicrobial, 37, 58, 81, 106, 171, 173
antimicrobial peptides, 106, 171
antimicrobial peptides and proteins, 171
antinociceptive, 118
antioxidant, 44, 46, 49, 60, 68, 79, 102, 103, 106, 113, 116, 117, 119, 126, 128, 169, 170, 172, 181
antioxidant defence, 79, 102, 103, 106
antiseptic, 106, 173
antiviral drugs, 99
anxiety, 150, 237, 238
anxiety disorder, 237, 238
apical membrane, 237
ApoAI, 118
ApoB, 118
ApoCIII, 120
apolipoprotein (Apo), 118
apoptotic, 58, 190
appetite, 193, 237

AQP1, 241, 243, 244
AQP2, 241, 243
AQP3, 241, 243, 244
AQP4, 243
AQP5, 243
AQP7, 243
AQP9, 244
Aquaphilus dolomiae, 166, 171, 173, 176, 178, 179, 183, 246, 254
aquaporin activity, 243
aquaporin-3, 253
aquaporins (AQPs), 241, 243, 244, 253
arachidonic acid, 38
arachidonic acid derivatives, 38
Argentina, 13
arginase 2, 105
arginine, 135
arm, 86, 101, 210
Armenia, 13
arsenic, 169, 174
arsenical, 82, 84, 108, 109, 169, 174, 182
arsenical-ferruginous, 82, 83, 84, 108, 109, 174, 182
arterial hypertension, 247
artery, 128
arthritis, 115, 116, 118, 119, 121, 126, 127, 128, 129
aseptic, 165
assessment, 32, 53, 54, 64, 69, 85, 86, 88, 100, 110, 136, 143, 157, 224
asthma, 31, 49, 54, 59, 62, 67, 78, 80, 84, 104, 111, 112, 134, 137, 156
astringent, 20
atherogenesis, 192
atherosclerosis, 218, 240, 241
athletes, 159, 160, 161, 214
atoms, 2, 3
atopic dermatitis, 166, 170, 174, 175, 179, 181, 182, 183, 231, 234, 254
atopic disease, 80
ATP, 138, 232, 237
audiometric, 77, 95, 97, 107
audiometric data, 77, 95, 97
audiometric normoacoustic curves, 95
auditory loss, 95
auditory tubal dysfunction, 76, 104
Austria, 13
autism, 237, 246
autoclaved tap water, 201
autoclaved water, 209
autoimmune disease, 118, 181
autoimmune diseases, 181
Avène®, 170, 171,179, 180, 183, 231, 232, 234, 235, 237, 240, 242, 243, 246, 250
average daily dose (ADD), 200
average daily gain, 207

B

B lymphocytes, 36
back pain, 120, 129
bacteria, 58, 78, 82, 84, 86, 87, 92, 99, 106, 194, 196, 199, 203, 205, 206, 207, 210, 225
bacterial infection, 201, 246
bacterium, 193, 220
Bacteroides, 197, 206, 208, 209, 210
Bacteroides sp., 209
Bacteroidetes, 191, 199, 200, 202, 206, 208, 217
balneo and mud therapies, 116
balneology, 26, 71, 129, 174, 180
balneophototherapy, 167, 168, 174, 180, 182
balneotherapy, 43, 62, 63, 66, 76, 116, 117, 118, 119, 120, 121, 124, 125, 126, 127, 128, 129, 130, 131, 165, 166, 167, 168, 173, 174, 175, 176, 178, 179, 181, 182, 183, 238, 251
Barnesiella, 206

barrier, 173, 175, 179, 185, 193, 198, 204, 219, 229, 246, 254
base, 14, 53, 135, 136, 137, 138, 142, 143, 144, 150, 152, 153, 156, 157, 159, 162
bases, 53, 136
basophil degranulation, 170
basophils, 80
bath, 8, 12, 116, 119, 121, 122, 126, 127, 130, 131, 175, 182, 183
bathing, 65, 120, 122, 126, 165, 167, 175, 181, 238
baths, 5, 24, 64, 65, 66, 94, 110, 118, 121, 122, 123, 124, 128, 131, 167, 172, 173, 180, 182
Batten disease (neuronal ceroid lipofuscinoses), 206, 225
Bdellovibrionales, 211
BDS, 33, 48
bedding, 226
Belgium, 13, 73, 194, 196, 258
beneficial effect, 2, 24, 105, 116, 120, 122, 144, 149, 159, 165, 172, 176, 204, 206, 232, 233
benefits, 44, 74, 77, 94, 97, 113, 115, 116, 117, 129, 172, 177, 178, 210
beta-endorphin, 117, 172, 181
beverages, 188, 242
bicarbonate (HCO_3^-), 7, 9, 10, 11, 12, 14, 15, 23, 68, 77, 89, 94, 95, 113, 117, 118, 120, 122, 123, 124, 126, 134, 136, 137, 138, 139, 143, 145, 146, 147, 148, 149, 157, 159, 162, 170, 171, 180, 198, 199, 202, 222, 228, 230, 234, 236, 247
bicarbonate- and sodium-rich, 148, 202
bicarbonate-calcium-magnesium, 77, 89
bicarbonated, 162, 231, 235, 236, 249
bicarbonate-fluorate-carbonic, 230
bicarbonate-rich, 138, 145, 202, 222
bicarbonate-rich, also enriched in sulphate, sodium, magnesium, calcium and iron, 202
bicarbonate-sodium-alkaline-lithic-fluorinated-silicated, 123
bicarbonate-sulphate, 121
bicarbonate-sulphur, 234
Bifidobacteriaceae, 202
Bifidobacterium, 192, 207, 210, 226
Bifidobacterium breve, 210
bilateral, 77, 93, 96, 122
bilateral OA of the knee, 122
bioactive materials, 175
bioavailability, 161, 238, 239, 242, 244, 245, 252, 254
biochemistry, 59, 61
biofilm, 86, 92
Bilophila, 197
biological activity, 227
biological fluids, 40
biological membranes, 228
biological responses, 60
biomarker, 34, 36, 38, 42, 50, 56, 58, 59, 60, 61, 128, 147, 154, 156, 205, 224, 251
biomarkers, 34, 38, 50, 56, 58, 59, 60, 128, 147, 154, 156, 205, 224
biomass, 31, 52
biomass particulate pollution, 31
biopsy, 78, 92
bisphosphonates, 238, 251
bisphosphonates transport, 238
bisulphide (HS^-), 16, 18, 19, 23
bivalent iron (Fe^{2+}), 7, 16, 17, 23
Blautia, 195
blockage, 80
blood, 22, 36, 65, 89, 106, 135, 138, 143, 145, 154, 162, 190, 193, 195, 202, 210, 211, 213, 215, 222, 224, 235, 238
blood plasma, 22

blood pressure, 154, 162, 190, 195, 211, 213, 215, 223
blood pressure reduction, 211
blood supply, 89, 106
blood urea nitrogen, 210
bloodstream, 193
BMD, 139, 140, 141, 144, 148, 149
BMI, 194, 195, 197, 205, 209
body acid load, 135
body adiposity, 192, 218
body composition, 224
body fluid, 135
body mass index (BMI), 194, 195, 197, 205, 209, 223
body temperature, 116, 210, 211
body weight, 192, 196, 197, 203
bonds, 2, 106
bone, vii, ix, 120, 133, 134, 135, 137, 138, 139, 140, 141, 144, 145, 146, 147, 148, 149, 151, 152, 153, 156, 157, 158, 159, 160, 161, 162, 163, 190, 214, 215, 223, 242, 252
bone cells, 138
bone disease, 134, 141, 157
bone form, 140
bone formation and resorptive markers, 140
bone fractures, 138, 144, 163, 242
bone health, vii, 133, 134, 135, 137, 139, 141, 144, 147, 148, 149, 152, 156, 157, 158, 159, 160, 161, 190
bone mass, 138, 139, 141, 145, 160
bone mass and size, 139
bone mass and strength, 141
bone metabolism, 134, 135, 137, 139, 141, 144, 146, 147, 149, 156, 159, 160, 161, 162, 214, 215, 223
bone microenvironment, 139
bone mineral content, 139, 158
bone mineral density (BMD), 138, 139, 140, 141, 144, 148, 149, 153, 157, 158, 162
bone resorption, 138, 141, 145, 158, 159, 161, 214, 252
bone surface density, 148
bone turnover, 139, 140, 144, 153, 156, 158
bone volume, 139, 148
bone volume density, 139
bone volumetric fraction, 148
Borg Dyspnoea Score (BDS), 33, 48
boron, 169, 173, 182, 243
bottled mineral water, 200, 201
bottled natural mineral waters, 4, 6, 7, 113
bottled water, 2, 3, 27, 142, 159, 212
bottled waters, 3, 27
boys, 85, 94, 96, 100
brain, 200, 237
Brazil, 13, 201
breakdown, 37
breast cancer, 151, 176, 184
breathing, 34
breathlessness, 33, 53
bromine, 66, 87, 96
bronchial, 32, 37, 45, 49, 54, 62, 63, 67
bronchial asthma, 49, 62, 63
bronchial dilation, 32
bronchial obstruction, 32, 37
bronchiolitis, 31
bronchitis, 37, 51, 56, 57, 58, 62, 63, 64, 65, 66, 67, 77
brushings, 88
BS ISO 21426:2018, 7, 23
Bulgaria, 13
bulimia, 238
bulimia nervosa, 238
burns, 163, 166, 176, 183
burns sequelae, 166, 176

butyrate, 204, 224, 229, 230, 231, 232, 248
butyrate transport, 229, 248
Butyricicoccus, 195

C

C. pneumoniae, 45
Ca^{2+}, 7, 10, 11, 12, 13, 23, 145, 146 147, 148, 230, 235, 236, 238, 239, 240, 242, 243
Ca^{2+} Mg^{2+}, 11, 12, 13
Ca^{2+} transport, 242
Caco-2 cells, 230, 231, 232, 233, 241, 245, 248
cadmium, 205
caecal, 209
caffeine, 142, 158
calcic, 160, 174
calcium (Ca^{2+}), 7, 9, 10, 11, 12, 13, 15, 16, 22, 23, 45, 77, 89, 100, 118, 120, 122, 123, 124, 128, 134, 135, 136, 137, 138, 139, 140, 141, 142, 143, 144, 145, 146, 147, 148, 154, 156, 157, 158, 159, 160, 161, 168, 169, 170, 171, 174, 180, 198, 199, 201, 202, 212, 214, 216, 230, 234, 235, 236, 238, 239, 240, 242, 243, 250, 252, 253
calcium and iron, 202
calcium and magnesium sulphate, sodium chloride, carbonic and ferruginous, 198
calorie, 134
calprotectin, 78, 85, 92
calvaria, 139
Campylobacter, 211
cancellous, 148, 160, 248
cancellous and cortical distal femur, 160, 248
cancellous distal femur, 148
cancer, 31, 134, 137, 151, 156, 171, 176, 184, 233, 235, 246, 248, 250
capillary, 106
carbogaseous, 16, 19, 20
carbohydrates, 233
carbon, 19, 20, 65, 78, 88, 109, 137, 243
carbon dioxide (CO_2), 7, 14, 15, 16, 19, 20, 23, 65, 78, 88, 89, 109, 137, 230, 236, 243
carbon dioxide-enriched (CO_2-enriched), 78, 88, 89, 109
carbonate, 15, 16, 66
carbonic acid, 20, 157
carbonic and ferruginous, 198
carcinogenesis, 172, 230, 232, 250
cardiovascular, 31, 35, 79, 118, 126, 128, 134, 137, 151, 162, 192, 218, 229, 233, 235, 247
cardiovascular disease, 35, 79, 134, 137, 151, 218, 235
cardiovascular diseases, 35, 79, 134
cardiovascular function, 126
cardiovascular risk, 118, 162, 192, 218, 247
cartilage, 117, 120, 128
cartilage degradation, 117
caspase-1, 192
CAT, 33, 46
catalase, 39, 172, 181
catecholamines, 127
catheter, 199
cation, 9, 10, 11, 12, 13, 122, 123, 147, 238
cations, 10, 122, 123, 147, 238
causality, 157
$CD8^+$, 121
cecum, 207
cell and intracellular membranes, 227
cell culture, 237
cell death, 44, 69

cell differentiation, 165, 175
cell extrusion, 199
cell growth, 169
cell infiltration, 79, 90
cell line, 45, 230, 231, 240, 241, 242
cell lines, 45
cell membrane, 228, 243
cell membranes, 228
cell wall, 193
cellular renewal, 169, 173
central nervous system, 237, 244, 251
cheese, 135
chemical, 1, 5, 6, 24, 25, 26, 31, 60, 75, 115, 116, 117, 129, 161, 165, 166, 168, 175, 177, 189, 213, 230, 235, 236, 239, 242, 244, 252
chemical agents, 32
chemical characteristics, 161, 168, 252
chemical effects, 117
chemical peel, 177
chemical properties, 166
chemicals, 213
chemiluminescence, 68, 113
chemokine, 37, 38, 58, 78, 79, 88, 89, 102, 109, 120, 171
chemokine receptor, 79, 102
chemokines, 37, 38, 58
chemotaxis, 59
chemotherapy, 176, 184, 204, 223
chemotherapy-induced neuropathic pain (CINP), 204, 223
child, 93
childhood, 93, 213
children, 80, 81, 84, 85, 93, 94, 95, 96, 98, 99, 100, 104, 106, 107, 109, 110, 112, 134, 137, 156, 158, 175, 211, 223, 226, 253
China, 81, 150
Chlamydia pneumoniae, 45, 69
chloride (Cl^-), 7, 9, 10, 11, 12, 13, 14, 15, 23, 65, 66, 78, 82, 83, 84, 85, 86, 87, 91, 92, 95, 97, 118, 120, 121, 122, 123, 134, 136, 146, 147, 148, 149, 152, 162, 170, 172, 174, 198, 199, 200, 221, 228, 230, 234, 236
chloride-sodium, 78, 84
chlorinated, 208
chlorination, 201
chlorine, 14, 113, 117, 124, 126
chlorine-sulphur-bicarbonate, 113, 117, 126
cholesterol, 195, 196, 197, 204, 215
chondrocyte, 126
Christensenellaceae, 202
christianity, 167
chronic active hepatitis, 240, 241
chronic back pain, 120, 129
chronic bronchopneumopathy, 46
chronic heart failure, 126
chronic inflammatory diseases, 90, 117
chronic inflammatory upper respiratory tract, 77, 94
chronic kidney disease, 136, 137, 150, 151, 152, 154, 155
chronic low-grade inflammation, 191, 218
chronic obstructive pulmonary disease (COPD), vii, xi, 29, 30, 31, 32, 33, 34, 35, 36, 37, 38, 39, 40, 41, 42, 43, 44, 45, 46, 47, 48, 49, 50, 51, 52, 53, 54, 55, 56, 57, 58, 59, 60, 61, 62, 65, 66, 68, 69, 70, 71, 107
chronic pain, 123
chronic rhinitis, 49, 79, 101, 108, 109
chronic rhinosinusitis (CRS), 44, 68, 69, 76, 77, 78, 79, 81, 82, 83, 84, 85, 86, 87, 90, 91, 104, 105, 108, 109, 110, 111, 112
chronic sinonasal disease, 77, 82, 108
chronic sinonasal inflammation, 79, 90
chronic sinonasal polyposis, 77, 88

chronic upper airways inflammatory status, 78, 95
chronic upper respiratory tract infections, 77, 101, 111
chronic wounds, 174, 177
chylomicra TG, 235
cicatrisation, 82, 176
cigarette smoke, 60
cigarette smoking, 31
ciliary motility, 86
ciliated cells, 78, 79, 83, 91
civilization, 167
CKD, 151
Cl^-, 7, 10, 11, 12, 13, 23, 148, 228, 230, 236
classification, ix, 2, 3, 6, 7, 10, 16, 22, 28, 220
cleaning, 177
cleansing action, 87, 104
climate, ix, 43, 68, 107
climate change, ix
climate therapy, 43, 68, 107
clinical evaluation score (CES), 79, 101, 102
clinical interventions, 105
clinical presentation, 99
clinical trials, 38, 97, 129
Clostridia sp., 208
Clostridiaceae, 201
Clostridiales, 196, 210
Clostridium, 195, 203, 206, 208, 211
Clostridium sensu stricto, 195, 203
cluster analysis, 35
cluster of differentiation, 197
CO_2, 7, 14, 15 16, 20, 23, 88, 89, 230
CO_2-enriched, 88, 89
coal, 63
coffee, 158
cognition, 237
cold, 8, 121, 125
cold mud baths, 121
coliform, 211
coliform contamination, 211
colitis, 198
collaboration, 94
collagen, 140, 147, 148
Colombia, 13
colon, 229, 230, 232, 235
colon cancer, 235
colon carcinogenesis, 230, 232
colonic mucosa, 199
colonisation, 208
colonization, 173, 175
colorectal cancer, 156, 233, 246, 248, 250
commercial, 200, 201, 207, 209, 230, 235, 245
common cold, 77
common symptoms, 89
communities, 207, 246
community, 168, 191, 200, 201, 207, 209, 222, 254
community structure, 209
comorbidity, 52, 55
compensation, 141
complement, 62, 178
complexity, 33
compliance, 81, 104, 145, 146
complications, 97
composition, 1, 5, 116, 135, 143, 146, 156, 161, 188, 189, 191, 199, 200, 201, 202, 203, 206, 209, 210, 211, 220, 222, 225, 230, 235, 236, 239, 246, 247, 254
compounds, 7, 15, 16, 42, 96, 98, 129, 209, 227, 228, 234
computed tomography, 118, 139
concept, vii, 1, 2, 4, 10, 166, 185, 218
conditioning, 146, 254
conductance, 247
conductive hearing loss, 93
congestion, 80, 106

connectivity, 141
connectivity density, 141
consensus, 158
constipation, 247
constituents, 4, 5, 9, 25, 166, 198, 213
consumption, vii, 78, 97, 102, 106, 108, 118, 122, 127, 133, 134, 136, 137, 141, 142, 143, 144, 148, 155, 159, 160, 161, 162, 188, 189, 190, 198, 199, 200, 201, 202, 205, 208, 209, 210, 213, 214, 222, 225, 233, 235, 239, 242, 247, 248, 255
contact dermatitis, 170, 174, 177
contaminant, 244
contamination, 211
content, iv, 6, 7, 9, 10, 50, 63, 67, 88, 129, 134, 135, 138, 142, 143, 144, 145, 146, 147, 149, 157, 175, 184, 203, 205, 245, 252
Contrex®, 231, 232, 238, 239, 240, 242
control group, 82, 83, 84, 85, 86, 87, 88, 89, 92, 95, 98, 142
controlled studies, 43, 122, 178
controlled trials, 130, 159, 174, 175, 176, 218, 250
controversial, 149, 223
cooking, 31, 244
cool, 8
COPD, 30, 31, 32, 33, 34, 35, 36, 37, 38, 39, 40, 41, 42, 43, 44, 45, 46, 47, 48, 49, 50, 51, 52, 53, 54, 55, 56, 57, 58, 59, 61, 65, 69, 70
COPD Assessment Test (CAT), 33, 46, 53
copper, 141, 169, 171, 173, 182, 205, 224
Coprococcus, 197
Coriobacteriaceae, 196
corneocyte, 172
coronary calcium score, 118
coronary heart disease, 66
correlation, 40, 41, 46, 54, 56, 85, 121, 124, 129, 193, 194, 195, 203, 210, 211, 246
correlation analysis, 195
correlations, 121, 203, 211, 246
cortical, 148, 160, 248
cortical distal femur, 148, 160, 248
cortical endosteal perimeter, 148
corticoids, 105
corticosteroid, 46, 47, 70, 83, 91, 93
corticosteroids, 47, 83, 91, 93
cortisol, 117
cosmetic, 166, 167, 177, 179, 181, 244, 253
cosmetics, 166, 167, 177, 179, 181, 244
cosmetology, 166, 178
cost, 97, 136
Costa Rica, 13
cough, 35, 47, 78, 99, 100
counterbalance, 135, 142, 146
covering, 199
C-reactive protein (CRP), 116, 124, 192
creatinine, 145
crenotherapy, 42, 43, 45, 47, 67, 69, 76, 109, 110
crises, 97
Croatia, 13
cross-sectional study, 139
CRP, 116, 124
CRS, 76, 77, 78, 79, 81, 82, 83, 84, 85, 86, 87, 90, 91, 104, 105
crust, 2, 3, 14, 15, 17, 87
crusts, 87
crystalline, 149
C-telopeptide, 138, 146
C-telopeptides, 146
C-terminal telopeptide of type I collagen, 140
C-terminal telopeptides, 145
culture, 139, 200, 207, 221, 254
culture medium, 221

cure, 25, 26, 74, 92, 93, 94, 104, 107, 110, 183, 188, 200, 234
cures, 25, 26, 74, 92, 93, 94, 183, 188
C-X-C motif chemokine receptor 4 (CXCR4), 79, 102, 108
Cyanobacteria, 200
cycles, 92
cycling, 161, 214
cyclooxygenase (COX), 38
cystathionine, 40
cysteine, 40, 135
cysteinyl-leukotrienes, 38
cytokine, 38, 70, 77, 101, 103, 106, 109, 116, 121, 126, 129, 170, 171, 204, 223
cytokines, 38, 101, 106, 109, 116, 121, 126, 129, 170, 204
cytology, 44, 68, 78, 79, 82, 83, 87, 88, 90, 92
cytology analysis, 88, 90
cytoplasm, 40
cytoplasmic, 40
cytoprotective, 116
Czech Republic, 13

D

damages, iv
danger, 205
DASH diet, 137
data analysis, 53
database, 162
decay, 21
decongestants, 83, 93
decontamination, 226
defence, 39, 58, 79, 102, 103, 106, 171, 229
deficiencies, 106, 213
deficiency, 168, 169, 190, 245
degradation, 117
Dehalobacteriaceae, 202
dental fluorosis, 203
deoxypyridinoline, 140, 145
deposits, 15, 194
depression, 22, 150, 237
depth, 124
dermatitis, 166, 169, 170, 174, 175, 177, 179, 181, 182, 183, 184, 231, 234, 254
dermatology, viii, 165, 166, 167, 168, 175, 177, 178, 179, 182, 183, 249, 257
Dermatology Life Quality Index, 175
Dermatophagoides Farinae, 86
Dermatophagoides Pteronyssinus, 86
dermatoses, 177, 185
destruction, 31, 35
detection, 34, 50, 60, 111
developed countries, 31
diabetes, 31, 134, 137, 153, 154, 155, 188, 189, 190, 201, 202, 213, 216, 217, 219, 222, 224, 225, 233, 234, 246, 248
diabetes-associated metabolic dysfunction, 190
diabetics, 81
diet, 75, 133, 134, 135, 136, 137, 138, 139, 140, 141, 144, 145, 150, 151, 152, 156, 158, 188, 191, 192, 196, 197, 199, 202, 207, 215, 216, 219, 220, 224
dietary acid load, 134, 135, 136, 138, 139, 140, 141, 142, 143, 144, 149, 150, 151, 152, 153, 154, 155, 156, 157, 158
dietary fat, 235
dietary intake, 135, 242
dietary supplementation, 250
diet-induced acid load, vii, 133, 134, 135, 137, 139, 141, 142, 144, 190
diet-induced obesity, 192, 220

differentiation, 120, 165, 175, 243, 244, 253
diffusion, 172
digestion, 235
digestive disorders, 199
dilation, 32
diploid, 172
direct observation, 193
Directive 2003/40/EC, 4, 25
Directive 2009/54/EC, 4, 5, 6, 25
disability, 120
discharge, 85
disclosure, 89, 92, 104
discriminant analysis, 197
disease activity, 118
disease model, 207
disease progression, 34, 38, 207
diseases, ix, 30, 34, 44, 60, 62, 74, 75, 76, 79, 80, 81, 88, 92, 99, 101, 102, 103, 104, 111, 115, 116, 117, 134, 135, 137, 142, 166, 168, 174, 191, 193, 200, 213, 216, 217, 220, 224, 246
disinfected water, 201
disorder, 59, 80, 169, 170, 174, 237
dissolved oxygen, 18
distilled water, 82, 83, 198, 203
distribution, 28, 228
diversity, 2, 166, 191, 200, 203, 204, 205, 206, 207, 209, 211, 221, 225
DNA, 58, 68, 113, 172, 181
DNA damage, 68, 113
donors, 54, 191, 217, 234
Dorea, 195
dorsal root ganglia, 204
dosage, 92, 149
douching, 87, 88
drainage, 106
drinking, 1, 5, 25, 142, 158, 160, 161, 167, 188, 189, 190, 198, 200, 201, 203, 204, 205, 206, 207, 208, 209, 210, 211, 212, 213, 214, 215, 221, 222, 223, 225, 226, 244, 245, 247, 252, 254
drinking habits, 188, 200, 210, 211
drinking mineral waters, 142
drinking water, 1, 5, 25, 160, 161, 188, 189, 198, 200, 201, 204, 205, 206, 207, 208, 209, 210, 211, 212, 213, 221, 222, 225, 226, 244, 245, 247, 254
drug therapy, 49
drugs, 49, 75, 89, 92, 103, 104, 122, 228
drugs consumption, 122
duration, 78, 91, 92, 98, 100, 103, 104, 149, 158
dusts, 32
dysbiosis, 191, 193, 216, 217
dyslipidaemia, 134, 137, 246
dyslipidemia, 223
Dysosmobacter spp, 194
Dysosmobacter welbionis, 194, 220
dyspnea, 53
dyspnoea, 33, 35, 36, 47, 49

E

E. coli, 198, 207
ear, ix, 74, 75, 76, 83, 93, 96, 97, 106
early and late responses, 80
EBC, 34, 38, 42, 46, 48
eclampsia, 169
ecology, 193
eczema, 166, 175
education, 131
efficacy, 43, 47, 49, 64, 66, 81, 83, 87, 90, 93, 96, 98, 99, 100, 104, 108, 109, 110, 112, 121, 128, 130, 131, 175, 183, 184, 185, 245, 247
effusion, 74, 76, 79, 93, 107, 110, 112
egg, 18

elastin, 37
elderly, 69, 81, 84, 86, 99, 101, 104, 108, 110, 111, 120, 129, 154, 156, 157, 158, 160
electrolysis, 209
electrolyte, 162, 190, 213, 230
electrolyte imbalance, 190
electronic structure, 21
electrons, 9
emergency, 80
emphysema, 31, 35, 51, 55, 57, 58, 67
encephalopathy, 169
endocrine, 127, 138, 172, 191, 193, 209, 216, 220
endocrine cells, 193
endocrine system, 127, 172
endoplasmic reticulum stress, 190, 215
endorphins, 127, 172
endoscopic, 77, 78, 83, 84, 88, 91, 108
endoscopic data, 78
endoscopic scores, 91
endoscopic surgery, 77, 88
endotoxaemia, 193
endotoxemia, 217
endotype, 36
end-stage renal disease, 151
endurance, 161, 214
energy, 139, 192, 205, 218, 229, 233
England, 168
enterocytes, 199, 231, 236, 237, 250
environment, 106, 124, 136, 178, 188, 199, 244
environmental conditions, 124
environmental factors, 191
enzyme, 38, 40, 42, 243, 251
enzymes, 38, 40, 251
eosinophil, 36, 38, 78, 79, 80, 82, 86, 87, 89, 91, 92
eosinophilia, 40, 54
eosinophilic, 40, 58, 80
eosinophils, 36, 38, 78, 79, 80, 82, 86, 87, 89, 92
eotaxin, 78, 89, 92
epidemic, 79
epidemiologic, 157
epidemiology, 111
epidermis, 173, 183, 237, 253
epidermolysis bullosa, 174, 177
epidermoside, 237
epidermoside transport, 237
epigenetics, 218
epilepsy, 158
epithelial and goblet cells, 87
epithelial cells, 37, 38, 40, 58, 60, 69, 88, 102, 198, 229, 233, 249
epithelial disruption, 199
epithelium, 106, 193, 199, 221, 229, 240, 251
equilibrium, 26, 135, 137
Erysipelotrichaceae, 197
erythrocytes, 240, 241
Escherichia coli, 198
ethmoid biopsy, 78
ethnicity, 151
Eubacterium, 206, 208
Eubacterium bioforme, 208
Europe, 81, 156, 167, 168
European League Against Rheumatism (EULAR), 123, 131
European Parliament, 4, 25
European Union, 3
Eustachian tube, 75, 106
Evian®, 231, 232, 238, 239, 241, 243, 245
evidence, ix, 55, 74, 81, 84, 94, 104, 107, 111, 116, 118, 119, 120, 126, 134, 135, 137, 139, 141, 142, 144, 146, 149, 150, 152, 160, 165, 189, 191, 192, 198
evolution, 92, 105

exacerbations, 31, 35, 38, 39, 41, 42, 54, 58, 59, 66
exclusion, 95
excretion, 136, 137, 138, 139, 140, 141, 143, 144, 145, 146, 148, 149, 152, 154, 158, 162, 227, 228, 238, 240, 242, 253
exercise, 33, 34, 48, 124, 131, 142, 159, 160, 161, 214
exercise performance, 159
exercise therapy, 124
exercise tolerance tests, 34
exercises, 122
exertion, 53
exhalation resistance, 102
exhaled breath condensate (EBC), 34, 38, 42, 46, 48, 54, 59, 61, 62, 71
exhaled nitric oxide (FeNO), 78, 79, 85, 89, 92
exocytosis, 235
expectoration, 56, 78, 100
experimental design, 92
exploitation, 4, 25, 166
exposome, 177, 185, 253
exposure, 31, 80, 84, 102, 149, 167, 203, 223, 232, 233, 244, 253, 254
extracellular matrix, 37, 38, 39, 58, 138
extracellular matrix proteins, 38, 138
extracts, 183
extremely hard, 22
extremely high in silicic acid, sodium, potassium, and hydrogen carbonate, 201
extrusion, 199

F

F^-, 7, 23, 148, 230, 233, 236
facial pain, 85
facial pressure, 81
faecal, 191, 192, 200, 201, 202, 203, 204, 205, 206, 207, 208, 209, 210, 211
faecal microbiota, 191, 200, 201, 202, 203, 208, 210, 211
Faecalibacterium, 192, 197, 204, 210, 211, 226
Faecalibacterium prausnitzii, 210, 211
faeces, 200, 207
families, 38, 201
family, 80, 97, 99, 199, 202, 204, 210, 232, 237, 253
family history, 80
family physician, 99
fasting, 154, 253, 254
fat, 129, 192, 194, 197, 201, 215, 219
fat mass, 196, 197
fat storage, 192
fatigue, 80, 123
fatigue impact scale, 123
fatty acid, 192, 193, 196, 219, 229, 235, 236, 237, 246, 250
fatty acids, 192, 219, 235, 237, 246, 250
fatty liver disease, 151, 155
Fe^{2+}, 7, 16, 17, 23
feces, 221
feed additives, 207
feed conversion, 207
female, 45, 47, 48, 82, 118, 119, 124, 128, 148, 160, 201, 202, 204, 207, 208, 209, 211, 231, 248
female rat, 148, 202
femoral neck, 140
femur, 140, 148, 248
FeNO, 78, 79, 85, 92
fermentation, 229
ferritin, 241, 245
ferruginous, 16, 17
FEV1, 32, 36, 47, 56
fibre, 141, 192, 229, 233

fibroblast, 119, 120, 128, 172, 181, 243, 253
fibroblast growth factor, 120
fibroblasts, 172, 181, 243, 253
fibromyalgia, 115, 116, 118, 123, 124, 126, 131
Fibromyalgia Impact Questionnaire (FIQ), 123
fibrosis, 37
Firmicutes, 191, 197, 199, 202, 204, 208, 217
fish, 135, 242
fixed residue, 6, 7, 8, 9, 10
flora, 208
fluctuations, 201
fluid, 42, 48, 88, 93, 109, 138, 210, 230, 246
fluoride (F^-), 7, 23, 122, 134, 141, 147, 148, 149, 162, 163, 198, 203, 222, 223, 230, 233, 234, 236, 249
fluoride and sodium, 198
fluorosis, 203
fluoxetine, 251
Fms related receptor tyrosine kinase 1 (FLT1), 79, 102
follow-up, 46, 83, 85, 86, 89, 92, 98, 100, 101, 103, 130, 131
food, 134, 135, 136, 144, 145, 188, 193, 205, 219, 229, 233, 235, 242, 244, 250
food additives, 244
food intake, 193, 219
food lipids, 235
food products, 205
forced expiratory volume in 1 second (FEV1), 32, 36, 47, 56
forced vital capacity (FVC), 32
forearm, 139
formation, 37, 58, 98, 138, 141, 154, 157, 158, 172, 236, 241, 244, 245, 247
fractures, 20, 138, 141, 144, 157, 158, 163, 242
fragility, 149
fragments, 127, 171
France, 8, 9, 13, 170, 172, 174, 198, 243
free fatty acid receptor 3, 193
free radicals, 171, 172
freezing, 22
frequency, 35, 77, 78, 91, 100, 101, 103
friendship, 79
fructose, 113, 160, 202, 214, 215, 248
fruits, 134, 135, 136, 140, 154, 242
full disease recovery, 78, 97
fumes, 31
functional, 37, 45, 64, 69, 84, 108, 115, 117, 119, 121, 122, 129, 170, 176, 182, 187, 227, 229, 246, 247, 257, 258
functional capacities, 122
functional capacity, 119, 121
functional changes, 37
functional mobility, 117
functional status, 121
fungi, 92
fungus, 106
FVC, 32

G

gallbladder, 249
gas composition, 188, 189, 198
gases, 24, 31
gastrectomy, 220
gastroesophageal reflux, 103
gastrointestinal tract, 191, 199, 225
gel, 91, 122, 130, 177
gene expression, 117, 120, 138, 244
gene expression modulation, 120
genera, 201, 209, 211
generalised OA, 122

genes, 79, 102, 103, 119, 128, 201, 244
genetics, 218, 222
genus, 199, 204, 206, 207, 208, 209, 210
Georgia, 13
Germany, 8, 13, 16
germ-free (GF), 192
Girard, 22, 28
Girard classification, 22
girls, 94, 96, 100
glucocorticoid, 70, 138, 159, 190, 215
glucocorticoids, 138
glucose, 190, 192, 193, 194, 195, 197, 204, 209, 215, 219, 226, 228, 231, 233, 234, 246, 248, 249
glucose and lipid metabolism, 193, 219
glucose regulation, 209, 226
glucose transport, 233
glucose uptake and metabolism, 190
glutamate, 136, 229, 247
glutathione, 39, 45, 69, 117, 172
glutathione peroxidase, 172
glycaemic control, 202
glycated haemoglobin (HbA1c), 205, 210
glycerol, 243, 244
glycoalbumin, 202, 210
glycolysis, 202
goblet, 37, 87, 88, 199
goblet cells, 87, 88, 199
GOLD, 31, 32, 41, 45, 48, 50, 56
Global Initiative for Chronic Obstructive Lung Disease (GOLD), 31, 32, 41, 45, 48, 50, 56
Greece, 13
growth, 116, 117, 120, 138, 169, 200, 207, 210, 225, 229
growth factor, 116, 138
growth hormone, 117, 138
guidelines, 44, 53, 56
gut, viii, 187, 188, 189, 191, 192, 193, 198, 199, 200, 201, 202, 204, 205, 206, 207, 208, 209, 210, 211, 212, 216, 217, 218, 219, 220, 222, 223, 225, 226, 246, 254
gut barrier permeability, 192
gut microbiota, viii, 187, 188, 189, 191, 192, 193, 198, 199, 200, 201, 202, 204, 205, 206, 207, 208, 209, 210, 211, 216, 217, 218, 219, 220, 222, 223, 225, 226, 246

H

H_2S, 16, 18, 19, 23, 38, 40, 41, 42, 44, 45, 70, 234
H_2SO_4, 205, 206, 209
H_2SO_4- and HCl-acidified water, 205
H_2SO_4-acidified water, 209
H_2SO_4-acidified drinking water, 205, 206
hair, 169
half-life, 21, 149
hand OA, 122
hard, 22
hardness, 7, 22, 213
harmony, 16
harvesting, 192
HCl, 205, 206, 207, 208, 209
HCl- or H_2SO_4-acidified drinking water, 205
HCl- or H_2SO_4-acidified water, 209
HCl-acidified drinking water, 205, 206, 207, 208
HCl-acidified water, 205, 207
HCO_3^-, 7, 10, 11, 12, 14, 15, 23, 143, 145, 146, 147, 148, 228, 230, 236
headache, 87
healing, 88, 92, 96, 97, 116, 166, 169, 173

health, vii, ix, xi, xii, 1, 2, 5, 7, 10, 11, 16, 24, 26, 27, 28, 29, 33, 41, 46, 48, 62, 64, 65, 67, 71, 74, 113, 134, 135, 137, 139, 141, 144, 147, 148, 149, 150, 152, 156, 157, 158, 159, 161, 188, 189, 191, 199, 200, 204, 210, 211, 212, 213, 221, 222, 225, 229, 232, 247, 248, 252, 253, 254, 257, 258, 259
health effects, 161, 229, 252, 253
health promotion, 74
health resort medicine, 1, 2, 5, 7, 10, 11, 16, 27, 71
health status, 33, 41, 46
healthy, 1, 41, 42, 54, 85, 88, 93, 113, 116, 117, 125, 126, 138, 139, 142, 143, 144, 145, 147, 148, 150, 152, 159, 162, 188, 191, 202, 209, 210, 218, 231, 232, 235, 238, 240, 241, 244, 251, 253
healthy individuals, 41, 116, 117, 144
hearing, 77, 93, 94, 95, 97, 98, 112
hearing damage, 95
hearing function, 93, 95
hearing impairment, 95
hearing loss, 77, 93, 94, 95, 98, 112
heart patients, 81
heartburn, 112
heat, 16, 117, 125, 127, 167, 172, 198
heavy metals, 205, 224
height, 140
helium, 2
hemochromatosis, 169
hepatitis, 241
heterogeneity, 91, 116, 124
high-calcium concentration rich in bicarbonate, 145
high-calcium concentration rich in sulphate and magnesium, 145
high fat, 223
high mineral content, 6
high sensitivity C-reactive protein, 192
high-bicarbonate, 143, 145, 146
high-calcium, 145, 146, 147, 160, 161, 214
high-calcium, high-sulphate, 146
highlands, 64
highly mineralised alkaline, 143
high-PRAL, 141, 143
high-sulphate, 145, 146, 147
hip, 122, 131, 139, 196, 197
hip circumference, 196, 197
hip OA, 122
histamine, 80, 170, 180
histidine, 135
histiocytes, 82
histone, 58, 70
histone deacetylase, 58, 70
history, 25, 35, 48, 188, 212
Hita tenryosui®, 241, 243, 244
homeostasis, 40, 42, 144, 150, 152, 162, 175, 189, 190, 192, 204, 205, 227, 228, 229, 232, 233, 234, 246, 248
homes, 31, 46, 211
homocysteine, 118, 128
homothermal, 8
hormone, 117, 127, 138, 190, 193, 194, 219
hormones, 127, 193
host, 14, 31, 37, 189, 191, 192, 193, 209, 218, 219, 246
host metabolism, 191, 192
hot, 8, 20, 21, 90, 117, 122, 126, 202
hot showers, 122
hot springs, 20, 90
household water, 211
HS^-, 16, 18, 19, 23
hue, 17
human, ix, 24, 40, 46, 68, 79, 85, 113, 115, 125, 127, 136, 166, 170, 172, 180, 181, 188, 191, 200, 209, 218,

220, 223, 226, 229, 230, 232, 233, 237, 240, 242, 243, 244, 246, 248, 250, 252, 253, 254
human activity, ix
human body, 136, 252
human health, 200, 233, 244
human skin, 171, 180, 181, 243
humid-hot inhalation, 95
humidity, 167
Hungary, 13, 118
hydrogen, 2, 14, 18, 38, 39, 60, 61, 69, 112, 119, 128, 135, 172, 188, 201, 204, 206, 223, 224, 243
hydrogen bonds, 2
hydrogen carbonate, 112, 201
hydrogen carbonate-rich, 112
hydrogen ions, 135
hydrogen peroxide, 39, 243
hydrogen peroxide (H_2O_2), 39, 198, 243
hydrogen sulfide, 60, 61, 69
hydrogen sulphide (H_2S), 16, 18, 19, 23, 38, 40, 41, 42, 44, 45, 70, 119, 128, 206, 234
hydrogen-rich, 204, 223, 224
hydrogen-rich drinking water, 204
hydrogen-water, 188, 223
hydropinic, 107, 117
hydrostatic pressure, 117
hydrotherapy, 26, 107, 123, 179, 183, 184, 188
hydrotherapy/balneotherapy, 123
hydroxide, 16
hydroxyproline, 147
hygiene, 74
hypercalciuria, 139
hypercholesterolaemic, 235
hypercholesterolemia, 252
hyperglycaemia, 207
hyperglycemia, 216
hyperkeratotic disorders, 170
hypernatremia, 170
hyperplasia, 37
hypersensitivity, 82
hypertension, 134, 137, 150, 151, 155, 223, 247
hyperthermia, 117, 126, 129
hypertonic, 22, 34, 54, 91, 92, 103, 105
hypertonic saline, 34, 54, 91
hypertonic saline solution, 91
hypertonic sodium chloride solutions, 92
hypertonic solutions, 91
hypertrophy, 79, 90
hypoacusis, 97
hypomelanosis, 169
hyposmia, 87
hypothermal, 8, 17, 20
hypothesis, 82, 98, 136
hypotonic, 22

I

I^-, 23
Iceland, 175, 182
ichthyosis, 166, 174, 177, 184
IDA, 245
identification, 55, 98, 227, 229, 246
identity, 166
idiopathic, 80
IFN, 77, 79
IgA, 44, 45, 69, 77, 83, 87, 88, 100, 108
IgE, 44, 69, 77, 80, 83, 86, 100, 108
IgG, 45, 83, 100
IgM, 83, 100
IL-1, 126
IL-10, 101
IL-17, 77, 101, 129
IL-1β, 77, 101, 116
IL-2, 44, 77, 101
IL-21, 77, 101
IL-23, 120
IL-3, 78, 89, 92

IL-4, 77, 101, 171, 175
IL-4R, 171
IL-5, 78, 89, 92
IL-6, 42, 77, 101, 116, 192, 196
IL-8, 38, 42, 77, 101, 121, 171, 198
ileum, 208
immersion, 125, 174
immune, 36, 39, 57, 60, 79, 80, 81, 90, 99, 100, 101, 102, 103, 105, 106, 107, 125, 170, 174, 178, 181, 191, 216
immune response, 39, 90, 99, 101, 106, 107, 181, 191
immune responses, 39, 181, 191
immune system, 36, 100, 125, 216
immune-regulatory, 81, 106
immunocompromised, 81
immunoglobulin (Ig), 44, 45, 63, 69, 77, 79, 80, 83, 86, 87, 88, 92, 103, 106, 108, 251
immunoglobulins, 92, 103, 106, 251
immunological, vii, 29, 64, 120, 165, 170
immunometabolism, 191
immunomodulation, 183
immunomodulatory, 44, 100, 170, 176, 179
immunosuppressive, 172
immunosuppressive agent, 172
immunosuppressive effect, 172
impaired quality of life, 120
improvements, 91, 92, 95, 122, 171, 192
impulsivity, 237
in vitro, 44, 46, 58, 105, 115, 116, 117, 125, 138, 170, 171, 172, 179, 180, 198, 230, 231, 232, 233, 236, 237, 240, 241, 243, 244, 245, 253
in vivo, 44, 115, 138, 170, 172, 198, 215, 240, 245
incidence, 81, 99, 118, 134, 135, 136, 202, 207, 208, 225, 235, 242
income, 31
increased workload, xiii
indifferent, 8
indirect effect, 251
individuals, 41, 83, 94, 101, 116, 117, 120, 140, 144, 192, 194, 217, 218
induced sputum, 34, 39, 45, 48, 54
inducible nitric oxide synthase, 105
induction, 69, 113, 214
infants, 221
infection, 35, 42, 45, 54, 69, 70, 77, 81, 93, 94, 99, 100, 101, 103, 106, 110, 111, 112, 193, 201, 246
infections, 35, 42, 77, 81, 94, 99, 100, 101, 103, 106, 110, 111, 112, 201
inferences, 45
inferior turbinate hypertrophy, 79, 90
inflammation, 34, 36, 37, 38, 39, 44, 48, 50, 54, 55, 56, 60, 61, 68, 69, 70, 71, 78, 79, 80, 81, 85, 90, 92, 93, 99, 102, 103, 106, 107, 108, 113, 118, 120, 121, 125, 170, 171, 175, 180, 192, 193, 194, 198, 205, 215, 216, 217, 218, 219, 220, 221, 224, 229, 246
inflammatory, 30, 35, 36, 37, 38, 39, 40, 42, 48, 54, 55, 56, 58, 59, 62, 77, 78, 79, 80, 81, 82, 88, 89, 90, 93, 101, 102, 105, 106, 115, 116, 117, 118, 120, 121, 124, 126, 129, 166, 170, 171, 176, 190, 192, 193, 199, 204, 221, 223, 234, 246, 247, 249
inflammatory and innate responses, 121
inflammatory and non-inflammatory rheumatic diseases, 124
inflammatory bowel disease, 234, 246, 249
inflammatory cells, 36, 37, 39, 56, 80
inflammatory disease, 35, 36, 37, 90, 116, 117, 118

inflammatory diseases, 116
inflammatory mediators, 37, 38, 54, 55, 80, 115, 120
inflammatory parameters, 30, 38, 48, 116
inflammatory responses, 120
inflammatory rheumatic diseases, 118
infrapatellar, 129
ingestion, 117, 133, 135, 140, 142, 143, 146, 147, 148, 149, 188, 190, 201, 211, 215, 233, 234
ingredients, 134, 250
inhalation, 30, 34, 43, 45, 48, 49, 66, 67, 68, 69, 70, 71, 89, 90, 100, 101, 102, 107, 108, 109, 110
inhalation resistance, 102
inhaler, 89
inhibition, 45, 58, 61, 69, 138, 180, 215, 232, 236, 240
inhibitor, 127, 190
initiation, 92
innate, 36, 37, 57, 79, 102, 103, 106, 129, 171, 178
innate immune response, 57, 79, 102, 103, 178
innate immunity, 37, 171
inorganic element, 228, 240
institutions, 255
insulin, 116, 137, 138, 154, 190, 192, 194, 196, 204, 215, 217, 219, 223, 234
insulin-like growth factor I (IGF-1), 138, 140, 141
insulin growth factor-1, 116
insulin resistance, 154, 192
insulin sensitivity, 192, 217
insulin signaling, 223
insulin signalling, 137, 215
insulitis, 207
integrins, 182
integrity, 106, 141, 151, 204, 205, 219
interference, 65
interferon (IFN), 79, 101
interferon-γ, 101
interleukin (IL), 37, 38, 42, 44, 58, 77, 78, 79, 89, 92, 101, 116, 120, 121, 126, 129, 171, 175, 192, 198
interleukin (IL)-18, 171
interleukin (IL)-1β, 77, 101, 116
interleukin (IL)-22/IL-22 receptor, 37
interleukin (IL)-3, 78, 89, 92
interleukin (IL)-6, 42, 77, 101, 116, 192, 196
interleukin-17, 77, 101, 129
interleukin-22 receptor, 58
intermediate mineral content, 6
intermittent, 78, 80, 84
intermittent asthma, 78, 84
intervention, 33, 34, 48, 82, 83, 85, 86, 89, 91, 94, 101, 103, 104, 125, 144, 145, 174, 184, 201, 204, 206, 209, 210, 226
intestinal, ix, 139, 141, 170, 180, 191, 193, 198, 199, 200, 204, 209, 216, 217, 219, 220, 221, 222, 224, 225, 229, 230, 231, 232, 233, 234, 235, 236, 237, 238, 239, 240, 241, 242, 244, 245, 246, 248, 249, 250, 251, 254
intestinal barrier, 191, 193, 204, 219, 220
intestinal epithelium, 193, 199, 221, 251
intestinal flora, 221
intestinal hormone peptide YY, 193
intestinal villi, 199
intestine, 233, 234, 235, 240, 249
intoxication, 245
intraoperative and postoperative biopsies, 82
iodide (I^-), 23, 66, 181

iodine, 44, 45, 47, 48, 69, 77, 86, 87, 96, 100, 108, 109, 110, 172
iodine bromide, 44, 69, 86, 87, 108
iodine-alkali-hydrogen-carbonic, 172
ion channels, 228
ion exchange, 209
ionic content, 6, 7, 9, 10, 11
ionisation, 26
ionising radiation, 21
ions, 3, 10, 14, 18, 22, 106, 118, 120, 134, 135, 143, 147, 180, 181, 209, 228, 236, 237, 241
Iran, 13
iris, 212
iron (Fe^{2+}), 2, 7, 16, 17, 23, 141, 169, 174, 199, 202, 205, 241, 244, 245, 254
iron transport, 245
iron-rich, 245
irradiation, 65, 180, 181, 204
irrigation, 68, 75, 82, 83, 84, 102, 108, 109, 111, 112
irrigations, 68, 75, 83, 84, 109, 111
irritability, 80
ISO 21426: 2018, 7, 23, 28
isotonic, 22, 46, 48, 82, 83, 84, 85, 86, 88, 91, 92, 96, 104, 109
isotonic saline, 46, 48, 86, 96, 104
isotonic solution, 91
isotope, 21
Israel, 13, 175
issues, 36, 74, 104, 212, 255
Italy, 6, 8, 9, 13, 16, 29, 45, 46, 47, 48, 82, 83, 84, 85, 86, 87, 88, 89, 90, 94, 95, 96, 100, 101, 108, 109, 167, 174, 258
itching, 80, 88, 89

J

Japan, 13, 153, 155, 201, 202, 243
jejunum, 201
joint capsules, 117
joint damage, 118
joint diseases, 117
joint mobility, 117
joints, 117, 119
Jordan, 62, 175

K

K^+, 148, 230, 235, 236, 240, 241, 252
K^+-ATPase, 240, 241
K^+-ATPase activity, 240, 241
K^+-pump, 240
keratin, 170
keratinocyte, 172, 173, 182, 232, 237, 240, 241, 242, 243, 244, 246, 253
keratinocytes, 172, 173, 232, 237, 241, 243, 244, 246
keratoses, 169
kidney, 134, 157, 210, 246
kidney and cardiovascular diseases, 134
kidney function decline, 210
kidney stones, 246
kidneys, 137
kill, 58
Kineothrix sp., 211
knee, 121, 122, 127, 129, 130
knee flexion, 121
knee OA, 121, 122
knee pain, 121
knees, 121
Koilonychia, 169

L

La Roche-Posay®, 171, 172, 174, 179
label indications, 6, 7
Lachnoclostridium, 206
Lachnospira, 197

Lachnospiraceae, 197, 204, 223
Lactobacillaceae, 201, 204
Lactobacilli, 207, 208
Lactobacillus, 197, 199, 204, 206, 207, 208, 209, 221
Lactobacillus gasseri, 197, 221
Lactobacillus sp., 208, 209
Lactococcus, 206
lactose, 252
lactulose, 231, 234, 249
Langerhans cells, 171, 180
laryngitis, 76, 78, 99, 103, 104, 112
laryngology, 99, 105
larynx, 99
laws, 26
L-cysteine, 40
LDL, 195, 197
lead, 134, 138, 204, 205, 227, 233, 255
lean, 192, 217
legislation, 1, 3, 4, 23, 25
leisure, 49
leisure time, 49
leptin, 121, 129, 190, 194, 196
Lequesne Algofunctional Index (LAFI), 121
lesions, 182, 199
leukocytes, 62, 124, 241, 244
leukotrienes (LTs), 38
Li^+, 23, 230
lifetime, 52, 153
ligand, 120, 138
light, 95, 98, 105, 177, 190
linear model, 197
lipemia, 249
lipid, 38, 113, 118, 126, 127, 172, 181, 190, 192, 193, 204, 219, 223, 224, 235, 236, 244, 249, 250, 253
lipid metabolism, 193, 219
lipid peroxidation, 172, 181
lipid profile, 118, 190, 204, 224
lipid transport, 235, 236
lipids, 127, 192, 244, 249, 250, 253
lipolysis, 194
lipopolysaccharide (LPS), 191, 193, 204, 220
lipoxins, 38
lipoxygenase (LOX), 38, 59
liquids, 24
lithium (Li^+), 23, 113, 169, 230
Lithuania, 13
liver, 134, 137, 151, 155, 191, 200, 221, 234, 235, 237, 248, 249, 252
liver cirrhosis, 200, 221, 234, 249
liver disease, 134, 137, 151, 155
living conditions, 142, 144
longitudinal study, 159
low mineral content, 6, 200, 214
low mineral water, 234, 249
low-bicarbonate, 143
low-calcium, 147, 161, 214
low-density lipoprotein (LDL), 120, 192, 195, 197, 215
lower respiratory tract infection, 35
low-grade, 120, 134, 139, 152, 159, 192
low-grade inflammation, 191, 192, 218
low-grade metabolic acidosis, 134, 152, 159
low-grade systemic inflammation, 120
low-PRAL, 141, 143
low-sulphate, 147
LTB_4, 38, 39, 49, 126
LTC_4, 38
LTD_4, 38
LTE_4, 38
lumbar spine, 140
lumen, 36, 106, 244
lung, 31, 32, 34, 35, 36, 37, 39, 40, 41, 42, 46, 47, 48, 51, 56, 57, 58, 59, 60, 64, 65, 70, 237
lung cancer, 31
lung disease, 34

lung function, 32, 35, 37, 41, 42, 46, 47, 48, 56
lung function tests, 32
lung parenchyma, 36, 37
lymphocytes, 36, 41, 44, 69, 82, 117, 170, 173
lysine, 135
lysozyme, 66

M

machinery, 138
macrophage, 36, 37, 38, 39, 41, 58, 59, 70, 105, 171, 194, 196
macrophage inflammatory protein, 171, 196
macrophages, 36, 37, 38, 39, 41, 58, 59, 70, 105, 194
magnesiac, 174
magnesium (Mg^{2+}), 7, 9, 10, 11, 12, 13, 15, 16, 22, 23, 77, 89, 100, 118, 120, 122, 134, 136, 142, 143, 144, 145, 146, 147, 148, 162, 168, 169, 174, 198, 199, 201, 202, 212, 213, 216, 230, 233, 234, 235, 236, 238, 241, 242, 247, 252
magnesium and bicarbonate, 145
magnesium-rich, 147
magnetotherapy, 122
magnitude, 98
majority, 93, 211, 228
malaise, 80
male, 40, 41, 45, 47, 48, 82, 138, 161, 198, 199, 201, 203, 205, 206, 207, 208, 209, 211, 214, 231
malignancy, 248
malondialdehyde, 172
management, 75, 93, 97, 111, 123, 124, 131, 152, 167, 175, 176, 183, 185, 238
manganese, 169, 173, 181, 182
mannitol, 231, 234, 249
mannitol transport, 234
Marina®, 240, 241, 251
markers, 85, 113, 125, 126, 139, 141, 142, 144, 145, 148, 153, 156, 158, 161, 192, 214, 218, 220
marketing, 4, 25
mass, 21, 139, 141, 196, 197
massages, 122
mast cell, 80, 86, 170, 180
mast cells, 86, 170
mastocytes, 78, 82
materials, 210
matrix, 127, 138, 194
matrix metalloproteinases (MMPs), 117, 120, 127
matter, iv, 198
measurements, 32, 49, 53, 200
meat, 135, 158, 242
mechanical effects, 117
mechanical pulmonary ventilation, 47
media, 93, 112
mediators, 30, 34, 37, 38, 55, 80, 81, 115, 120, 220
medical, xiii, 2, 5, 25, 66, 71, 74, 75, 81, 95, 103, 107, 168, 179, 188, 234, 246
medical history, 75, 107
Medical Hydrology, 1, 2, 24, 25, 26, 28, 71, 179, 189, 221, 258
medical Spas, 5
medication, 81, 89, 121
medicine, ix, x, 2, 26, 61, 71, 76, 111
Mediterranean diet, 134, 137, 156
medium mineral, 8, 9, 123
medium mineralisation, 8, 9, 123
medium-high-bicarbonate, 143
medium-PRAL, 143
medullary volume, 148
Melgaço®, 11, 20, 230, 231, 232, 233, 234

membrane, viii, 94, 209, 227, 228, 229, 236, 237, 240, 243, 246, 250, 252, 253
membrane fluidity, 243
membrane transport, viii, 227, 228, 229, 237, 240, 246
membrane transporter, viii, 227, 228, 229, 237, 246
membranes, 227, 228, 236, 243, 252, 253
memory, 237
men, 82, 83, 88, 89, 99, 140, 153, 155, 157, 161, 209, 214, 224, 252
menopause, 202
mental health, 156
mesothermal, 8
meta-analysis, 52, 102, 111, 150, 151, 155, 157, 162, 218, 250
metabolic acidosis, 134, 136, 138, 139, 142, 152, 159, 242
metabolic disease, 189, 191, 193, 216, 217, 224, 246, 254
metabolic diseases, 191, 216, 217, 224, 246
metabolic disorders, 189, 193, 202, 216, 219, 220
metabolic dysfunction, 190, 191, 193, 255
metabolic health, 188, 189, 191, 199, 204, 211, 212
metabolic health and disease, 188, 189, 211, 212
metabolic pathways, 220
metabolic syndrome, 35, 108, 113, 127, 134, 137, 154, 155, 188, 192, 197, 200, 201, 202, 204, 213, 214, 215, 217, 221, 222, 224, 247
metabolism, 42, 134, 135, 137, 139, 141, 144, 146, 147, 149, 156, 159, 161, 162, 188, 190, 191, 192, 199, 206, 209, 214, 215, 216, 217, 223, 225, 228, 244, 248, 250, 255
metabolites, 191, 193, 202, 219
metabolome, 202
methodology, 92
methylation, 40
Mg^{2+}, 7, 10, 11, 12, 13, 23, 145, 146, 147, 148, 230, 233, 236, 238, 241, 242
mice, 46, 70, 192, 194, 198, 200, 201, 204, 205, 206, 207, 208, 209, 215, 216, 217, 219, 220, 225
microbial cells, 191
microbial communities, 221
microbial community, 222
microbial metabolites, 193, 219
microbicidal, 37
microbiological, 5, 84
microbiomes, 40
microbiota, 188, 189, 191, 192, 193, 194, 195, 196, 197, 198, 199, 200, 201, 202, 203, 204, 205, 206, 207, 208, 209, 210, 211, 216, 217, 218, 219, 220, 221, 222, 223, 224, 225, 226, 246, 254
micronised nasal douche, 85, 97
micronised nasal wash, 94
microorganism, 166, 175, 246
microorganisms, 166, 175
microparticles, 101
microstructural properties, 144, 148
microvilli absorption, 199
middle ear disturbances, 77, 94
middle ear infection, 93
middle ear with effusion, 93
migration, 171, 173, 182
milligrams, 9
mineral, iii, vii, viii, ix, 1, 3, 4, 5, 6, 8, 9, 20, 23, 25, 26, 27, 28, 47, 65, 68, 70, 84, 86, 92, 99, 100, 106, 107, 108, 113, 116, 117, 118, 120, 121,

122, 123, 124, 125, 126, 127, 129, 130, 131, 133, 134, 135, 137, 138, 139, 142, 143, 144, 145, 146, 147,148, 149, 151, 155, 156, 158, 159, 160, 161, 162, 165, 166, 167, 168, 169, 170, 172, 174, 177, 179, 180, 181, 183, 184, 188, 189, 190, 198, 199, 200, 201, 202, 209, 210, 211, 213, 214, 215, 216, 221, 222, 227, 228, 229, 230, 231, 232, 233, 234, 235, 236, 238, 239, 240, 242, 243, 245, 246, 247, 248, 249, 250, 251, 252, 253, 254, 255
mineral and thermal waters, 5
mineral content, 5, 92, 137, 139, 142, 144, 158, 166, 172, 230
mineral deficiency, 168, 169, 170, 190
mineral water, iii, vii, viii, ix, 1, 2, 3, 4, 5, 6, 7, 8, 9, 10, 11, 16, 17, 18, 19, 23, 24, 25, 26, 27, 28, 30, 48, 68, 70, 100, 106, 107, 108, 113, 116, 117, 118, 120, 122, 124, 125, 126, 127, 130, 133, 134, 135, 137, 138, 142, 143, 144, 145, 146, 147, 148, 149, 155, 156, 159, 160, 161, 162, 165, 166, 167, 168, 170, 171, 172, 173, 174, 175, 176, 177, 178, 179, 180, 181, 183, 184, 188, 189, 190, 198, 199, 200, 201, 202, 210, 213, 214, 221, 222, 227, 228, 229, 230, 231, 232, 233, 234, 235, 236, 238, 239, 240, 242, 243, 245, 246, 247, 248, 249, 250, 251, 252, 253, 254, 255
mineral water consumption, vii, 106, 108, 118, 127, 133, 134, 137, 142, 144, 155, 189, 190, 202, 213, 247, 255
mineralisation, 9, 121, 138, 141
mineralization, 28, 252
mitochondria, 40
mitochondrial, 40, 190, 216
mitochondrial biogenesis, 190, 216
mitogen, 44, 117
MMP13, 120
MMPs, 117
mobility, 117, 224
models, 118, 179, 198, 247
modern society, 75
modifications, 82, 238
modified Borg dyspnoea scale, 33
moisture, 175
moisture content, 175
molar concentration, 7, 22
mole, 22
molecular weight, 9
molecules, 2, 22, 38, 39, 40, 106, 243
monocyte, 171, 196
monocyte chemoattractant protein, 171
monolateral or bilateral OME, 77, 96
mononuclear cells, 46, 80, 117
morbidity, 31, 32, 34, 51, 52, 79, 128
morning stiffness, 119
Morocco, 13
mortality, 31, 34, 51, 56, 155, 233
motif, 79, 102, 120
mRNA, 194, 196
mucociliary clearance, 91, 106, 108
mucociliary transport time, 77, 82, 87, 90, 91
mucolytic, 44
mucosa, 75, 80, 87, 105, 199, 201, 221
mucosa-adhered, 201
mucosal, 77, 81, 82, 83, 85, 88, 90, 92, 106, 250
mucosal inflammation, 81
mucosal recovery, 77, 83, 92
mucous, 240
mucus, 37, 77, 88, 91, 106, 193, 219, 230
mucus content, 88
mucus hypersecretion, 37

mud bath, 117, 120, 121, 126, 127, 130 172
mud packs, 117, 119, 120, 122, 124
mud therapy, 43, 64, 116, 122, 124
mud bath therapy, 117, 127
mud bathing therapy, 124, 131
multicellular organisms, 205
muscle, 40, 56, 117, 141, 193
muscle shape and mass, 141
muscle spasm, 117
muscle tone, 117
mutant, 206
mycosis fungoides, 174

N

Na^+, 7, 10, 11, 12, 13, 148, 228, 230, 233, 234, 235, 236, 237, 240, 241, 252
Na^+ Ca^{2+}, 11, 12, 13
Na^+ Ca^{2+} Mg^{2+}, 11, 12, 13
Na^+ Mg^{2+}, 11, 12
NaCl, 134, 136, 159
Naftusia®, 240, 251
nail, 169
nasal, 44, 68, 69, 74, 76, 77, 78, 79, 80, 81, 82, 83, 84, 85, 86, 87, 88, 89, 90, 91, 93, 96, 99, 100, 101, 103, 104, 108, 109, 110, 111, 112
nasal adapter, 85, 86, 101
nasal blockage and discharge, 81
nasal blood supply, 89
nasal brushings, 88
nasal ciliary motility, 78, 91
nasal cytology, 44, 68, 78, 79, 82, 83, 87, 90
nasal cytology data, 79, 87
nasal discharge and blockage, 80
nasal diseases, 79
nasal endoscopic surgery, 74, 76, 83, 104
nasal functional endoscopic surgery, 77, 82
nasal immune response, 90
nasal inflammation, 78
nasal itch, 78, 100
nasal lavage, 88, 104
nasal lavage fluid, 88
nasal mucociliary clearance, 77
nasal mucociliary transport time, 79, 83, 100, 103
nasal mucosa appearance, 87
nasal mucosa congestion, 87
nasal mucosal recovery, 77, 92
nasal mucus content, 77, 91
nasal obstruction, 85, 87, 88
nasal patency, 89
nasal polyp, 76, 77, 78, 79, 81, 85, 87, 90, 104
nasal polyposis, 76, 77, 81, 87, 104
nasal resistance, 77, 83, 90, 91
nasal respiratory flow, 77, 90, 91
nasal secretion, 87, 104, 109
nasal spray, 87, 90
nasal symptoms, 80, 85, 89
National Health and Nutrition Examination Survey, 136, 140
natural killer cell, 173, 253
natural mineral water, vii, ix, 1, 2, 3, 4, 5, 6, 7, 8, 9, 10, 11, 16, 17, 18, 19, 24, 25, 27, 30, 43, 48, 161, 165, 166, 167, 168, 170, 171, 172, 173, 174, 175, 176, 177, 178, 212, 221, 247, 248, 252, 253
natural mineral water types, 3, 4
natural science, 224
natural water, 2, 14, 22, 28, 200
nebulisation, 45, 47, 96
nebulised, 101
necrosis, 79, 85, 116, 171, 190, 197
negative correlation, 40, 41, 124
neoplasm, 105

nerve, 117
nervous system, 237
net acid, 136, 143, 150, 152, 253
net endogenous acid production (NEAP), 134, 136, 138, 139, 140, 141, 153, 154
neurobiology, 250
neurocognitive deficits, 80
neurodegenerative disorders, 125, 244
neuronal ceroid lipofuscinoses, 206
neurons, 238
neuropathic pain, 204, 223, 238
neuropeptides, 172
neurotransmission, 251
neutral, 8, 10, 207, 208, 209
neutral drinking water, 208, 209
neutral pH drinking water, 208, 209
neutral water, 207, 208
neutrophil, 36, 37, 38, 39, 58, 59, 68, 78, 84, 86, 113, 121, 222
neutrophil and spore counts, 78, 86
neutrophil count, 84
neutrophil extracellular traps (NETs), 37, 58
neutrophil-derived proteases, 37
neutrophilia, 36
neutrophils, 30, 36, 37, 38, 41, 42, 56, 58, 78, 80, 82, 87
NF-κB (nuclear factor kappa-light-chain-enhancer of activated B cells), 190
nitric oxide (NO), iv, 25, 60, 76, 79, 82, 83, 84, 85, 89, 103, 105, 112, 145, 147, 163, 209, 243
nitric oxide synthase, 105
non-acidified drinking water, 205, 206
non-acidified tap water, 205
non-acidified water, 207
non-alcoholic, 134, 137
non-alcoholic fatty liver disease, 134, 137
nonallergic chronic rhinosinusitis, 44, 68, 109
nonallergic CRS, 77, 83, 84
nonallergic rhinitis, 80, 103
non-communicable diseases, 134, 135, 137, 142
non-infectious rhinitis, 80
non-*Lactobacilli*, 208
non-obese diabetic, 207, 225
non-pharmacological, viii, 49, 74, 81, 87, 91, 96, 103, 104, 123, 124, 131, 187
non-pharmacological treatments, 123
non-polar, 2
non-smokers, 41, 52, 102
non-sulphurous, 44, 49, 121, 122
non-sulphurous water baths, 122
normal development, 237
normal saline, 48
North America, 156, 168
nose, 75, 76, 81, 83, 99
noxious particles, 31
n-telopeptides, 147
nuclear factor kappa B subunit 1 (NF-KB1), 79, 102
nuclei, 2
nucleus, 2
nutrient, 133, 134, 138, 144, 188, 212, 213, 228, 246, 248
nutrients, 133, 134, 138, 144, 188, 213, 228, 246
nutrition, 142, 150, 177

O

obese, 134, 137, 156, 192, 217, 218
obesity, 134, 137, 155, 188, 189, 192, 193, 197, 201, 202, 216, 217, 218, 219, 220, 221, 222, 224, 233, 246, 248
objective examination, 77, 87, 91

objectivity, 98
obsessive-compulsive disorder, 237
obstruction, 32, 37, 41, 56, 57, 85, 87, 88, 89
obstructive lung disease, 64, 65
obstructive polyposis, 79, 90
occupational, 31, 52, 80
occupational exposure, 31, 52
occurrences, 100
oedema, 106, 171
oesophageal, 62
old, 40, 41, 45, 46, 47, 48, 74, 98, 207
oleic acid, 236
olfactory threshold, 83
oligometallic, 124
oligomineral, 8, 9
OME, 76, 77, 78, 79, 93, 94, 95, 96, 97, 104
OME with deafness, 78, 95
oocytes, 241, 243
operational taxonomic units (OTUs), 210, 211
oral glucose tolerance test (OGTT), 194, 197, 209
order, 30, 45, 49, 83, 97, 99, 124, 167, 210, 211, 228
organ, 41, 191, 216, 220, 227, 228, 246
organic and inorganic dusts, 32
organic compound, 228, 229, 231
organic compounds, 231
organism, 2, 8, 24, 106, 171
organs, 105, 191
ORL, 74, 75, 76, 96, 101, 103, 104, 105, 107, 110
osmosis, 209
osteoarthritis (OA), 115, 116, 117, 118, 119, 120, 121, 122, 123, 127, 128, 129, 130, 131, 158
osteoblast, 138, 149
osteoblasts, 138
osteocalcin, 147
osteoclast, 138, 157
osteomalacia, 169
osteoporosis, 134, 140, 141, 144, 149, 157, 158, 160, 162, 238, 242, 252
osteoporotic fractures, 141, 158
otitis media, 74, 76, 79, 93, 97, 107, 110, 112
otitis media with effusion (OME), 74, 76, 77, 78, 79, 93, 94, 95, 96, 97, 104, 107, 110, 112
otology, 93, 105
otorhinolaryngology (ORL), vii, xi, 44, 73, 74, 75, 76, 77, 96, 101, 103, 104, 105, 107, 110, 257, 258
ovariectomised, 148, 202
ovariectomy, 148
overall mineralisation, 8
overlap, 31
overtime, 83
overweight, 156, 192, 194, 196, 218
oxalate, 136
oxidation, 14, 18, 40, 61
oxidation products, 118
oxidative stress, 38, 39, 45, 46, 59, 60, 70, 204, 214, 223, 229
oxygen, 40, 61, 173, 184
ozone, 4, 25

P

paediatric recurrent upper respiratory tract infections, 100
pain, 81, 85, 115, 116, 117, 119, 120, 121, 122, 123, 124, 125, 130, 131, 172, 223, 238, 251
pain control, 117
pain improvement, 115
pain intensity, 119
pain management, 251
pain medication, 121
pain threshold, 117, 123, 172

painful symptomatology, 122
pancreatic cancer, 156
pancreatic islets of Langerhans, 190
pancreatitis, 234, 249
Parabacteroides, 195, 206, 208
parallel, 100, 147, 197
paranasal sinuses, 81
Parasutterella, 195
parathyroid, 138, 161, 190, 214, 252
parathyroid hormone (PTH), 138, 141, 144, 145, 146, 147, 190
parenchyma, 36, 37
parents, v
paronychia, 169
participants, 119, 140, 141, 142, 143
pathogenesis, 36, 38, 46, 55, 57, 111, 203
pathogens, 37
pathological, 35, 37, 38, 75, 90, 95, 97, 149, 182, 219
pathology, 30, 57, 67, 74, 97, 102
pathophysiological, 60, 228
pathophysiological roles, 60
pathophysiology, 111, 129, 191
pathway, 2, 38, 58, 59, 60, 61, 192, 193, 212, 215, 216, 219, 225
pathways, 38, 58, 59, 60, 61, 192, 193, 212, 219, 225
Pedras Salgadas®, 11, 20, 230, 231, 232, 233, 234
Pelagibacterium, 203
peloid therapy, 65, 66, 121, 129
pelotherapy, 64, 65, 167, 174
peptide, 106, 109, 171, 172, 193
peptides, 106, 109, 171, 172
perennial, 44, 79, 80, 90
perennial allergic rhinitis, 44, 79, 90
peripheral blood, 46, 54, 117
peripheral blood mononuclear cell, 46, 117
permeability, 106, 192, 219, 234, 243, 249
permission, iv
permit, 245
peroxidation, 38, 172
persistent, 30, 31, 35, 79, 80, 90, 99, 176
persistent allergic rhinitis, 79, 90
persistent cough, 99
pH, 14, 15, 17, 18, 19, 20, 38, 42, 49, 61, 62, 135, 136, 137, 138, 140, 142, 143, 145, 146, 147, 148, 152, 156, 184, 188, 189, 205, 206, 207, 208, 209, 211, 224, 225, 226, 228
phagocytosis, 58
pharmaceutical, 209
pharmacological, viii, 5, 6, 74, 80, 82, 84, 90, 92, 93, 97, 98, 99, 103, 104, 123, 131, 168, 171, 174, 178, 187, 190
pharmacological agents, 168
pharmacological treatment, 74, 81, 99, 174, 178
pharmacotherapy, 126
pharyngeal or laryngeal diseases, 76, 103
pharyngitis, 76, 77, 78, 79, 90, 93, 99, 101, 102, 103, 104, 108, 111
pharyngology, 99, 105
pharynx, 99, 101
phenotype, 30, 35, 40, 50, 55, 61, 80, 191, 192
phenotypes, 30, 35, 50, 55, 80, 191
Philadelphia, 224
phobia, 81
phosphate, 137, 145
phosphorous, 135
phosphorus, 135, 148
phototherapy, 174
phylum, 191, 200, 205
physical activity, 143

physical exercise, 48, 142
physical properties, 116
physical therapy, 121
physical-chemical analysis, 6
physicians, x, 167
physiological, 5, 6, 8, 60, 90, 94, 98, 100, 104, 106, 125, 138, 198, 212, 228, 237, 245, 253
physiology, 209
phytate, 135
phytochemicals, 134, 141
phytoestrogens, 141
pilot study, 66, 96, 110, 130, 131, 181, 196, 213
placebo, 45, 46, 47, 48, 49, 89, 92, 104, 119, 161, 173, 175, 176, 182, 196, 204
placenta, 237
plant proteins, 135
plasma cells, 78, 82
plasma membrane, 237, 243, 252
plasmocytes, 82
platelets, 238
playing, 94
plethysmography, 32
pneumatic otoscopy, 97
pneumoconiosis, 63
pneumonia, 69
Poland, 13
polar, 2, 243
Politzer insufflation, 94, 95, 96, 106
pollen, 84
pollution, 5, 31, 52, 177, 244
polydipsia, 234
polymorphonuclear cells, 44
polyps, 77, 78, 79, 83, 85, 90
polyuria, 234
population, 52, 82, 88, 93, 94, 99, 102, 104, 136, 149, 153, 165
Portugal, x, xii, 13, 20, 26, 27, 29, 73, 115, 133, 165, 187, 227, 255, 257, 258, 259
positive correlation, 46
postmenopausal, 140, 141, 145, 147, 148, 158, 160, 161, 162, 214, 231, 235, 249
postnasal drip, 99
postprandial triglyceride (ppTG), 231, 232, 235, 250
potassium (K^+), 118, 120, 122, 136, 137, 142, 146, 148, 152, 154, 201, 230, 235, 236, 240, 241, 251, 252
potential renal acid load (PRAL), 134, 136, 137, 138, 140, 141, 143, 145, 146, 147, 149, 150, 152, 154, 155, 158, 253
preparation, iv
prevalence rate, 80
prevention, 66, 74, 76, 99, 107, 144, 189, 192, 200, 219, 232, 242, 250
Prevotella, 192, 208, 210
Prevotella copri, 210
Prevotella loescheii, 208
primary airways infections, 78, 97
probe, 234
probiotic, 179, 192, 218
probiotics, 218
procollagen I amino-terminal propeptide, 148
procollagen type I N propeptide, 140
prodiabetogenic diet, 207
producers, 204
profibrogenic, 190
progenitor cells, 57
prognosis, 96
pro-inflammatory, 80, 101, 116, 119, 128, 192, 223
pro-inflammatory cytokines, 116
pro-inflammatory genes, 119, 128
project, 67

prolactin, 127
proliferation, 39, 117, 173, 193, 229, 244
prophylaxis, 110, 247
prostaglandin, 38, 116
prostaglandin E2, 116
prostaglandins (PGs), 38
protection, 113, 126, 185, 204, 214
protective role, 172, 203, 224
protein oxidation, 113, 118, 126
proteins, 37, 38, 120, 135, 138, 140, 171, 173, 193, 227, 228, 237, 243
Proteobacteria, 191, 193, 199, 200, 202, 220
protons, 2
pruritus, 173, 175, 176, 183
Pseudoflavonifractor capillosus, 210
psoriasis, 166, 169, 170, 174, 175, 180, 182, 183
Psoriasis Area Severity Index (PASI), 174
psychosocial, 33
public health, 153, 189, 201, 245
public policy, 52
pure water, 22
purified water, 200
purity, 5, 166

Q

quality of life (QoL), 31, 32, 33, 41, 48, 78, 79, 85, 91, 94, 97, 120, 122, 130, 173, 178, 184
quantification, 88, 93
questionnaire, 32, 33, 53, 121, 123
Questionnaires for Symptoms and Quality of Life, 32

R

radiation, 167, 172, 174, 177, 182, 223
radiation dermatitis, 174
radicals, 171, 173
radioactive, 16, 21, 69, 79, 90, 110
radiodermatitis, 176
radiotherapy, 176
radon (Rn), 16, 21, 23, 64
randomised, 33, 45, 46, 47, 48, 49, 70, 82, 83, 84, 87, 88, 89, 90, 96, 100, 108, 109, 110, 112, 121, 122, 123, 140, 141, 143, 145, 146, 147, 174, 175, 176, 178, 184, 196, 197, 204, 209, 210, 221, 235, 249
randomised controlled trials (RCTs), 33, 174
rating scale, 53
ratio, 9, 15, 19, 32, 33, 42, 61, 118, 191, 203, 205, 207, 217, 234
reactant, 188
reaction medium, 188
reactions, 14, 21, 86
reactive oxygen species (ROS), 39, 60, 117
reactivity, 90
receptor, 37, 58, 79, 102, 120, 138, 171, 178, 190, 193, 204, 219, 241, 243, 253
receptors, 243
recognition, ix, 144
recommendations, iv, 94, 123, 131
recovery, 76, 77, 82, 92, 95, 97, 104, 169, 173, 239
recovery process, 104
rectum, 201
recurrent rhinosinusitis, 77, 87
recurrent upper respiratory tract, 78, 100, 106, 110
redox, 39, 61, 105, 106, 107, 113, 115, 117, 125, 190, 205, 214

reflux, 42, 62, 99, 102, 103
regeneration, 55
regulatory T cells, 121
rehabilitation, ix, 65, 66, 74, 107, 126, 176, 183
reinforcement, 193
relapses, 97
relatively low in magnesium, 201
relaxation, 49
relevance, 45, 46, 85, 92, 94, 96, 98, 135, 144, 188, 190, 207, 228, 246
relief, 105
remission, 176
remodelling, 37, 39, 106, 139, 144, 148, 162
renal calculi, 169
renal tubular acidosis, 136
renewal, 169, 173, 199
repair, 39, 79, 102, 103, 120
requirements, 4, 25, 28, 234
researchers, x
residue, 1, 6, 7, 8, 9, 10, 17, 209
residues, 17, 209
resistance, 70, 77, 82, 83, 84, 90, 91, 102, 105, 106, 108, 154, 192, 194, 201, 224
resolution, 87
resorption pit, 138
resorptive marker, 138
resources, ix
respiration, 39
respiratory disorders, 44
respiratory tract abnormalities, 78, 84
respiratory tract disease, 81
response, 35, 41, 49, 68, 80, 92, 104, 113, 127, 138, 150, 155, 159, 180, 200, 201, 222, 249, 250, 254
responsiveness, 54
restoration, 106, 241
reticulum, 190, 215, 243
reverse osmosis, 209
reverse osmosis-treated water, 209
rheumatic diseases, vii, 115, 116, 117, 118, 124, 126, 127, 128
rheumatoid arthritis (RA), 115, 118, 119, 120, 126, 127, 128
rhinitis, 44, 49, 69, 74, 76, 77, 78, 79, 80, 81, 85, 86, 89, 90, 91, 99, 101, 103, 104, 107, 108, 109, 110, 111
rhinogenic deafness, 77, 93, 94, 97, 110
rhinomanometric, 77, 87, 91, 102
rhinomanometric data, 77, 91, 102
rhinorrhoea, 80, 87, 89
rhinosinusitis, 44, 74, 78, 79, 81, 87, 93, 99
rhinovirus infection, 45
rich in bicarbonate, 145, 147
rich in calcium, 145
rich in calcium and sulphate, 145
rich in calcium, magnesium and bicarbonate, 145
rich in chloride, fluoride and sodium, 198
rich in sulphate and magnesium, 145
rich in sulphide ion, 122
richness, 135, 150, 200, 203, 209, 210, 226
risedronate, 232, 239, 251
risk, 5, 31, 32, 50, 52, 54, 80, 81, 93, 99, 118, 119, 128, 138, 141, 143, 144, 150, 151, 153, 154, 155, 156, 157, 162, 192, 202, 203, 213, 218, 221, 223, 225, 233, 235, 245, 247
risk factors, 31, 52, 80, 150, 202, 203
risks, 119, 143, 221
Rn, 16, 23
rodents, 209
Rokko®, 241, 243
Romania, 13, 121
Romboutsia, 195
root, 134, 135, 204
roots, 134, 135

ROS, 39
rosacea, 177
Roseburia, 197, 203, 204
routes, 234
Ruminococcaceae, 203, 204, 210, 211
Ruminococcus, 192, 195
Ruminococcus2, 195
Russia, 13

S

safety, 66, 74, 105, 123, 158, 247
saline, 23, 34, 46, 48, 50, 54, 87, 88, 91, 111, 118, 120, 128, 182
saline water, 23, 118, 120
salinity, 224
Salmonella, 211
salso-bromo-iodine, 77, 86, 87, 88, 96, 97, 109, 110
salt bath, 121
salt-bromine-iodic, 87
salt-bromide-iodine, 45, 47, 48, 49, 77, 100, 101
salt-rich saline water, 118
salts, 15, 86, 91, 136, 182, 233, 245
saltwater, 175, 180
salty-earthy-alkaline, 79, 101
satiety, 193
sauna, 43, 64, 127
scaling, 171
scars, 176, 183
SCFA, 203
school, 93, 94
scientific knowledge, 198
scientific method, ix, 5, 74
scientific papers, 168
scope, 50
seasonal, 78, 80, 84, 109, 112, 127
seasonal allergic rhinitis, 78, 84, 109, 112
seborrheic, 166, 169, 174, 177
seborrheic dermatitis, 169, 174, 177
sebum, 184
secondary effects, 105
secretion, 87, 101, 193, 198, 204, 230
security, 188, 189, 211
sediment, 224
seed, 96
segmented filamentous bacteria (SFB), 199, 208
selenium, 142, 168, 169, 171, 181, 182
self-control, 213
sensation, 8, 84, 105
sense of smell, 81, 85
senses, 105
sensitivity, 46, 70, 192, 196, 249
sensitization, 131
sensor, 40, 61
sequencing, 254
serotonin, 232, 237, 250, 251
serotonin transport, 232, 237, 250, 251
serum, 41, 44, 61, 63, 69, 108, 126, 127, 129, 143, 155, 215, 223
serum bicarbonate, 143
services, 23, 28, 85
severity, 32, 36, 39, 42, 61, 78, 80, 100, 103, 174, 175, 198
sex, 86
SGRQ, 33, 42, 48, 53
sham, 202
shape, 141, 222
shock, 188
short-chain fatty acids (SCFAs), 192, 193, 202, 204, 219
side effects, 84, 85, 88, 89, 91, 92, 100, 102, 245
signaling pathway, 37, 215
signalling, 60, 137, 190, 192, 193, 215, 219
signals, 216, 220
signs, 88, 93
silica, 142

silicate, 15, 168
silicium, 170, 171
silicon, 243, 244, 245, 254
sinonasal diseases, 74, 79, 92
sino-nasal 5 (SN5), 78, 79, 85, 91
sino-nasal outcome test (SNOT), 79, 90, 91
sinuses, 81, 99
sinusitis, 74, 76, 77, 79, 81, 93, 101, 104, 108
Sirt1-AMPK-PGC1-α, 190
sirtuin 1, 190, 215
skin, 117, 165, 166, 167, 168, 169, 170, 171, 172, 173, 174, 175, 176, 177, 178, 180, 181, 183, 184, 185, 237, 243, 244, 253
skin barrier, 169, 173, 177, 185
skin carcinogenesis, 172
skin diseases, 166, 168, 174, 175, 178
skin disorders, 167, 176, 178
skin explants, 172
skin exposome, 167, 177
skin inflammation, 175
sleep deprivation, 177
small intestine, 240, 251
smokers, 41, 42, 47, 48, 52, 55, 56, 61, 70, 83, 102
smoking, 31, 47, 48, 52, 57, 70, 84, 102, 104, 109, 158, 177, 209
smooth muscle, 40, 56
smooth muscle cells, 40
sneezing, 80, 88, 89
SO_4^{2-}, 7, 10, 12, 13, 23, 145, 146, 148, 230, 233, 236, 242
social costs, 31
social development, 94
social impact, 78, 100, 103
sodium (Na^+), 7, 9, 10, 15, 61, 65, 66, 78, 81, 82, 83, 84, 85, 86, 87, 91, 92, 95, 97, 113, 118, 120, 121, 122, 123, 134, 137, 138, 144, 145, 146, 147, 148, 152, 156, 162, 170, 172, 174, 190, 198, 199, 200, 201, 202, 203, 213, 214, 221, 228, 230, 234, 235, 236, 240, 249, 251
sodium bicarbonate-rich, 138, 145
sodium chloride (NaCl), 65, 82, 83, 84, 85, 86, 87, 91, 92, 95, 97, 118, 120, 121, 122, 134, 136, 148, 149, 152, 159, 162, 170, 198, 199, 221
sodium chloride bath, 65, 121
sodium-bicarbonate-alkaline, 120
sodium-bicarbonated, 162, 235, 249
sodium-bicarbonate-fluorate-carbonic, 230
sodium chloride, bicarbonate, calcium, magnesium, sulphate and iron-rich, 199
sodium-chloride-sulphate, 86
sodium-glucose cotransporter 2, 190
sodium-rich, 113, 148, 149, 162, 174, 202, 214
sodium-rich carbonated, 148, 162
sodium-rich, magnesiac, calcic, sulphate-rich and chloride-rich, 174
soft, 22
solid state, 24
solubility, 16, 20, 205
solution, 14, 22, 46, 48, 82, 83, 84, 85, 86, 87, 88, 91, 94, 96, 98, 100
Spa, vii, 11, 12, 17, 21, 26, 45, 46, 47, 48, 49, 62, 66, 68, 69, 74, 76, 82, 83, 84, 85, 86, 87, 88, 90, 94, 95, 97, 100, 103, 107, 110, 113, 115, 116, 117, 118, 120, 121, 122, 123, 124, 126, 127, 128, 129, 130, 131, 176, 180, 182, 212, 214, 221, 234
Spa therapy, 68, 74, 76, 86, 90, 94, 95, 97, 103, 107, 110, 113, 116, 117, 118, 119, 120, 121, 122, 123, 124, 126, 127, 128, 129, 130, 131, 212, 214

Spain, 1, 8, 13, 16, 17, 24, 25, 28, 123, 199, 258
Spatone®, 241, 245
species, 39, 60, 61, 117, 192, 200, 204, 207, 208, 210, 226
species richness, 200, 210, 226
specific bone surface, 148
specific compounds, 16
specific nonseasonal rhinitis, 86
speleotherapy, 43, 66
spine, 139
spirometry, 32, 35, 47, 48, 53
spondyloarthritis, 118
spore, 78, 86
Sprague-Dawley rats, 113, 214, 215
spray, 75, 86, 87, 88, 91, 108, 166, 177
spring, 13, 20, 21, 160, 179, 180, 198
sputum, 34, 35, 36, 37, 39, 40, 41, 45, 48, 54, 56, 58, 59, 61, 63
St George's Respiratory Questionnaire (SGRQ), 33, 42, 48, 53
stability, 166, 177, 185
standard deviation, 40, 85, 141, 200
standard error, 41, 94
Stanford Health Assessment Questionnaire (HAQ), 121
Staphylococcus, 84, 173, 175, 179, 181, 201, 222, 254
Staphylococcus aureus, 84, 173, 175, 179, 181, 222, 254
starch, 204
stars, 2
state, 2, 16, 18, 42, 45, 74, 91, 119, 123, 129, 206, 254
steam hot-vapour inhalation, 86
sterile, 48
steroids, 47, 48, 81, 83, 84, 94, 99, 103
stimulation, 138, 245
stomach, 237
storage, 192
stress, 39, 46, 59, 60, 125, 150, 173, 177, 190, 214, 215
stress response, 125
strong mineralisation, 8
strongly mineralised, 9
structural model index, 148
structure, 1, 24, 58, 149, 193, 199, 204, 209, 252
structuring, xiii
style, 105, 247
subgroups, 10, 93, 98, 104
substance, 2, 22, 170
substrate, 49
subthermale, 8
succession, 225
succinate, 193
sulfate, 68, 198, 225, 247
sulfhydric, 19
sulfur, 61, 67, 68, 131, 225
sulphate (SO_4^{2-}), 7, 9, 10, 12, 13, 14, 23, 85, 86, 100, 118, 120, 122, 123, 143, 145, 146, 147, 148, 172, 174, 198, 199, 200, 201, 202, 206, 230, 233, 234, 236, 242, 245, 253
sulphate and iron-rich, 199
sulphate-bicarbonate-calcium, 122
sulphate-calcium-magnesium-fluoride, 122
sulphated, 94, 116
sulphated mineral-medicinal waters, 116
sulphate-rich and chloride-rich, 174
sulphate-sodium-chloride, 85
sulphide, 18, 19
sulphur, 16, 18, 19, 40, 45, 100, 110, 113, 117, 119, 125, 126, 128, 135, 168, 170, 173, 177, 206, 234
sulphur bath, 119, 128, 131
sulphurous, 27, 43, 44, 45, 47, 49, 68, 70, 74, 76, 77, 78, 82, 83, 84, 94, 95, 96, 99, 100, 105, 107, 108, 109, 110,

113, 117, 118, 121, 122, 125, 130, 213
sulphurous water baths, 122
sulphurous-arsenical-ferruginous, 82, 83, 84, 108, 109
sulphurous-salty-bromic-iodic, 84
sulphurous-sodium-chloride-bicarbonate-alkaline, 95
sulphurous-sulphate-calcium-magnesium, 100
sulphurous-sulphated-bicarbonate-calcic, 94
sulphur-rich, 168, 170, 173, 177
sulphur-salt-calcium-magnesic, 45
Sun, 70, 155, 220, 223
superoxide anion ($O_2^{-\bullet}$), 39
superoxide dismutase, 39, 79, 102, 172
superoxide dismutase 2 (SOD2), 79, 102
superoxide radical ($O_2^{-\bullet}$), 46, 119
supplementation, 160, 192, 194, 203, 204, 210
surfactant, 39
surgical, 75, 93, 97, 98, 190
surgical intervention, 93
surveillance, 222
survival, 138, 188
sustainable development, ix
swollen joints, 119
symptom, 31, 32, 33, 36, 44, 46, 47, 48, 49, 50, 77, 78, 79, 80, 85, 86, 87, 89, 91, 93, 100, 101, 103
symptoms, 31, 32, 33, 36, 44, 46, 47, 48, 49, 77, 78, 80, 85, 86, 87, 89, 91, 93, 100, 101, 103
synaptic transmission, 246
syndrome, 63, 118, 131, 155, 213
synergistic effect, 124, 167
synovial, 118, 127
synovial fluid, 127
synoviocytes, 119, 128
synovium, 120
synthesis, 2, 42, 106, 170
systemic lupus erythematosus, 118
systemic sclerosis, 118
systolic blood pressure, 210
systolic blood pressure (SBP), 210

T

T cells, 121
T helper type (Th), 80, 101, 171, 175
T lymphocytes, 36, 44, 117, 170
Tannerella, 206, 207
tap water, 1, 25, 199, 200, 201, 202, 205, 206, 208, 209, 211, 221, 238, 239, 243, 246
target, 41, 45, 151, 156, 219
target organs, 45
taxa, 197, 200
taxonomy, 24
techniques, 32, 254
technologies, 179
teeth, 169
telomere length, 124
telomere shortening, 124
temperature, 1, 2, 7, 8, 16, 20, 83, 116, 118, 120, 121, 122, 210
tender joints, 119
tendons, 117
Tenericutes, 200, 208
tepid, 8
terminals, 238
testing, 98, 142, 233
testis, 237
Tests for Analysis of Lung Inflammation, 34
texture, 177
Th1, 101, 171
Th17, 171
Th2, 80, 101, 171, 175
thalassotherapy, 167, 174

The 6-Minute Walk Test, 34
therapeutic agents, 5
therapeutic effect, ix, 65, 70, 100, 121, 129, 130, 166, 173, 175, 183, 229
therapeutic effects, ix, 65, 100, 130, 166, 173, 183, 229
therapeutic interventions, 75
therapeutic properties, 17, 23, 174, 189
therapeutic use, 166, 168, 169, 170, 174, 189
therapeutics, 60
therapy, 43, 49, 63, 64, 65, 67, 68, 74, 75, 76, 79, 81, 85, 86, 90, 93, 94, 95, 96, 97, 99, 100, 102, 103, 104, 105, 107, 108, 110, 111, 113, 116, 117, 118, 120, 121, 123, 124, 126, 127, 128, 129, 130, 131, 167, 168, 172, 176, 177, 183, 184, 190, 212, 213, 214, 219
thermal bath, 94, 110, 118, 172, 173
thermal effects, 117
thermal treatment, 45, 76, 83, 91, 98, 102, 104
thermal water, vii, 27, 29, 30, 38, 43, 44, 45, 47, 48, 49, 60, 68, 69, 70, 71, 73, 74, 75, 76, 77, 78, 79, 82, 83, 84, 85, 86, 87, 88, 89, 90, 91, 92, 94, 95, 96, 97, 98, 99, 100, 101, 102, 103, 104, 105, 106, 107, 108, 109, 110, 111, 112, 113, 116, 117, 124, 129, 130, 166, 167, 168, 170, 171, 172, 174, 177, 179, 180, 181, 184, 185
thermoregulation, 188
thioredoxin, 39
threats, 212
throat, 75, 76, 83, 99
thromboxanes (TXs), 38
tight junction proteins, 193
tinea capitis, 173
tinea corporis, 173
tinea versicolor, 173, 169
tissue, 37, 79, 102, 103, 120, 127, 149, 194, 227, 228, 246, 248
tissue homeostasis, 248
tissue repair, 79, 102, 103, 120
tissue repair and acute and chronic inflammatory responses, 120
TLR2, 171
TLR4, 79, 102, 171
TLR5, 171
TNF, 77, 78, 79, 85, 92, 101, 190, 194, 196, 197
TNF-α, 77, 78, 85, 92, 101, 190, 194, 196
tobacco, 102, 177
tobacco smoking, 177
tolerability, 86, 89, 94, 100, 112
toll-like receptor (TLR), 79, 102, 171, 204
tonsillitis, 77
topical antibiotics, 81
total antioxidant capacity, 118
total cholesterol (TC), 195, 196, 197
total glutathione, 117
total nasal resistance, 82, 84
total nasal respiratory flow, 82
total pyridinoline, 145
total symptom score (TSS), 77, 78, 79, 85, 89, 91, 101, 102
total thiols, 117
toxic effect, 205
toxicity, 105, 168, 169, 223, 224
toxicity disorders, 168, 169
trabecular bone pattern factor, 148
trabecular bone score, 141
trabecular number, 141, 148
trabecular separation, 141
trabecular spacing, 148
trabecular thickness, 148
trace elements, 5, 166, 182, 247
trachea, 99
transducer, 61

transforming growth factor-β, 121
transmission, 192
transplants, 191, 192
transport, 28, 77, 79, 82, 83, 87, 90, 91, 100, 103, 227, 228, 229, 231, 232, 236, 237, 240, 241, 242, 243, 244, 248, 249, 250, 251
transport processes, 243
treatment, 4, 25, 33, 43, 44, 45, 46, 47, 48, 49, 56, 62, 63, 66, 67, 69, 74, 75, 76, 81, 82, 83, 84, 85, 86, 87, 88, 89, 90, 91, 92, 93, 94, 95, 96, 97, 98, 99, 100, 101, 102, 103, 107, 108, 109, 110, 111, 117, 119, 126, 130, 131, 149, 162, 166, 167, 174, 175, 176, 178, 181, 182, 183, 184, 189, 194, 195, 196, 197, 198, 199, 201, 202, 207, 234, 238, 243, 244, 245, 252
Treponema, 211
trial, 28, 70, 86, 98, 121, 123, 126, 128, 129, 130, 131, 143, 159, 184, 197, 204, 209, 210, 221, 224
triglyceride, 124, 155, 194, 195, 197, 232, 235, 250
triglycerides (TG), 194, 195, 197, 235
trimethylamine-N-oxide (TMAO), 191
tubal dysfunction, 78, 94, 97
tumour necrosis factor (TNF), 77, 78, 79, 85, 92, 101, 116, 171, 190, 194, 196, 197
Turicibacter, 203, 206
Turkey, 13, 123
turnover, 58, 139, 140, 144, 153, 156, 158, 170
twins, 192, 200, 217
tympanic effusion, 93
tympanic membrane, 94
tympanogram, 77, 96, 97
tympanogram data, 77, 97
tympanometry, 97
type, 6, 17, 48, 50, 75, 76, 80, 82, 83, 84, 88, 91, 92, 96, 97, 119, 120, 134, 136, 137, 138, 147, 149, 153, 165, 167, 171, 200, 202, 206, 207, 213, 216, 220, 225, 233, 246, 252
type 1 diabetes (T1D), 207, 208, 213, 225
type 2 diabetes (T2D), 134, 137, 153, 202, 213, 216, 219, 233, 246
type-1 collagen C-telopeptide, 147
types, 1, 4, 15, 31, 36, 39, 81, 91, 92, 103, 177, 200, 201, 222, 237, 254
tyrosine, 79, 102

U

Ukraine, 13
ultrasound, 122, 153, 184
ultrasound therapy, 122
ultraviolet (UV) radiation, 167, 169, 172, 174, 181, 182
Unclassified Bdellovibrionales, 203
Unclassified Ruminococcaceae, 203
United Kingdom, 13, 189, 200
United States, 8, 13, 154, 167, 179
universe, 3
upper airways, 75, 78, 90, 95, 106
upper respiratory tract, 44, 68, 74, 75, 77, 78, 88, 94, 99, 100, 101, 102, 103, 106, 107, 110, 111
upper respiratory tract disease, 44, 74, 75, 88, 102, 111
upper respiratory tract infections, 77, 99, 101, 103
upper respiratory tract inflammations, 44, 68, 107
uranium, 15
urea, 243
urea nitrogen, 210
Uriage-les-Bains®, 172, 181

urine, 40, 136, 137, 141, 143, 145, 152, 234
urolithiasis, 137, 247
USA, 12, 13, 81
UV radiation, 167, 169, 172, 174, 181, 182
UVA radiation, 172, 181
UVB radiation, 169, 172, 174, 182
UVA+UVB radiations, 172

V

vaccine, 244
vacuole, 243
vacuole and endoplasmic reticulum membranes, 243
valence, 9, 18
validation, 53, 64
vapour inhalation, 87, 90
vapour jet, 95
variables, 188, 194, 212
vascular trophic, 44
vasoactive intestinal peptide, 170, 180
vasoconstriction, 61
vasodilation, 61
vasodilatory, 44
vasomotor, 79, 80, 89, 90
vasomotor rhinitis, 79, 89, 90
vegetables, 102, 134, 135, 136, 140, 153, 154
Venezuela, 13
ventilation, 47, 70, 93
very cold, 8
very hard, 22
very hot, 8
very low mineral content, 6, 142
very mineralised, 9
very soft, 22
very weak mineralisation, 8, 9
vessels, 126, 171
Vibrio, 211
Vichy®, 11, 12, 20, 21, 172, 181, 185, 198, 241, 244, 253
Vidago®, 230, 231, 232, 233
viruses, 99
visceral adiposity, 192
visceral fat, 201
viscosity, 106
visual analogue score (VAS), 77, 78, 79, 83, 89, 92, 100, 119, 121, 123
vitamins, 134, 141
vitiligo, 174, 177
Vittel®, 12, 231
VLDL, 235
Volcic®, 231
volunteers, 202

W

waist and hip circumferences, 197
waistline, 195
waist-to-hip, 205
waking, 210
warm, 8, 46, 83, 90, 100, 101
warm inhalations, 83
warm or thermal, 8
warm vapour inhalations, 100, 101
Washington, 26
waste, 188, 210
wastewater, 26
water, ix, 1, 2, 3, 4, 5, 8, 10, 14, 15, 16, 18, 20, 21, 22, 23, 25, 26, 27, 30, 38, 42, 43, 44, 45, 47, 48, 49, 68, 69, 70, 71, 74, 76, 77, 78, 79, 82, 83, 84, 85, 86, 87, 88, 89, 90, 91, 92, 94, 95, 96, 97, 100, 101, 103, 104, 105, 106, 107, 108, 109, 110, 111, 112, 113, 116, 117, 118, 121, 122, 123, 125, 127, 129, 130, 131, 134, 142, 143, 144, 145, 147, 148, 149, 150, 157, 159, 161, 162, 163, 165, 166, 167, 170, 171, 172, 174, 175, 177, 179,

180, 181, 182, 183, 184, 185, 188, 189, 190, 198, 199, 200, 201, 202, 203, 204, 205, 206, 207, 208, 209, 210, 211, 212, 213, 214, 215, 216, 221, 222, 223, 224, 225, 226, 230, 231, 232, 233, 234, 235, 236, 237, 238, 239, 240, 241, 242, 243, 244, 245, 246, 248, 249, 250, 251, 252, 253
water baths, 121, 122, 123, 124, 167, 182
water consumption, 144, 160, 188, 189, 198, 199, 208, 210, 248
water exercises, 122
water ingestion, 135, 188, 215
water intake, 113, 125, 144, 188, 189, 210, 211, 213, 226, 253
water intake volume, 188, 189, 210
water mineral/ion, 188, 189, 198
water permeability, 241, 243, 253
water pH, 188, 189, 208, 226
water quality, 200, 211, 222
water resources, ix
water security, 188, 189, 210, 211
water substance, 1
weak mineralisation, 8, 9
wealth, ix
weight gain, 201, 203, 207, 209
well-being, 33, 238
wells, 166
Western Ontario and McMaster Universities Arthritis Index (WOMAC), 121, 122, 130
westernised, 134, 136, 191
white adipose tissue browning, 192
whole-body mud application, 120
women, 52, 82, 83, 88, 89, 99, 117, 118, 119, 120, 122, 123, 127, 139, 141, 142, 143, 145, 147, 148, 150, 152, 153, 155, 157, 158, 160, 161, 162, 184, 200, 202, 204, 210, 214, 221, 224, 231, 235, 240, 242, 247, 249, 253
wood, 31
wood smoke inhalation, 31
workers, 63, 82, 84, 86, 87, 94, 101, 209
World Health Organization (WHO), ix, 55, 112, 189, 190, 212, 213, 221, 252
worldwide, 30, 31, 71, 79, 81, 166
wound healing, 108, 184

X

xerosis, 175, 176, 183

Y

young, 98, 101, 111, 146, 155, 161, 209, 214, 231, 235, 240, 252, 253
young adults, 235
young women, 155, 240, 253

Z

zinc, 141, 168, 170, 171, 173, 182

Β

β-carboxy-terminal telopeptide of collagen, 148
β-defensin-2 (hBD-2), 37, 78, 79, 85, 92, 171